Advances in Food Science and Technology

Scrivener Publishing
100 Cummings Center, Suite 541J
Beverly, MA 01915-6106

Publishers at Scrivener
Martin Scrivener (martin@scrivenerpublishing.com)
Phillip Carmical (pcarmical@scrivenerpublishing.com)

Advances in Food Science and Technology

Edited by

Visakh P. M., Sabu Thomas, Laura B. Iturriaga, and Pablo Daniel Ribotta

Scrivener Publishing

WILEY

Co-published by John Wiley & Sons, Inc. Hoboken, New Jersey, and Scrivener Publishing LLC, Salem, Massachusetts.
Published simultaneously in Canada.

For general information on our other products and services or for technical support, please contact our Customer Care Department within the United States at (800) 762-2974, outside the United States at (317) 572-3993 or fax (317) 572-4002.

Wiley also publishes its books in a variety of electronic formats. Some content that appears in print may not be available in electronic formats. For more information about Wiley products, visit our web site at www.wiley.com.

For more information about Scrivener products please visit www.scrivenerpublishing.com.

Cover design by Russell Richardson

Library of Congress Cataloging-in-Publication Data:

ISBN 978-1-118-12102-3

Printed in the United States of America

10 9 8 7 6 5 4 3 2 1

Contents

Preface xi
List of Contributors xv

1 Food Chemistry and Technology 1
Visakh P. M., Sabu Thomas, Laura B. Iturriaga and Pablo Daniel Ribotta
1.1 Food Security 1
1.2 Nanotechnology in Food Applications 4
1.3 Frozen Food and Technology 5
1.4 Chemical and Functional Properties of Food Components 7
1.5 Food: Production, Properties and Quality 8
1.6 Safety of Enzyme Preparations Used in Food 10
1.7 Trace Element Speciation in Food 11
1.8 Bio-nanocomposites for Natural Food Packaging 13
References 14

2 Food Security: A Global Problem 19
Donatella Restuccia, Umile Gianfranco Spizzirri, Francesco Puoci, Giuseppe Cirillo, Ortensia Ilaria Parisi, Giuliana Vinci and Nevio Picci
2.1 Food Security: Definitions and Basic Concepts 20
2.2 Main Causes of Food Insecurity 27
2.2.1 Social Issues 28
2.2.2 Economic Issues 36
2.2.3 Environmental Issues 41
2.3 The Food Insecurity Dimension 50
2.3.1 Current Situation at Global Level 50
2.3.2 The Food, Financial and Economic Crisis and Their Implications on Food Security 55

2.3.3 The Last Concern: Food Prices Volatility 65
2.3.4 The Food Sector Numbers: Trends in Global Food Production and Trade 72
2.4 Conclusions 93
References 95

3 Nanotechnology in Food Applications 103
Rui M. S. Cruz, Javiera F. Rubilar, Igor Khmelinskii and Margarida C. Vieira
3.1 What is Nanotechnology? 103
3.2 Food Formulations 105
3.3 Food Packaging 107
3.3.1 Enhanced Barrier Properties 107
3.3.2 Active Packaging 112
3.3.3 Intelligent Packaging 114
3.4 Regulation Issues and Consumer Perception 115
Acknowledgements 116
References 116

4 Frozen Food and Technology 123
Elisabete M.C. Alexandre, Teresa R.S. Brandão and Cristina L.M. Silva
4.1 Introduction 124
4.2 Treatments: Pre-freezing 125
4.2.1 Fruits and Vegetables 125
4.2.2 Fish Products 127
4.2.3 Meat Products 128
4.3 Freezing Process 129
4.4 Freezing Methods and Equipment 131
4.4.1 Freezing by Contact with Cold Air 131
4.4.2 Freezing by Contact with Cold Liquid 135
4.4.3 Freezing by Contact with Cold Surfaces 135
4.4.4 Cryogenic Freezing 136
4.4.5 Combination of Freezing Methods 137
4.4.6 Innovations in Freezing Processes 137
4.4.7 Food Products and Freezing Methods 139
4.5 Effect of Freezing and Frozen Storage on Food Properties 142
4.5.1 Physical Changes 142
4.5.2 Chemical Changes 143
4.5.3 Microbiological Aspects 145

4.6 Final Remarks 146
References 147

5 **Chemical and Functional Properties of Food Components** **151**
Campos-Montiel R.G., Pimentel-González D.J. and Figueira A.C.
5.1 Introduction 151
5.2 Functional and Chemical Properties of Food Components 152
5.2.1 Functional Foods: Historical Perspective and Definitions 152
5.2.2 Legislation on Functional Food Claims 153
5.2.3 Classification of Functional Foods 161
5.2.4 Functional Properties of Food Components 162
5.3 Nutritional Value and Sensory Properties of Food 168
5.3.1 Nutritional Value of Food 169
5.3.2 Sensory Properties of Food 172
5.4 Postharvest Storage and Processing 174
5.4.1 Bioactive Compounds Postharvest 174
5.5 Conclusion 177
Acknowledgements 178
References 178

6 **Food: Production, Properties and Quality** **185**
Yantyati Widyastuti, Tatik Khusniati and Endang Sutriswati Rahayu
6.1 Introduction 185
6.2 Food Production 186
6.3 Factors Affecting Production and Improvement of Food 187
6.3.1 Soil and Climate 187
6.3.2 Population and Income Per Capita 188
6.3.3 Technology 188
6.3.4 Plant Source Foods 191
6.3.5 Animal Source Foods 193
6.4 Food Properties 196
6.5 Food Quality 197
References 199

7	**Regulatory Aspects of Food Ingredients in the United States: Focus on the Safety of Enzyme Preparations Used in Food**	**201**
	Shayla West-Barnette and Jannavi R. Srinivasan	
	7.1 Introduction	202
	7.2 Regulatory History of Food Ingredients: Guided by Safety	202
	7.3 Scientific Advancement as Part of the Regulatory History of Enzyme Preparations	206
	7.4 Safety Evaluation of Enzyme Preparations	216
	7.4.1 Identity of the Enzyme	216
	7.4.2 Manufacturing Process and Composition	219
	7.5 Conclusion	223
	Acknowledgements	223
	References	223
8	**Trace Element Speciation in Food**	**227**
	Paula Berton, Estefania M. Martinis and Rodolfo G. Wuilloud	
	8.1 Introduction	228
	8.2 Implications of Toxic Elements Speciation for Food Safety	230
	8.2.1 Arsenic	231
	8.2.2 Mercury	234
	8.2.3 Tin	235
	8.2.4 Chromium	236
	8.2.5 Cadmium	237
	8.3 Elemental Species and Its Impact on the Nutritional Value of Food	238
	8.3.1 Selenium	238
	8.3.2 Iron	240
	8.3.3 Cobalt	241
	8.3.4 Zinc	242
	8.4 Elemental Species in Food Processing	243
	8.5 Potential Functional Food Derived from Health Benefits of Elemental Species	246
	8.5.1 Selenium	246
	8.5.2 Iron and Zinc	247

8.6 Analytical Methods for Food Elemental Speciation Analysis 249
8.6.1 Species Separation 249
8.6.2 Species Detection: Elemental and Molecular 253
8.7 Conclusions 256
References 257

9 Bionanocomposites for Natural Food Packing 265
Bibin Mathew Cherian, Gabriel Molina de Olyveira, Ligia Maria Manzine Costa, Alcides Lopes Leão, Marcia Rodrigues de Morais Chaves, Sivoney Ferreira de Souza and Suresh Narine
9.1 Introduction 266
9.2 Natural Biopolymer-based Films 267
9.2.1 Polysaccharide Films 268
9.2.2 Protein Films 270
9.3 Modification of Film Properties 274
9.3.1 Natural Nanoreinforcements 274
9.3.2 Cellulose-based Nanoreinforcements 275
9.3.3 Starch Nanocrystals/Starch Nanoparticles 282
9.3.4 Chitin/Chitosan Nanoparticles 283
9.3.5 Plant-Protein Nanoparticle 285
9.3.6 Plasticizers 286
9.3.7 Clays 288
9.3.8 Active Agents 290
9.4 Environmental Impact of Bionanocomposites Materials 290
9.4.1 Safety and Toxicology 291
9.4.2 Biodegradability and Compostability 293
9.5 Conclusions and Future Perspectives 294
References 294

Index 301

Preface

"Advances in Food Science and Technology" summarizes many of the recent technical research accomplishments in the area of food science and technology, such as food security as a global problem, nanotechnology in food application, frozen food and technology food: production, properties & quality, trace element speciation in food, bionanocomposites for food packing application etc. It is written in a systematic and comprehensive manner and recent advances in the developments in food science area and food technologies are discussed here in detail. Therefore, the content of the current book is unique. It covers an up-to-date record on the major findings and observations in the field of food science and food technology and it is intended to serve as a "one stop" reference resource for important research accomplishments in this area. The various chapters in this book are contributed by prominent researchers from industry, academia and government/private research laboratories across the globe. This book will be a very valuable reference source for university and college faculties, professionals, post-doctoral research fellows, senior graduate students, food science technologists and researchers from R&D laboratories working in the area of food science.

The first chapter on food chemistry and technology gives an overview of the area of food science and technology such as food security a global problem, nanotechnology in food application, frozen food and technology food: production, properties & quality, trace element speciation in food, bionanocomposites for food packing application. This chapter is very essential for the beginners in these fields since it provides a basic yet thorough understanding of the food science field.

The following chapter provides an overview on food security as a global problem. The first part of this chapter reviews food security: definitions and basic concepts, main causes of food insecurity including social issues, economic issues, environmental issues and later in the chapter, the authors explain the various aspects of the food insecurity dimension such as current situation at global level, financial and economic crisis and their implications on food security Lastly, they look at food prices volatility, food sector numbers: trends in global food production and trade.

A survey on nanotechnology in food application is tackled in the third chapter. The authors concentrate on the importance of nanotechnology in food science, applications and also address some of the challenges. This chapter also brings out new innovative methods for food formulations and novel applications such as food packaging, enhanced barrier, active packaging, and intelligent packaging.

The fourth chapter on frozen food and technology comprises several subtopics. The first topic looks at pre-freezing treatments of different food products such as fruits, vegetables, fish, and meat products. In the another topic, the authors explain about the freezing methods and equipment such as freezing by contact with cold air, freezing by contact with cold liquid, freezing by contact with cold surfaces, cryogenic freezing and combination of freezing methods. The last section of this chapter, the authors explain the effect of freezing and frozen storage on food properties such as physical changes, chemical changes, microbiological aspects

The following chapter on chemical and functional properties of food components provides the basic understanding of food components, nutritional value and sensory, post harvest storage and processing. This chapter gives an overview of functional and chemical properties of food components with some subtopics such as functional foods: historical perspective and definitions, legislation on functional food claims, classification of functional foods and functional properties of food components.

Another chapter examines the new aspects on food production, food properties and food quality. In this chapter the authors mainly focus on the food production factors sSuch as, soil, climate, population, income and technology, plant source foods and animal source foods.

The following chapter is based on regulatory aspects of food ingredients in the United States with the focus on the safety of enzyme preparations used in food. The authors explain the various aspects such as regulatory history of food ingredients, scientific advancement as part of the regulatory history of enzyme preparations, safety evaluation of enzyme preparations, identity of the enzyme and manufacturing process and composition.

In the chapter on trace element speciation in food, the authors discuss the implications of toxic elements such as arsenic, mercury, tin, chromium, cadmium on speciation for food safety. Elements such as selenium iron, cobalt, zinc, impact on the nutritional value of food are also discussed. Moreover, the authors examine the analytical methods for food elemental speciation analysis, species separation and species detection.

The book concludes with a chapter on bionanocomposites for natural food packing which discusses the natural biopolymer-based films such as polysaccharide films and protein films. Sections are given over to the modification of film properties such as natural nanoreinforcements, cellulose-based nanoreinforcements, starch nanocrystals/starch nanoparticles, chitin/chitosan nanoparticles, plant-protein nanoparticle, plasticizers, clays and active agents. The chapter concludes with a section on the environmental impact of bionanocomposites materials, their safety and toxicology, biodegradability and compostability.

The editors of this unique volume would like to express their sincere gratitude to all the contributors of this book, who made excellent support to the successful completion of this venture. We are grateful to them for the commitment and the sincerity they have shown towards their contributions in the book. Without their enthusiasm and support, the compilation of this book could not have been realized. We would like to thank all the reviewers who have taken their valuable time to make critical comments on each chapter. We also thank the publisher Scrivener-Wiley for recognizing the demand for such a book, and for realizing the increasing importance of the area of food science and technology.

Visakh. P. M
Sabu Thomas
Laura B.Iturriaga
Pablo Daniel Ribotta
January 1, 2013

List of Contributors

Elisabete Alexandre obtained her PhD in food science and technology from the College of Biotechnology, Portuguese Catholic University, Porto, Portugal, in 2011. She is currently working on chemical and physical phenomena in foods during processing. She has authored 2 book chapters, published 6 articles in referred international journals and co-authored 17 communications in scientific meetings.

Paula Berton is a PhD student in analytical chemistry, and is Laboratory Instructor at the National University of Cuyo, Mendoza, Argentina. She has co-authored 13 papers and 2 book chapters. Her research is focused on the use of ionic liquids for microextraction-based analytical methodologies for elemental speciation analysis.

Teresa R.S. Brandão is a chemical engineer with a PhD in biotechnology from the College of Biotechnology, Portuguese Catholic University. She is a researcher at the Centre for Biotechnology and Fine Chemistry of the Portuguese Catholic University. Her research interests have been focused on food processing, modelling quality and safety attributes of food products with emphasis in statistical experimental design procedures. She authored 8 book chapters, published 45 articles in referred international journals and-co-authored more than 80 communications in scientific meetings.

Bibin Mathew Cherian is a scientist in the Department of Natural Resources at São Paulo State University. He has a PhD in chemistry, MSc in analytical chemistry and BSc in industrial chemistry, chemistry and mathematics. He is active in the field of biobased nanoreinforcments, nanocomposites, nanomedicine, membranes and medical implants.

Ligia Maria Manzine Costa is a PhD scholar at the Federal University of ABC. She has an MSc in materials engineering and a BSc in chemistry. Her research interests include electrospinning, polymeric nanofibers, resorbable polymers, bacterial cellulose, natural rubber latex.

Marcia Rodrigues de Morais Chaves is a faculty member at the University of Sagrado Coração. She has a PhD in chemical engineering, MSc in materials engineering and a BSc in chemistry. Her research interests are in cellulose separation from different vegetable fiber sources and agro-industrial waste, as well on fiber-composite polymers and environmental aspects of these materials.

Giuseppe Cirillo received his PhD in 2008 from the University of Calabria, Italy. He is currently in a post-doctoral position at the same university and a visiting researcher at IFW Dresden, Germany, working on polymeric nanotechnologies and biomaterials. He is the author and co-author of more than 60 publications and the co-editor of the book *Antioxidant Polymers*.

Rui M.S. Cruz holds a PhD in biotechnology-food science and engineering. He works in the area of food preservation, particularly in active packaging to improve food products quality and extend shelf-life. He has published 12 peer-reviewed papers, 6 book chapters and 1 book edition, and he is also a reviewer for several scientific journals in the area of food science and technology.

Gabriel Molina de Olyveira is a PhD scholar at the Federal University of ABC. He has an MSc and BSc in materials engineering. He has experience in the rubber industry and manufacturing plastic packaging. His research interests include bioelectrochemistry, bionanotechnology, bionanocomposite and bionanomedicine.

Sivoney Ferreira de Souza is a PhD scholar at the Federal University of ABC. She has an MSc in energy in agriculture and BSc in chemical engineering. Her research interests include nanostructured materials especially cellulose nanofibers in biomedical application.

Ana Cristina Figueira is a coordinating professor of chemistry at the University of the Algarve, Portugal. Her scientific interests are in food chemistry with a focus on food authenticity and the study of bioactive components of food and food by-products. She has co-authored 1 book, 7 book chapters and 11 scientific papers.

Igor Khmelinskii holds a PhD and Habilitation in chemistry. He has authored more than 150 peer-reviewed papers and 5 book chapters. His research interests include food analysis, photophysics, photochemistry, magnetic field effects, and climate change.

Tatik Khusniati is a senior food microbial biochemist, awarded as PhD from Hokkaido University, Japan in 2008. For the past 18 years she has been developing more intensive dairy food-microbial biochemistry research. She has a number of publications both in national and international journals in relation to dairy microbiology.

Alcides Lopes Leão is a Professor of College of the Agricultural Sciences at São Paulo State University. He has PhD in forestry, MSc in energy in agriculture and a BSc in agricultural engineering. He is the co-founder of ONG INFO, and International Natural Fibers Organization, based in Amsterdam, the Netherlands. He is active in the field of composites, natural fibers, recycling, biomass energy and agricultural and municipal garbage.

Estefanía Martinis holds a post-doc position at the National University of Cuyo, Argentina. She is the co-author of 14 publications and 1 book chapter. She works in the field of development of analytical methods for toxic elements determination at trace levels using functionalized nanomaterials and ionic liquids.

Rafael Germán Campos Montiel is a researcher at the Autonomous University of Hidalgo State, Argentina and has experience in extraction of bioactive compounds from microorganisms and plants used as additives in foods. He has published 3 books, 8 chapters and 11 scientific papers in several journals. He has also worked in the Hidalgo state government solving food industries problems.

Suresh Narine is the Ontario Research Chair in Green Chemistry and Engineering and NSERC/GFO/ERS Industrial Research Chair in Lipid Derived Biomaterials, is a professor of physics and astronomy and chemistry at Trent University and Director of the Trent

Centre for Biomaterials Research in Canada. He has a PhD in food science, a MSc in condensed matter physics and a BSc in chemical physics.

Ortensia Ilaria Parisi obtained her PhD in environment, health and eco-friendly processes with a thesis on "Polymeric Materials for Biomedical Applications: Synthesis and Characterisation". Her research interests are in the areas of biomaterials, molecularly imprinted polymers, graft polymers, functional polymers, stimuli responsive hydrogels as well as functional foods and nutraceutics. She is author of more than 40 publications regarding the above-mentioned topics.

Nevio Picci received his degree in chemistry in 1975 from the University of Pisa and he is currently full professor in pharmaceutical technology at the University of Calabria, Italy. His research interest involves the application of functional polymers, biomaterials and nanotechnologies in biomedical, pharmaceutical and food sciences. He is the author and co-author of more than 150 publications.

Diana Pimentel is a researcher at the Autonomous University of Hidalgo State, Argentina and has experience in food technology with specific expertise encapsulating bioactive compounds and probiotics. She has published 16 scientific papers in several journals. She has received Pan-American and Latin-American awards for her pioneering contributions recognized by international companies like Bimbo and Kellogs.

Francesco Puoci earned his BS in chemistry from the University of Calabria in 1999 and his PhD in 2002. His research activities focus on the synthesis of polymeric functional materials for pharmaceutical and technological applications as well as functional foods and nutraceutics.

Endang Sutriswati Rahayu is a senior lecturer at the Faculty of Agricultural Technology, Gadjah Mada University, Yogyakarta, Indonesia. She received her PhD in agricultural chemistry from the University of Tokyo, Japan in 1991. Her research and publications are mainly related to lactic acid bacteria (fermented foods and probiotics) and food safety (foodborne fungi and mycotoxin). She belongs to several professional associations such as the Asian Federation

Society for Lactic Acid Bacteria and the Indonesian Society for Lactic Acid Bacteria, Microbiologist, and Food Technologist.

Javiera F. Rubilar is a researcher at the Department of Chemical Engineering and Bioprocesses of the Pontificia Universidad Católica de Chile. She holds a PhD in chemistry and has published 3 peer-reviewed papers. In 2011 she won third place in the best research presentation award at the ISEKI Food conference.

Donatella Restuccia is an assistant professor of commodity sciences at the Department of Pharmacy and Health and Nutrition Sciences of the University of Calabria. Research activity is principally focused on food quality and safety evaluation and in particular on the determination of natural contaminates and bioactive compounds in foods. She is the author or co-author of about 60 publications.

Cristina L.M. Silva is a chemical engineer with PhD in Biotechnology from the College of Biotechnology, Portuguese Catholic University. She is an associate professor at the College of Biotechnology and a senior researcher at the Centre for Biotechnology and Fine Chemistry of the Portuguese Catholic University. She is the leader of a research team involved in thermal and non-thermal food processing, focusing on process optimisation and development of strategies for food quality and safety. She has authored 11 book chapters, published 80 articles in referred international journals and co-authored more than 150 communications in scientific meetings.

U. Gianfranco Spizzirri received his PhD from the University of Calabria in 2005. His research is focussed on the synthesis of polymeric functional materials for technological applications. Particular interest is devoted to development of specific experimental protocols in the evaluation of active components in nutraceutical supplements and food matrices. He is the author and co-author of more than 50 publications.

Jannavi Srinivasan is a review chemist in the FDA's Office of Food Additive Safety. Her expertise includes bioengineered crops and enzymes added to food. She has a PhD from Wayne State University Detroit. She was a postdoctoral fellow at University of Michigan and has worked for ten years in the industry.

Margarida C. Vieira is a Professor Coordinator (PhD) and Head of the Department of Food Engineering (ISE-UAlg) since 2009. Her main research area is innovative technologies for food preservation. She has published 16 peer-reviewed papers, 10 book chapters and edition of 2 books. In 1999 she won the first place in the Product Development Division's Poster Competition at the IFT Annual Meeting.

Giuliana Vinci is an associate professor of commodity science at the Department of Management of Sapienza University of Rome. The author of several publications (150) in national and international journals relating food quality, food security and sustainable development.

Shayla West-Barnette is a consumer safety officer in FDA's Office of Food Additive Safety where she serves on the Enzyme Review Team as well as a microbiology reviewer. She holds a bachelor's degree in biology from Bennett College and a PhD in microbiology and immunology from Wake Forest University.

Yantyati Widyastuti is a highly distinguished animal nutritionist. She obtained her PhD from Tokyo University of Agriculture, Japan in 1989. She is a leader of animal nutrition research group and head of Applied Microbiology laboratory in the Research Center for Biotechnology, Indonesian Institute of Sciences. She has published a number of papers in several international journals.

Rodolfo Wuilloud is a Professor at the National University of Cuyo and Researcher at the National Council for Scientific and Technical Research (CONICET) of Argentina. He is the author of 79 papers and 3 book chapters. His research focuses on development of analytical methods for elemental speciation based on microextraction techniques using ionic liquids and solid-phase preconcentration.

1

Food Chemistry and Technology

State of the Art, New Challenges and Opportunities

Visakh P. M.[1,2], Sabu Thomas[1,2], Laura B. Iturriaga[3] and Pablo Daniel Ribotta[4]

[1]Centre for Nanoscience and Nanotechnology, Mahatma Gandhi University, Kottayam, Kerala, India
[2]School of Chemical Sciences, Mahatma Gandhi University, Kottayam, Kerala, India
[3]Institute of Chemical Sciences, Faculty of Agronomy, National University of Santiago del Estero, Santiago del Estero, Argentina
[4]Department of Science and Technology, National University of Córdoba, Córdoba, Argentina

Abstract

This chapter presents a brief account of the various categories of food chemistry and technology along with the different parameters associated with them. Included in the discussion of food chemistry and technology are such issues as food security, nanotechnology in food applications, frozen food and technology, chemical and functional properties of food components, the production, properties and quality of food, safety of enzyme preparations used in food, trace element speciation in food, bionanocomposites for natural food packing, etc.

Keywords: Food security, nanotechnology, frozen food, functional properties of food components, food production, trace element speciation in food, food packing

1.1 Food Security

Nutritional status in food consumption is generally identified by three indicators: calorie, protein, and fat intake while food

Visakh P. M., Sabu Thomas, Laura B. Iturriaga, and Pablo Daniel Ribotta (eds.) Advances in Food Science and Technology, (1–18) © 2013 Scrivener Publishing LLC

consumption is mainly related with domestic food production and food imports achieved by international trade. The concept of food security has developed over the past three decades. Concerns about food security up to the end of the 1970s were mostly directed at the national and international level and concerned the ability of countries to secure adequate food supplies. It was only later that the level of analysis shifted to include a focus on food security at local level, even down to households and individuals [1].

Definitions of food security identify the outcomes of food security and are useful for formulating policies and deciding on actions, but the processes that lead to desired outcomes also matter. Most current definitions of food security therefore include references to processes as well as outcomes and, taken together, these processes constitute the complexity of the food system.

A variety of factors, both internal and external, affect the food security of a country, and straightforward explanations for world hunger should be treated with caution. Food security is, in fact, a multifaceted concept that goes far beyond the number of people that can be sustained by the earth's limited food resources, to encompass a broad range of aspects which are, however, related in some fashion to two basic causes: insufficient national food availability and insufficient access to food by households and individuals. Population growth over the past century has been accompanied by enormous increases in food production [2].

Among economic issues related with food insecurity, neglect of agriculture and world trade rules are the most severe. Despite the evidence that investment in agriculture results in growth and poverty reduction, spending on agriculture as a share of total public spending in developing countries fell by half between 1980 and 2004 [3]. By 2050 it is estimated that the world will need to increase food production by 70 percent to feed a larger, more urban, and, it is hoped, wealthier population [4, 5]. The Green Revolution, and "industrialized" agriculture more generally, has often been associated with problems of environmental degradation and pollution [6].

Trade and financial factors have been also considered as a driving force in food crisis. Although fundamental factors were clearly responsible for shifting the world to a higher food price equilibrium in the years leading up the 2008 food crisis, there is little doubt that when food prices peaked in June of 2008, they soared well above the new equilibrium price. By March 2009, prices of staple grains had fallen by 30 percent from their peak in May 2008, while energy prices fell by around 50 percent, before stabilizing and then increasing again. At the moment, the global food prices remain high, partly due to increasing fuel prices, and the World Bank's Food Price Index is around its 2008 peak. However, the current global food price situation seems to possess both similarities and differences with 2008 [7]. It is similar in four respects. First, global grain stocks are low, driven by lower production. Second, higher oil prices have impacted agricultural commodity prices, and the recent events in the Middle East and North Africa add to the current uncertainty. Crude oil prices underpin production costs of agricultural products relying on fertilizers and petroleum, in particular in developed and emerging economies and transport costs in many developing countries

The Eastern European countries, after recording bumper crops in 2008, were unable to sustain potential growth in the subsequent years, and the 2010 drought led to substantially reduced levels of crop production in the region. On the contrary, Latin America and the Caribbean suffered weather-related production shortfalls in 2008 but recovered in 2009 and 2010. In Asia, growth in food production remained strong throughout the last decade, generally in the range of 2–4 percent per year, although they faced a slowdown in 2009 and 2010. Production failed to grow in 2009 in sub-Saharan Africa, which had seen growth in the range of 3–4 percent per year over the previous decade, while the region registering the slowest growth in food production in recent years is Western Europe. Production did increase in 2007 and 2008 under the effect of high prices and reduced set-aside requirements in the European Union, but declined by around 2 percent in 2009 as a result of lower prices and unfavorable weather conditions. In this regard, the prospect for an expansion in grain production in 2011 is particularly related with the expectation of a return to regular climatic conditions firstly in the Russian Federation, after last year's devastating dryness. Encouragingly, the country has announced the lifting of its export ban from July 2011 and weather permitting, excellent crops are also anticipated in Ukraine. However, other important producing regions (Europe and North America) are now facing difficult weather situations which eventually, may hamper yields.

1.2 Nanotechnology in Food Applications

Nanotechnology is an important tool that is influencing a large number of industrial segments. The food industry is investing in mechanisms and procedures to use nanotechnology to improve production processes and produce food products with better and more convenient functionalities [8].

One of the functions of food packaging is to increase the shelf life of foods, protecting it from microbial and chemical contamination and other factors, such as oxygen and light. The use of nanotechnology in food packaging is a promising application aimed at achieving longer shelf life of food products, rendering them safer [9]. In 2006, about 400 companies around the world included in the agricultural and food industry segment actively invested in the research and development of nanotechnology, and by 2015 this is expected to happen in more than 1,000 companies [10].

The use of nanomaterials in food formulations has the potential to produce stronger flavorings, colorings, and nutritional additives, and also improve production operations, lowering the costs of ingredients and processing [11]. Nestlé reported that they recognize the potential of nanotechnology to improve the properties of food and food packaging. However, the company declares no research in the field of nanotechnology [12].

New solutions can be provided for food packaging through the modification of the permeability behavior of the packaging systems. Some of these include: enhanced barrier (mechanical, microbial and chemical), antimicrobial, and heat-resistance properties [13, 14]. In the late 1980s, the concept of polymer-clay nanocomposites (PCN) was developed and first commercialized by Toyota [15], but only since the late 1990s have works been published on the development of PCN for food packaging [16].

There are different forms to improve the plastic materials' barrier. One of them is the incorporation of clays or silicates in the polymer matrix. These layered inorganic solids have drawn the attention of the packaging industry due to their availability, low cost, significant enhancements and relatively simple processing [17].

Controlled release of active and bioactive compounds in food packaging applications, and nanoencapsulation of functional added-value food additives are other possible applications [18, 19]. Metal and metal oxide nanoparticles and carbon nanotubes are the nanoparticles most used for the development of active packaging with antimicrobial properties [20].

Silver is the most common nanoadditive used in antimicrobial packaging, with several advantages such as strong toxicity to a wide range of microorganisms, high temperature stability and low volatility [21].

Several mechanisms were proposed to explain the antimicrobial properties of silver nanoparticles. The adhesion to the cell surface, degrading lipopolysaccharides and forming "pits" in the membranes, largely increasing permeability [22], penetration inside bacterial cell, damaging DNA; and releasing antimicrobial Ag^+ ions by Ag-nanoparticles dissolution [23] are some of the proposed hypotheses.

1.3 Frozen Food and Technology

Freezing is one of the oldest and most frequently used processes for long-term food preservation. Nowadays, the freezing process is strongly implemented worldwide, being one of the most common preservation methods used for all kinds of commercialized foods: fruits (whole, puréed or as juice concentrates) and vegetables; fish fillets and seafood, including prepared dishes; meats and meat products; baked goods (i.e., bread, cakes, pizzas); desserts and an endless number of precooked dishes [24].

Food preservation by freezing occurs through different mechanisms. When temperature is lowered below 0°C, there is a reduction in the microbial loads and microbial activity; therefore, the deterioration rate of foods decrease. Freezing temperatures affect biological materials in various ways depending on their chemical composition, microstructure and physical properties. The low temperatures also have a strong impact in enzymatic activity and oxidative reactions that help products avoid deterioration. In addition, with ice crystal formation, less water will be available to support deteriorative reactions and microbial viability [25, 26].

Upon placing the food (whole or in pieces) in solutions of high sugar or salt concentration, the water inside the food moves to the concentrated solution and, simultaneously, the solute from the concentrated solution is transferred into the food. Osmotic concentration of fruits and vegetables prior to freezing improves their quality in terms of color, texture and flavor, and the combination of this treatment with partial air drying requires less energy consumption than air drying alone [27, 28].

The freezing process involves four main stages: (i) pre-freezing stage – sensible heat is removed from the product, reducing the temperature to the freezing point; (ii) super-cooling – temperature falls below the freezing point, which is not always observed; (iii) freezing – latent heat is removed and water is transformed into ice (i.e., crystallization) in all product; (iv) sub-freezing – the food temperature is lowered to the storage temperature.

There are many factors that will determine the success of the freezing operation. Freezing methods and type of equipment used, composition and shape of product to be frozen, packaging materials, freezing rates and ice crystallization, product moisture content, specific heat, heat transfer coefficients and packaging, are examples of factors that will determine freezing efficiency and product quality.

In cryogenic freezing the food is in direct contact with the refrigerant through three different ways: (i) the cryogenic liquid is directly sprayed on the food in a tunnel freezer, (ii) the cryogenic liquid is vaporized and blown over the food in a spiral freezer or batch freezer, or (iii) the food product is immersed in cryogenic liquid in an immersion freezer. However, the most common method used is the direct spraying of cryogenic solutions over the product while it is conveyed through an insulated tunnel [29].

Jalté *et al.* [30] studied the effects of pulsed electric fields pretreatment on the freezing, freeze-drying and rehydration behavior of potatoes, and concluded that the quality and rehydration of the samples improved. LeBail *et al.* [31] reviewed the application of high pressure in the freezing and thawing of foods. Alizadeh *et al.* [32] froze salmon fillets by pressure shift freezing and verified that ice crystals were smaller and more regular than the ones obtained with conventional freezing methods.

During freezing, changes in temperature and concentration (due to ice formation) play an important role in enzymatic and nonenzymatic reactions rates. Ice crystals may release the enclosed contents of food tissues, such as enzymes and chemical substances, affecting the product quality during freezing and frozen storage. The main chemical changes verified during freezing and frozen storage are related to lipid oxidation, protein denaturation, enzymatic browning and degradation of pigments and vitamins.

Freezing is one of the oldest and most common processes used in food preservation and one of the best methods available in the food industry. There are several methods and various equipment that can be used and adapted according to the different types of foods. Freezing usually retains the initial quality of the products. However, during freezing and frozen storage, some physical, chemical and nutritional changes may occur. To avoid this impact on fresh products, mainly in fruits and vegetables, some pretreatments may be required to inactivate enzymes and microorganisms.

1.4 Chemical and Functional Properties of Food Components

The concept of functional foods has spread around the world and has become increasingly popular [33–35]. However, at present, an internationally accepted definition for functional foods is inexistent.

A worldwide accepted classification for the functional foods that have been developed and are available can't be found, to date. Some have, however, suggested a common classification based on the functional foods' origin or modification [36–39]. Polyphenols are classified into phenolic acids, flavonoids, and less commonly into stilbenes and lignans. Many studies have focused on the antioxidant activities of flavonoids. Although several flavonoids are highly efficacious free radical scavengers *in vitro*, there is little information on the importance of dietary flavonoids as antioxidants *in vivo*, or evidence for such activity *in vivo*. Moreover, there have been few studies on phenolic acids compared to the number of studies on flavonoids, despite the high content of phenolic acids in fruits, cereals, and some vegetables [40].

Factors included in physical properties that may be affected by food processing such as shape, color, size, surface condition, texture, freshness, total solids, etc., can change the appearance of the product. In biological terms, we can talk about total bacteria, total coliform bacteria, total mold, free of pathogenic microorganisms, etc.; in sensory aspects, flavor, aroma, taste, texture, etc., are involved; finally, in the chemical properties are included the nutritional value, moisture content, functional value, pH, chemical contaminants and food additives, etc. Food composition is determined by proximate analysis of carbohydrate, lipid, and protein contents, as well as minerals and vitamins. Actually, researchers have focused on further evaluation of amino-acid content and its quality, fatty and acid profiles, simple and complex carbohydrates, soluble and insoluble fibers, and other content like functional additives such as antioxidants, known as nutraceutical ingredients

Nowadays there is a lot of research involved in the improvement of the nutritional value of foods. One of the topics that is more useful in the development and improvement of the nutritional value of foods is the soybean. Soybean is a good substitute since it is a good source of protein (about 40%), edible oil of high quality that is cholesterol free (about 21%) and carbohydrate (34%) [41]. It is one of the most promising foods in the world, available to improve the diet of millions of people. Cereals are the most important source of food and have a significant impact in the human diet throughout the world. Since the 90s, in India and Africa, cereal products comprise 80% or more of the average diet, 50% in Central and Western Europe, and between 20–25% in the US [42]. Cereals like maize, rice, millet and sorghum can supply sufficient qualities of carbohydrate, fat, protein and many minerals, but diets consisting primarily of cereals are high in carbohydrate and deficient in vitamins and protein. The sensory characteristics of foods, especially appearance, texture, and flavor influence the food purchasing decisions of consumers. Therefore, a major concern is to increase the nutritional composition of products without negatively compromising the sensory qualities [43].

1.5 Food: Production, Properties and Quality

Most production of food comes from land, although there is great potential for the sea to provide various seafoods. From land, food production traditionally is closely related to agriculture and generally refers to cultivation of plants or crops and rearing of animals. Their productivity is strongly affected by the genotype of plants or crops and animals. Food production is faced with a very difficult situation relating to climate change all around the world. The impact of climate change is very severe and includes an increase in temperature. Drought affects all stages of crop growth and development, since absorption of nutrients from the soil is influenced by temperature condition and moisture. Soil and climatic conditions including the physical, chemical and biological properties of soil, the rates at which nutrients are supplied, and applied fertilizer affect the growth of crops and their product.

Certain regions suffer from increased incidents of heat waves and droughts without the possibility for shifting crop cultivation [44]. The physiological responses of crops suggest that they will grow faster, with slight changes in development, such as flowering and fruiting, depending on the species. Changes in food quality in a warmer and high CO_2 situation are to be expected. These include, for example, decreased protein and mineral nutrient concentration as well as altered lipid composition [45]. Organic farming is a method in agriculture based on ecology and naturally occurring biological processes. By this technology the perception among consumers is that organically produced crops possess higher nutritional quality. Herencia *et al.* [46] found that organic crops showed higher phosphorus and dry matter content and lower nitrogen and nitrate content than conventional crops. They also found crops with opposite trends in nutrient content depending on cultivation cycle. This seems to indicate that conditions in which the crop was developed is more influential than the type of fertilization. The limitation of fertilization applied in organic farming can lead to an available nitrogen shortage for plants and possibly less nitrogen content.

Fruits and vegetables are rich in minerals and vitamins which serve an array of important functions in the body. Vitamin A maintains eye health and boosts the body's immunity to infectious diseases. B vitamins are necessary for converting food into energy. Folate, one of the most common B vitamins can also significantly reduce the risk of neural tube birth defects in newborns and contribute to the prevention of heart disease. Vitamin C and vitamin E are important micronutrients in fruits and vegetables that serve as powerful antioxidants that can protect cells from cancer-causing agents. Vitamin C, in particular, can increase the body's absorption of calcium and iron from other foods. Calcium is an essential mineral for strong bones and teeth, while low iron levels can lead to anaemia, one of the most severe nutrition-related disorders. Many fruits and vegetables are also very high in dietary fiber, which can help move potentially harmful substances through the intestinal tract and lower blood cholesterol levels. Much fruit and vegetable potency is believed to also come from substances known as phytochemicals. Phytochemical antioxidants from fruits, vegetables and legumes can significantly inhibit the development of cardiovascular disease. Combinations of phytochemical antioxidants from different plant categories such as fruits, vegetables and legumes may possess complementary cardiovascular disease fighting activities [47].

Since more attention is being paid to the role of food in human health and in food safety and security [48, 49], secondary metabolites content is a factor which must be considered during the assessment of agricultural systems. Antioxidants and probiotics have recently attracted the attention of consumers and the food industry because of their potential health benefits. The natural dietary antioxidants in fruits, vegetables and legumes promote vascular health. The different food categories possess different bioactive compounds with various antioxidant capacities.

1.6 Safety of Enzyme Preparations Used in Food

Since ancient times, enzymes have been used in the preparation of various foods such as cheese, yogurt, bread, and alcoholic beverages [50]. Although these uses have spanned thousands of years, scientific understanding of how enzymes function did not formally develop until the 19th century [50]. One of the earliest observations of enzyme activity occurred in 1814, when Kirchoff noted the decomposition of starch by germinated barley [51]. In 1833, the first clear observance of a specific enzyme-catalyzed reaction was made by Puyen and Persey, who found that a precipitate from malt extract contained a heat-stable substance that could convert starch to sugar [52].

During the early 1950s, a committee led by James Delaney held hearings to address the use of food ingredients [53]. In a report based on these hearings, the committee estimated that nearly 840 ingredients were used in food. Of these, only about 420 were considered safe, and many had never been evaluated for safety. This report, along with the incidents of chemical contamination of food that occurred in 1954 and 1958, prompted Congress to amend the 1938 Act with the 1958 Food Additives Amendment. It is generally accepted that pathogenic microorganisms would not be used in the production of enzymes intended for use in food [54]. A nonpathogenic microorganism is one that is very unlikely to produce disease under ordinary circumstances [55].

1.7 Trace Element Speciation in Food

Enzymes are ubiquitous in nature and have been used in foods and in food processing for millennia. In response to changes in consumer demand, new developments in molecular biology and manufacturing technologies have paved the way for faster, more efficient routes in food enzyme manufacturing and in the production of food using enzymes. These new developments have also allowed for adjustment of enzyme properties to manufacturing conditions, and production of enzyme preparations that contain lower levels of undefined contaminants from the production process. The Food and Drug Administration (FDA) has continuously adjusted its regulatory procedures to keep up with these evolving technologies. However, regardless of the technology used to manufacture food enzymes, safety has been, and will always remain, at the core of the FDA's evaluations.

Food safety depends not only on the determination of total levels, but also on the speciation of trace elements occurring in foodstuffs. Thus, the biochemical and toxicological properties of a chemical element critically depend on the form in which it occurs in food [56, 57]. Human exposure to metal compounds in the general environment is usually greater through food and drink than through air [58]. Elemental species can be present in food due to anthropogenic or natural sources. In the first case it is a result of external contamination because of environmental pollution, food processing or leaching from packaging materials. In the second case it results from an endogenous synthesis by a plant or an animal (methylmercury or organoarsenic species) [59]. The role of elemental speciation and speciation analysis in human health hazard and risk assessment is critical for several toxic heavy metals and metalloids like arsenic (As), mercury (Hg), tin (Sn), chromium (Cr) and cadmium (Cd). For all of these elements, some considerations regarding their sources, presence in food and toxicity are reviewed in the following sections.

Arsenic (As) occurs in food as inorganic, as well as organic, compounds. Toxicity varies greatly between individual species. In general, organic As compounds are significantly less toxic than inorganic As compounds. Mobility in water and in body fluids largely determines species toxicity. It is reported that the toxicity conforms to the following order (highest to lowest toxicity): arsines

> inorganic arsenites > organic trivalent compounds (arsenooxides) > inorganic arsenates > organic pentavalent compounds > arsonium compounds > elemental As [60, 61]. For organic species, generally, the toxicity decreases as the degree of methylation increases [62].

Mercury (Hg) is one of the most toxic elements impacting human health. Because of its high bioaccumulation, Hg is among the most highly bioconcentrated trace metals in the human food chain. For example, predatory fish can have up to 106-fold higher Hg concentrations than ambient water and up to 95% of this Hg can be in the form of methylmercury [63]. The chemical form of Hg controls its bioavailability, transport, persistence and impact on the human body. All Hg species are toxic, while organic Hg compounds are generally more toxic than inorganic species. Tin (Sn) is one of the essential elements at trace levels involved in various metabolic processes in humans. It may be introduced into food either as inorganic or as organotin compounds. Most of the inorganic Sn compounds are nontoxic because of their low solubility and absorption [64]. However, organic Sn compounds are mostly toxic [65].

Canned foods, such as tomato sauce and fruit juices, are known to contain high concentrations of Sn. Other sources of Sn are cereal grains, dairy, meat, vegetables, seaweed and licorice. When inorganic Sn is introduced to foodstuff, there is a possibility of it turning into an organic Sn compound [66]. Additionally, dietary exposure to organotin compound may result from the consumption of organotin-contaminated meat and fish products. The butyltin and phenyltin compounds accumulate within the marine food chain, eventually accumulating in aquatic food products such as fish, oysters, and crab. Chromium (Cr) is extensively used in the chemical industry as a catalyst, pigment, and other applications such as metal plating. As a result, different species of Cr can be released into the environment (soil, surface, and ground waters) and are then available to humans (67).

Cadmium (Cd) is mainly present in foodstuffs as inorganic Cd salts. Because organic Cd compounds are unstable, Cd can be found in all types of food, and particularly high amounts occur in organs of cattle, seafood, and some mushroom species. This metal is found in all parts of food plants, but in animals and humans it is found in liver, kidney, and milk.

Food is the primary source of essential elements for humans. To exert an effect, essential elements must be bioavailable from food, i.e., available both for absorption and for subsequent utilization by the body. On the other hand, essential elements can also be toxic if taken in excess. The margin between deficiency and toxicity can be narrower for some elements (iron and selenium) than for others (cobalt or zinc).

Selenium (Se) is an essential trace element for man and animals. It is an integral part of the antioxidant enzymes (gluthatione peroxidase and iodothyronine deiodinase) which protect cells against the effects of free radicals formed during normal oxygen metabolism.

Iron is the most abundant transition metal in the human body (4–5 g in a human adult of 70 kg weight) and its deficiency is the most frequent nutritional problem in the world. It is an essential element required for growth and survival because it is involved in a broad spectrum of essential biological functions such as oxygen transport, electron transfer and DNA synthesis.

1.8 Bio-nanocomposites for Natural Food Packaging

Bio-nanocomposites are groups of polysaccharides (e.g., starch, cellulose), proteins (e.g., soy protein isolates, gelatin), and polyesters (e.g., polyhydroxyalkanoates, PHAs), among others. Materials obtained only with the raw material properties are unsatisfactory. To this end, some additives are needed for the polymer matrix to improve its mechanical properties (tensile strength, elongation and modulus), water absorption (solubility, vapor barriers, swelling), and morphology (homogeneity, porosity). Further study opens the possibility to add package active agents with antibacterial, antiviral, antioxidants, among others, called active packaging.

Nanomaterials used in the cultivation, preparation, storage and packaging of food and drink has enabled the obtainment of products with better characteristics such as materials for the controlled release of medicines and agrochemicals, containers with higher mechanical strength and antimicrobial properties, smart packaging capable of preserving food for longer periods of time, among others [68]. Nanotechnology is increasingly being used in agriculture, food processing, and food packaging. Nanomaterials as nanoparticles, nano-emulsions and nano-capsules are found in agricultural chemicals, processed foods, food packaging and food contact materials, including food storage containers, cutlery and chopping boards. Despite rapid developments in food nanotechnology, little is known about the occurrence, fate, and toxicity of NPs [69]. Nanotechnology for food packing is based on organic and inorganic nanomaterials added into a polymer matrix. Nanoparticles such as metals and metal oxides, cellulose nanofibers, chitin and chitosan, and exfoliated clay are used as mechanical reinforcing, barriers to gas diffusion, and antimicrobial additives [70].

Nanoparticles of Ag, ZnO, TiO_2 and SiO_2 are commonly used in food plastic wrapping in a polymer-based nanocomposite. These NPs present excellent UV blocking and gas diffusion barrier, but the main characteristic of their use is antimicrobial action. Food packaging materials are an express source of pollution due to the high amount disposed of in the world environment. The problem is aggravated since these materials are usually made from non-biodegradable and non-renewable sources, such as petroleum-based polymers.

Biocomposite materials based in starch, cellulose and chitin/chitosan are biodegradable, and are a suitable alternative to the petroleum-based polymer materials for food packaging [71]. However, these materials are more sensitive to physico-chemical degradation and are suitable to be attacked by microorganisms. Thus, additives are incorporated in these materials to increase the mechanical, chemical and biological resistance.

Nanoparticles are increasingly used as additives in food packaging and food contact materials due to their antimicrobial property. After use, these materials need to be discarded into the environment. The effect on the biodegradability and compostability is related to the microbial toxicity of NPs. The biodegradation process occurs through microorganisms. The use of antimicrobial additives (e.g., Ag, TiO_2, ZnO, and SiO_2) on a large scale may be hazardous to the microbes in the environment [72, 73]. Thus, the biodegradation process will be severely compromised, and it may be completely inhibited, affecting the decomposition of these materials in landfills and composting units.

References

1. E. Clay. Food security: Concepts and measurement. In *Trade reforms and food security: Conceptualising the linkages*. Rome: Food and Agriculture Organization of the United Nations (FAO), 2002.

2. L.T. Evans. *Feeding the ten billion: Plans and population growth*. Cambridge, UK: Cambridge University Press. 1998.
3. H. Jiang. Rising agricultural commodity prices: How we got here and where do we go. Office of Global Analysis. Foreign Agricultural Service. Washington, DC: USDA. 2008.
4. X. Irz, L. Lin, C. Thirtle, S. Wiggins. Agricultural productivity growth and poverty alleviation. *Devel. Pol. Rev.* 19:449–466, 2001.
5. N. Majid. Reaching millennium goals: How well does agricultural productivity growth reduce poverty? Employment Strategy Papers, 2004 No. 12. Geneva, Switzerland: International Labor Organization. 2004.
6. P.L. Pingali, P.A. Roger, eds. *Impact of pesticides on farmer health and the rice environment*. Laguna, Philippines: IRRI, 1995.
7. World Bank. DC2011-0002. Responding to global food price volatility and its impact on food security. Development Committee. Washington, DC: World Bank, 2011.
8. M.C. Roco. Nanoscale science and engineering for agriculture and food systems. Washington: National Planning Workshop, 2002.
9. S. Neethirajan, and D.S. Jayas. Nanotechnology for the food and bioprocessing industries. *Food and Bioprocess Technology* 4:39–47, 2011.
10. T. Joseph, and M. Morrison. Nanotechnology in agriculture and food: A Nanoforum report. Institute of Nanotechnology, 2006.
11. G. Miller, and R. Senjen. Out of the laboratory and onto our plates. Nanotechnology in food and agriculture. Friends of the Earth Report, 2008.
12. C. Shaffer. Is food nanotech withering on the vine? *Food Quality* 2011.
13. A.L. Brody. Case studies on nanotechnologies for food packaging. *Food Technology* 102–107, 2007.
14. Q. Chaudhry, M. Scotter, J. Blackburn, B. Ross, A. Boxall, L. Castle, R. Aitken, and R. Watkins. Applications and implications of nanotechnologies for the food sector. *Food Additives and Contaminants* 25(3), 241–258, 2008.
15. J. Collister. Commercialization of polymer nanocomposites. In R. Krishnamoorti and R.A. Vaia, eds. *Polymer nanocomposites: Synthesis, characterization and modeling*. Washington: American Chemical Society, 2002.
16. S. Ray, A. Easteal, S.Y. Quek, and X.D. Chen. The potential use of polymer-clay nanocomposites in food packaging. *International Journal of Food Engineering* 2(4), article.5, 2006.
17. H.M.C. de Azeredo. Nanocomposites for food packaging applications. *Food Research International* 42, 1240–1253, 2009.
18. A. Fernandez, S. Torres-Giner, and J.M. Lagaron. Novel route to stabilization of bioactive antioxidants by encapsulation in electrospun fibers of zein prolamine. *Food Hydrocolloids* 23(5), 1427–1432, 2009.
19. A. Lopez-Rubio, E. Sanchez, Y. Sanz, and J.M. Lagaron. Encapsulation of living bifidobacteria in ultrathin PVOH electrospun fibers. *Biomacromolecules* 10, 2823–2829, 2009.
20. J.M. Lagaron, and A. Lopez-Rubio. Nanotechnology for bioplastic: Opportunities challenges and strategies. *Trends in Food Science and Technology*. doi:10.1016/j.tifs.2011.01.007, 2011.
21. H.M.C. de Azeredo. Nanocomposites for food packaging applications. *Food Research International* 42, 1240–1253, 2009.

22. I. Sondi, and B. Salopek-Sondi. Silver nanoparticles as antimicrobial agent: A case study on *E. coli* as a model for Gram-negative bacteria. *Journal of Colloid Interface Science* 275, 177–182, 2004.
23. J.R. Morones, J.L. Elechiguerra, A. Camacho, K. Holt, J.B. Kouri, J.T. Ramirez, and M.J. Yacaman. The bactericidal effect of silver nanoparticles. *Nanotechnology* 16(10), 2346–2353, 2005.
24. P.J. Fellows. Freezing. In *Food processing technology: Principles and practice*, P.J. Fellows, ed. Woodhead Publishing Limited and CRC Press LLC: Cambridge, England, 418–451, 2000.
25. R.P. Singh, and D.R. Heldman. Food Freezing. In *Introduction to food engineering*, R.P. Singh and D.R. Heldman, eds. Academic Press, Elsevier: California, USA, 501–541, 2009.
26. D.R. Heldman, and R.P. Singh. Thermodynamics of food freezing. In *Food process engineering*, D.R. Heldman and R.P. Singh, eds. AVI Publishing Company, INC.: Westport, Connecticut, 158–215, 1981.
27. M.S. Rahman, and J. Velez-Ruiz. Food preservation by freezing. In *Handbook of food preservation*, M.S. Rahman, ed. CRC Press, Taylor & Francis Group: Boca Raton, USA, 635–665, 2007.
28. A. Collignan, A.L. Raoult-Wack, and A. Themelin. Energy study of food processing by osmotic dehydration and air-drying. *Agricultural Engineering Journal* 1(3): 125–35, 1992.
29. M.F. North, and S.J. Lovatt. Freezing methods and equipment. In *Handbook of frozen food processing and packaging*, D.-W. Sun, ed. CRC Press, Taylor and Francis Group: Boca Raton, USA, 199–210, 2006.
30. M. Jalté, J.-L. Lanoisellé, N.I. Lebovka, and E. Vorobiev. Freezing of potato tissue pre-treated by pulsed electric fields. *LWT – Food Science and Technology* 42(2): 576–580, 2009.
31. A. LeBail, D. Chevalier, D.M. Mussa, and M. Ghoul. High pressure freezing and thawing of foods: A review. *International Journal of Refrigeration* 25(5): 504–513, 2002.
32. E. Alizadeh, N. Chapleau, M. de Lamballerie, and A. Le-Bail. Effect of different freezing processes on the microstructure of Atlantic salmon (Salmo salar) fillets. *Innovative Food Science & Emerging Technologies* 8(4): 493–499, 2007.
33. Y. Yang. Scientific substantiation of functional food health claims in China. *The Journal of Nutrition* 138, 1199S–1205S. 2008.
34. A. Ikeda, A. Moraes, G. Mesquita. Reflections on trends and opportunities of functional foods. *Revista P&D Engenharia de Produção* 8(2), 40–56. 2010.
35. N. Sutar, P.P. Sutar, D. Mohapatra. New Horizons in functional food sector: An Indian perspective. *J. Dairying, Foods & H.S.* 29 (3/4):166–172. 2010.
36. S. Kaur, M. Das. Functional foods: An overview. *Food Science and Biotechnology* 20 (4), 861–875. 2011.
37. L. Kotilainen, R. Rajalahti, C. Ragasa, E. Pehu. Health enhancing foods: Opportunities for strengthening the sector in developing countries. Agriculture and Rural Development Discussion Paper 30. The International Bank for Reconstruction and Development/The World Bank 2006.
38. M. Klimas, C. Brethour, D. Bucknell. Introduction and background in *International market trends analysis for the functional foods and natural health*

products industry in the United States, Australia, the United Kingdom, and Japan. March 17, p. 3. Nutri-Net Canada, Ontario, Canada. 2008.

39. I. Siró, E. Kápolna, B. Kápolna, A. Lugasi. Functional food. Product development, marketing, and consumer acceptance – A review. *Appetite* 51:456–467. 2008.
40. G.E. Castillo, S.I. Martínez. *Manual de fitoterapia.* Elsevier Masson, pp 29–38. Clifford, 1999.
41. S.R. Singh, K.O. Rachie, K.E. Dashiell. *Soybeans for the tropics: Research, production and utilization.* John Wiley and Sons Ltd, Chichester, UK, pp 230. 1987.
42. I.C. Onwueme, T.D. Sinha. Field Crop Production in Tropical Africa. Michael Health Ltd. Reigate Survey RH2 9EL, Technical Centre for Agricultural and Rural Cooperation, CTA. p. 190–192. 1991.
43. R. Bou, R. Codony, A. Tres, E.A. Decker, F. Guardiola. Dietary strategies to improve nutritional value, oxidative stability, and sensory properties of poultry products. *Critical Reviews in Food Science and Nutrition,* 49:800–822. 2009.
44. J.E. Olesen, M. Trnka, K.C. Kersebaum, A.O. Skjelväg, B. Seguin, P. Peltonen-Sainio, F. Rossi, J. Kozyra, F. Micale. Impacts and adaptation of European crop productivity systems to climate change. *Europen Journal of Agronomy* 34:96–112, 2011.
45. F.M. DaMatta, A. Grandis, B.C. Arenque, M.S. Buckeridge. Impact of climate changes on crop physiology and food quality. *Food Research International* 43:1814–1823, 2010.
46. J.F. Herencia, P.A. Garcia-Galavi., J.A.R. Dorado, and C. Maqueda. Comparison of nutritional quality of the crops grown in an organic and conventional fertilized soil. *Scientia Horticulturae* 129:882–888, 2011.
47. S.Wang, J.P. Melnyk, R. Tsao, and M.F. Marcone. How natural dietary antioxidants in fruits, vegetables and legume promote vascular health. *Food Research International* 44:14–22, 2011.
48. A. Hoisington, M.M. Manore, C. Raab. Nutritional quality of emergency foods. *J. American Dietetic Assoc.* 111:573–576, 2011.
49. P. Combris, R. Goglia, M. Henini, I.G. Soler, M. Spiteri. Improvement of the nutritional quality of foods as a public health tool. Public Health doi: 19.1016/j.puhe, 2011.07.004.
50. O. Kirk, T.V. Borchert, and C.C. Fuglsang. Industrial enzyme applications. *Current Opinion in Biotechnology* 13:345–351, 2002.
51. H. von Euler. *General chemistry of the enzymes.* Wiley, 1912.
52. G.A. Tucker, and L.F.J. Woods. *Enzymes in food processing.* Springer Netherlands, 1995.
53. F.H. Degnan. Rethinking the applicability and usefulness of the GRAS concept. *Food and Drug Law Journal* 46:553–582, 1991.
54. M.W. Pariza, and E.A. Johnson. Evaluating the safety of microbial enzyme preparations used in food processing: Update for a new century. *Regulatory Toxicology and Pharmacology* 33:173–186, 2001.
55. M.W. Pariza, and E.M. Foster. Determining the safety of enzymes used in food-processing. *Journal of Food Protection* 46:453–468, 1983.
56. L. Ebdon. *Trace element speciation for environment, food and health.* Royal Society of Chemistry: Great Britain, 2001.
57. S.T. Omaye. *Food and nutritional toxicology.* CRC Press: 2004.

58. G. Nordberg, B.A. Fowler, M. Nordberg, L. Friberg. *Handbook on the toxicology of metals*, 3rd ed. Academic Press: Burlington, p. 992, 2007.
59. P. Szefer, J.O. Nriagu. *Mineral components in foods*. CRC Press/Taylor & Francis: 2007.
60. I. Komorowicz, D. Baralkiewicz. Arsenic and its speciation in water samples by high performance liquid chromatography inductively coupled plasma mass spectrometry –Last decade review. *Talanta* 84 (2):247–261, 2011.
61. B.K. Mandal, K.T. Suzuki. Arsenic round the world: A review. *Talanta* 58(1):201–235, 2002.
62. M. Leermakers, W. Baeyens, M. De Gieter, B. Smedts, C. Meert, H.C. De Bisschop, R. Morabito, P. Quevauviller. Toxic arsenic compounds in environmental samples: Speciation and validation. *TrAC Trends in Analytical Chemistry* 25(1):1–10, 2006.
63. K. Leopold, M. Foulkes, P. Worsfold. Methods for the determination and speciation of mercury in natural waters – A review. *Analytica Chimica Acta* 663(2):127–138, 2010.
64. M. Nordberg, G.F. Nordberg. Toxicology and biological monitoring of metals. In *General and applied toxicology*. John Wiley & Sons, Ltd: 2009.
65. R. Cornelis, J.A. Caruso, H. Crews, K.G. Heumann. *Handbook of elemental speciation II - Species in the environment, food, medicine and occupational health*. John Wiley & Sons Ltd.: Chichester, Vol. 2, p. 767, 2005.
66. Y.-H. Li, H. Long, F.-Q. Zhou. Determination of trace tin by catalytic adsorptive cathodic stripping voltammetry. *Analytica Chimica Acta* 554(1-2):86–91, 2005.
67. N. Unceta, F. Séby, J. Malherbe, O. Donard. Chromium speciation in solid matrices and regulation: A review. *Analytical and Bioanalytical Chemistry* 397(3):1097–1111, 2010.
68. G. Miller, and R. Senjen. Nanotechnology in food and agriculture. In *Nano meets macro: Social perspectives on nanoscience and nanotechnology*. Pan Stanford Publishing, p.417–444, 2010.
69. S.B. Sekhon. *Nanotechnology, Science and Applications* Vol.3, p. 1, 2010.
70. P. Das, M.A. Xenopoulos, C.J. Williams, Md.E. Hoque, and C.D. Metcalfe. *Environmental Toxicology and Chemistry* Vol. 31, p. 122, 2012.
71. V. Siracusa, P. Rocculi, S. Romani, M. Dalla Rosa. *Trends in Food Science & Technology* Vol. 19, p. 634, 2008.
72. D. Sharma, J. Rajput, B.S. Kaith, M. Kaur, S. Sharma. *Thin Solid Films* Vol. 519, p. 1224, 2010.
73. C. Levard, E.M. Hotze, G. Lowry, G.E. Brown, Jr. *Environmental Science and Technology* Vol.46, p. 6900, 2012.

2

Food Security: A Global Problem

Donatella Restuccia[1], Umile Gianfranco Spizzirri[1], Francesco Puoci[1], Giuseppe Cirillo[1], Ortensia Ilaria Parisi[1], Giuliana Vinci[2] and Nevio Picci[1]

[1]University of Calabria, Department of Pharmacy, Health and Nutritional Sciences, Rende (CS), Italy
[2]Sapienza University of Rome, Department of Management, Rome, Italy

Abstract

Food security is fundamentally about achieving reliable access to adequate, affordable and nutritious food supplies sufficient to avoid chronic hunger, crisis hunger and stunted development. Chronic hunger afflicts hundreds of millions of people. Latest figures from the Food and Agriculture Organization (FAO) estimate that nearly 1 billion people are undernourished worldwide, suffering food insecurity. Roughly 15 percent of humanity is considered hungry or malnourished, especially women. The majority of the hungry (65 percent) are in India, China, the Democratic Republic of Congo, Bangladesh, Indonesia, Pakistan and Ethiopia. The number has been increasing at a rate of almost four million per year since the second half of the 1990s, rendering the goal of the 1996 World Food Summit–to halve the number of undernourished people, 815 million at that time by 2015–far-fetched. Also the first Millennium Development Goal (MDG) falls short of food security aspirations in seeking only to reduce by half the proportion of the world's population experiencing hunger. Among the driving factors affecting food security, productivity is surely a crucial aspect; on the other hand, there are many other factors behind food insecurity to be analyzed comprised of social, environmental and economic issues. Moreover, unexpected events can contribute to global access to safe and stable food supplies. This happened in particular from 2003–2009, when a food price crisis followed by the financial crisis and global economic recession pushed the number of hungry and undernourished people in the world to unprecedented levels. In the first half of 2010, world agricultural commodity markets appeared to enter calmer times. Prices of food and

Visakh P. M., Sabu Thomas, Laura B. Iturriaga, and Pablo Daniel Ribotta (eds.) Advances in Food Science and Technology, (19–102) © 2013 Scrivener Publishing LLC

agricultural commodities remained high, but had nevertheless declined from the peaks of 2008, and the world economy was emerging from recession. However, there are growing concerns about high market volatility partly exacerbated by many governments uncoordinated policy actions intended to ensure adequate supplies on domestic markets. This chapter will discuss food security concepts and main causes, and data about levels and trends in global hunger will be presented. Moreover, trends in food prices, production and trade will also be evaluated in the context of recent developments in the global economy and agricultural markets.

Keywords: Food security, social issues, economic aspects, environment, economic crisis, food prices, volatility, food production, food trade

2.1 Food Security: Definitions and Basic Concepts

Food security, or rather insecurity, is at the heart of food crises and food-related emergencies. The great concern about this issue induced FAO to reaffirm its vision of a food-secure world in May 2007 at the 33rd Session of the Committee on World Food Security where it was declared that:

> *"FAO's vision of a world without hunger is one in which most people are able, by themselves, to obtain the food they need for an active and healthy life, and where social safety nets ensure that those who lack resources still get enough to eat."* [1]

This statement represents a further evolution of the definition of food security adopted at the World Food Summit in November 1996, stating that:

> *"Food security exists when all people at all times have physical or economic access to sufficient safe and nutritious food to meet their dietary needs and food preferences for an active and healthy life."* [2]

It follows that global food security as defined by FAO requires that all people have access to adequate supplies of safe, nutritious food of their own choice for healthy living. The widely accepted World Food Summit definition underlines the multidimensional nature of food security as it involves food accessibility, availability, utilization, and stability. Equitable access to food refers to both access to the supply (or availability) of food and to the entitlement to food, i.e., the resources, both financial and natural, and human ability to obtain food [3]. Food availability is the physical presence of food in the area of concern through all forms of domestic production, commercial imports and food aid. Food availability might be aggregated at the regional, national, district or community level and is determined by:

- production: food produced in the area;
- trade: food brought into the area through market mechanisms;
- stocks: food held by traders and in government reserves;
- transfers: food supplied by the government and/or aid agencies.

Food access concerns a household's ability to acquire adequate amounts of food, through one or a combination of own home production and stocks, purchases, barter, gifts, borrowing and food aid. The following are some examples:

- own production – crops, livestock, etc.;
- hunting, fishing and gathering of wild foods;
- purchase at markets, shops, etc.;
- barter – exchange of items for food;
- gifts from friends/relatives, community, government, aid agencies, etc.

In some cases, food may be available but not accessible to certain households if they cannot acquire a sufficient quantity or diversity of food through these mechanisms.

Food utilization refers to a household's use of the food to which they have access, and an individual's ability to absorb and metabolize the nutrients. In fact, food may be available and accessible but certain household members may not benefit fully if they do not receive an adequate share of the food in terms of quantity and diversity, or if their bodies are unable to absorb food because of poor food preparation or sickness. Food utilization includes aspects like:

- the ways in which food is stored, processed and prepared, including the water and cooking fuel used, and hygiene conditions;
- feeding practices, particularly for individuals with special nutrition needs, such as babies, young children, the elderly, sick people, and pregnant or lactating women;

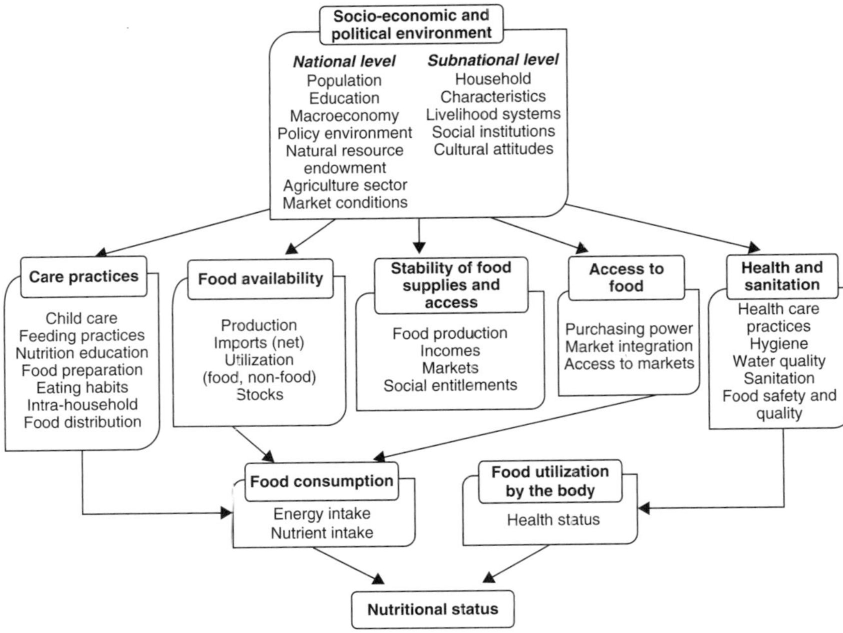

Figure 2.1 Conceptual framework of possible causes of low food consumption and poor nutritional status.

- the sharing of food within the household, and the extent to which this corresponds to individuals' nutrition needs – growth, pregnancy, lactation, etc.;
- the health status of each member of the household.

The conceptual framework that gave operational meaning to FAO's food security definition is depicted in Figure 2.1 [4].

Broadly defined, food security includes health and nutrition outcomes (such as malnourishment and anthropometric measures of food insecurity) and consumption outcomes (nutrient intake). Health and nutritional outcomes are direct results of consumption outcomes. Nutritional status in food consumption is generally identified by three indicators: calorie, protein, and fat intake, while food consumption is mainly related with domestic food production and food imports achieved by international trade. Agricultural potential (including both agronomic aspects and resources management) is an important prerequisite for long-term food supply or production [5]. Relevant policies can be applied to improve agricultural potential through proper investment. Trade and trade policies (regional and global) also influence both national and international food availability and the cost of food imports at the national level (including food aid). In addition to food supply obtained by production and trade, food consumption is also affected by food distribution within the country with discrepancies between urban and rural areas. Keeping all these aspects in mind, the sequential approach of examining 1) food consumption; 2) production, import, and distribution; and 3) agricultural potential, can help to distinguish outcomes of food security (food consumption) from determinants and future potential (food production, import, and distribution), providing more targeted policy recommendations.

As food insecurity occurs when food is either unavailable and/or where there is a lack of entitlement to food, it generally appears in two basic forms:

- *Transitory food insecurity*: This generally refers to extreme cases of hunger caused by war, flooding, drought, crop failure, pest infestations, and loss of purchasing power in farming communities and market failures through high food prices. Such problems can also trigger production and subsistence food crises threatening a populations access to food.
- *Chronic food insecurity*: Long term and deep-rooted food insecurity is largely driven by endemic poverty. People are subject to a daily problem of poor diet through an inability to achieve their basic nutritional requirements, either because they are unable to buy it or to produce it for themselves.

In cases of food insecurity, once basic caloric needs are met, a second stage of food concerns addresses safety and healthfulness. This safety dimension involves securing food supplies free from contamination, adulteration or food-borne diseases, and healthy foods that reduce the influence of diet-based diseases and promote well-being. While the poorest face chronic or crisis hunger anchored largely in commodity supplies and prices, safety and wellness are related to changes occurring in the global food economy.

Today, food insecurity expresses itself in three ways. At the most extreme level people face chronic food insecurity. Another large number of people live on less than 1.25 USD per day, mostly in rural areas and mostly dependent on farming for their incomes.

While their subsistence-oriented economies mean that they are not chronically hungry, they are vulnerable to food crises brought on by civil disorder, natural disaster or politically-imposed famine. The third group, primarily comprised of women and children, faces nutrient deficits that stunt physical and mental development while increasing vulnerability to disease. All three extract a terrible human price through both suffering and lost productivity. Some 8 million people die each year of hunger-related causes, and more than half of these are children. Millions more reach adulthood with impaired physical and mental abilities, constraining their ability to support themselves, their families and their communities [6]. Moreover, food crises affecting individual countries further shock and destabilize the food security status of part of or the entire population (the newly food-insecure) and worsen it for those who were already food-insecure prior to the emergency (the chronically food-insecure) [7]. FAO's Global Information and Early Warning System on Food and Agriculture (GIEWS) monitors and disseminates information on countries in crisis requiring external assistance for food (Figure 2.2).

As can be seen from Figure 2.2, food crises can be triggered by a number of factors—natural or human-induced. If the emergency is natural, it may be described as either sudden or slow-onset, and if it is human-induced it may be the result of socio-economic problems or war/conflict. The total number of recorded emergencies in recent years is far higher than in the 1980s. Since the mid-1980s, the general trend has been towards an increase in the number of countries affected by emergencies. The number of human-induced emergencies seems to have increased the most, with war/conflict accounting for most of them.

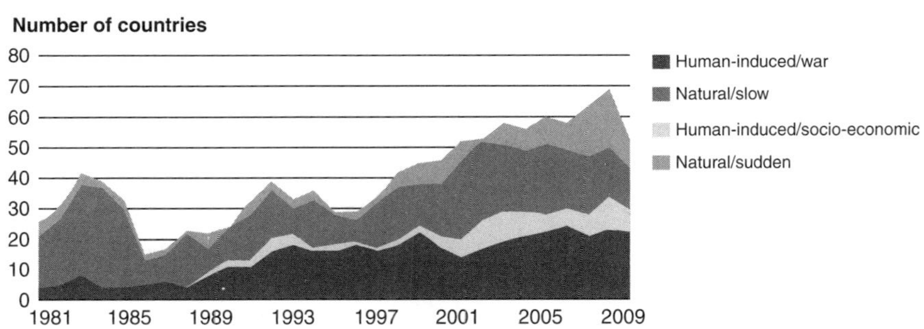

Figure 2.2 Emergencies (by type) in countries requiring assistance, 1981 to 2009. Source: FAO.

The concept of food security has developed over the past three decades. Concerns about food security up to the end of the 1970s were directed more at the national and international level, and concerned the ability of countries to secure adequate food supplies. It was only later that the level of analysis shifted to include a focus on food security at the local level, even down to households and individuals [3]. Moreover, in a more general analysis, alongside security and safety has emerged the new concern of sustainability as the ability of one generation to meet its food needs without compromising the ability of future generations to meet theirs. Its economic component must ensure the continued profitability of farming, while its social component must make both those who farm and those who leave farming better off [8].

Definitions of food security identify the outcomes of food security and are useful for formulating policies and deciding on actions, but the processes that lead to desired outcomes also matter. Most current definitions of food security therefore include references to processes as well as outcomes and, taken together, these processes constitute the food system in its complexity. The performance of the food system determines whether or not food security is achieved (Figure 2.3).

Definition of functioning of food systems has helped as well to show both desired food security goals and what needs to happen to bring these about. In this regard, it has been stated that: "Food systems encompass: (i) activities related to the production, processing, distribution, preparation and consumption of food; and (ii) the outcomes of these activities contributing to food security (food availability, with elements related to production, distribution

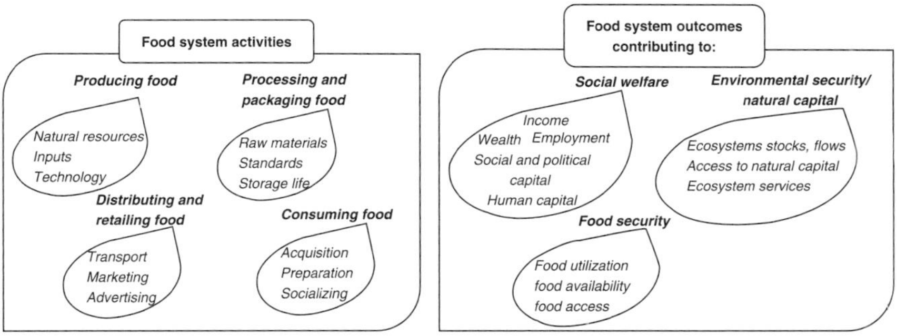

Figure 2.3 Food system activities and food security outcomes.

and exchange; food access, with elements related to affordability, allocation and preference; and food use, with elements related to nutritional value, social value and food safety). The outcomes also contribute to environmental and other securities (e.g., income). Interactions between and within biogeophysical and human environments influence both the activities and the outcomes [9]. The sum of all the processes in a food system is sometimes referred to as a food chain and a variety of processes along a food chain need to occur in order to bring about food security. The main conceptual difference between a food system and a food chain is that the system is holistic comprising a set of simultaneously interacting processes, whereas the chain is linear containing a sequence of activities that need to occur for people to obtain food. The concept of the food system is useful for scientists investigating cause and effect relationships and feedback loops, and is important for the technical analyses that underpin policy recommendations. However, when communicating the findings of such investigation it is often easier to use the concept of the food chain. A food system comprises multiple food chains operating at the global, national and local levels. Some of these chains are very short and not very complex, while others circle the globe in an intricate web of interconnecting processes and links.

The food security status of any household or individual is typically determined by the interaction of a broad range of agro-environmental, socio-economic and biological factors [10]. As with the concepts of health or social welfare, there is no single, direct measure of food security. However, the complexity of the food security problem can be simplified by focusing on three distinct but interrelated dimensions: aggregate food availability, household food access, and individual food utilization. Depending on their mandates and the aims of their assessment, different agencies have developed diverse approaches to assess food security [11–13]. However, the theory behind each approach is based on the same underlying concept. This concept incorporates issues of availability and access to food, and acknowledges that, in an emergency, people may adopt a variety of coping strategies in response to food insecurity. The concept also includes issues around vulnerability, and sees famine as a process, comprising distinct stages [14]. Methodologies are also similar, and largely depend on secondary information sources and rapid-assessment techniques, such as interviews, focus groups and proportional piling [14, 15]. The main differences between agencies' approaches stem from their different objectives, and the different ways the information is analyzed to determine whether the population in question is food insecure. For some agencies the main aim is to assess risks to livelihoods, as well as to lives. In their food-security assessments they consider a variety of interventions that protect livelihoods (food aid, de-stocking and fodder distribution, cash-for-work, seeds and tools distributions, etc.). To estimate the severity of food insecurity, the analysis of shifts in food entitlements, coping strategies and nutritional status are accomplished. On the other hand, the food-economy approach, which is widely used to estimate food-aid needs is also common [16]; to evaluate the severity of food insecurity it judges the size of the food deficit. For example, the FAO's easy-to-use measure of undernourishment has the advantage that it is calculated every year in a consistent way for all countries. It is based on the distribution of the dietary energy supply within a country's population and two benchmarks have been assessed for measuring hunger. The first indicator is the "minimum dietary energy requirement." This naturally varies by age and sex so that a weighted average is calculated for each country based on its population profile (typically this average for light activity is just below 2,100 kilocalories per day) while the second indicator is the proportion of children under five years who are underweight in relation to their age. This measure is used to estimate the number and proportion of undernourished annually. Results are reported as a 3 year moving average to the Committee on World Food Security and the annual FAO publication: the State of Food Insecurity in the World (SOFI). Anyway, measuring food and nutrition insecurity is a multidimensional problem that requires accounting for both short- and long-term food and nutrition insecurity, as well as considering chronic, transitory, and periodic food and nutrition insecurity. Measures of household food and nutrition security, such as those based on surveys of dietary intake, must be compared with adequacy norms. Finally, the use of potential substitute indicators such as real wage rates, employment, price ratios, migration flows, changes in consumption structure, incidence of illness, and so forth may be appropriate at times [17].

2.2 Main Causes of Food Insecurity

A variety of factors, both internal and external, affects the food security of a country and straightforward explanations for world hunger should be treated with caution. Food security is, in fact, a multifaceted concept that goes far beyond the number of people that can be sustained by the earth's limited food resources, to encompass a broad range of aspects which are however related in some fashion to two basic causes: insufficient national food availability and insufficient access to food by households and individuals. In particular, food security is strictly related with issues like population growth, control and mobility, resource distribution, consumption patterns, agricultural production, climate change, environmental degradation, socio-economic status, development, trade relations, land ownership tights, access to microfinance and to healthcare services. Moreover, the problems of inequity are further exacerbated by internal conflict and war which can dislocate rural and farming communities, while vulnerability is also increased due to natural or human-induced disasters. All these aspects can be broadly classified in social, economic and environmental issues.

2.2.1 Social Issues

2.2.1.1 Poverty, Income Distribution and Changing Patterns of Food Consumption

There is evidence that amounts of suitable food are being produced in the world today, although not available to all, and the fundamental hunger problem today relies more on income distribution, rather than food shortages [18]. This is because hungry people seem to be too poor to buy food, while, at the same time, obesity and chronic illnesses associated with excessive food intake are becoming a serious problem in developed countries [19, 20]. Among social issues, in fact, poverty is undoubtedly a fundamental cause of hunger (poor households are unable to purchase food despite its availability) and, at the same time, it is equally one of its consequences as undernourished families are less able to work or learn to their full potential. About 40% of the world's population—2.6 billion people—live on less than 2.00 USD per day, with 1.4 billion of them living on less than 1.25 USD per day. About 925 million people lack sufficient purchasing power to access even enough calories to sustain a medium level of physical activity.

As stated above, taking a long-term perspective, hunger and inadequate access to food are not just a matter of food scarcity or high food prices; these are only some of its immediate symptoms. Food insecurity is critically linked to poverty and low incomes, more than agricultural production [21]. In many past cases of famine in certain countries, overall production or availability of food was often a poor predictor of the amount of food that the poor segments of the population could acquire. For example, Africa as a continent has not been able to increase its agricultural production to face population growth and this led to periods of decline or stagnation in its food and total agricultural outputs per capita. However, even in countries and regions that have performed better and now have food surpluses (e.g., much of South Asia), hunger and malnutrition are still widespread. Although many Asian consumers are rapidly diversifying and enriching their diets, leading to a sustained surge in demand for livestock products, fruits, vegetables and vegetable oils, and some feed grains, over 500 million other Asians go hungry, and in South Asia (as in Central America, Near East and North Africa, sub-Saharan Africa and across the Commonwealth of Independent States countries), the actual number of hungry people continues to grow [7]. These people do not have the means to buy sufficient food to meet basic food needs, and desperately need better livelihood opportunities highlighting that past patterns of growth have been insufficient or have failed to adequately benefit the poor. A poor nation may increase its food production, national food self-sufficiency and economic growth to lift itself upward in the poverty statistics, but wide sections of its people may remain food insecure because other factors that affect their access to the food are not considered in economic indicators [22, 23]. In other words, development indices that focus on increased production of food alone are weak instruments to evaluate food distribution between populations and within populations which are mainly related with people's incomes. In most developing countries, large segments of both the rural and urban populations are poor, and a large share of their money is devoted to buy food [24, 25]. In development economics this is of course a reflection of the Engel curve, to the extent that lower income households have a higher share of food in their expenditures in comparison with higher income households. Moreover, when incomes start to rise, most of the first increments are spent for food, firstly to access enough calories to overcome hunger and then to upgrade the quality of diets. It follows that successful poverty reduction would have the double effect of achieving the humanitarian goal of reducing hunger but, at the same time, causing an increase in consumption of agricultural products. The world demand for food, in fact, is expected to double in the first half of the 21st century; half of that growth should come from population growth and half from growth in purchasing power of low-income consumers [26]. Consumers of rich countries have now been joined by millions of newcomers from China, India, and other developing countries, where rapid economic growth has led to increasing incomes for the new urban middle class, creating new food demands and changing consumption that mimics the patterns of rich countries. The new consumers of the global South are shifting to diets rich in meat and dairy products. This is confirmed by the UN Inter-agency Report on the International Assessment of Agricultural Knowledge, Science and Technology for Development [27]. Global demographic changes and changing patterns of income distribution over the next 50 years are expected to lead to an increased general demand for food, as well as different patterns of food consumption (meat and dairy products in particular). In this regard, it is predicted that global cereal demand will increase by 75% between 2000 and 2050, while global demand for meat doubles during that same period. The increase in demand for the latter also implies an additional increase in feedstock demand. Hence, the growing demand for other foodstuff, such as meat and dairy products, creates knock-on effects on the demand for certain crops like maize, and it is noteworthy that more than three-quarters of this growth in demand for both cereals and meat will be achieved by developing countries [28].

2.2.1.2 *Population Growth and Urbanization*

The world's population reached six billion people just before the turn of the millennium and the most up-to-date estimates suggest that global population will increase by another 2.5 billion to a total of 9.2 billion in 2050. Most of this increase will be in less developed regions of the world where population is projected to rise from 5.4 billion now to 7.9 billion in 2050. An important contextual factor, however, is how much the rate of global population increase has slowed from its peak during the 20th century. Population growth reached its fastest rate in 1963, at 2.19% a year. Today, the growth rate has almost halved, to 1.15%. It continues to decline and is projected to fall below 1% in 2020 and to less than 0.5% by 2050. Long-term projections now suggest that the world's population will stabilize at just above ten billion in the year 2020 [29]. The global picture, then, contradicts the Malthusian nightmare of population exponential growth. But this is not to overlook the real demographic challenges that still lie ahead. Principal among these is that while the global picture shows population growth slowing down significantly, almost all of the remaining projected growth will take place in developing countries. A comparison of the world's most populous countries in 2007 and as projected in 2050 illustrates the point (Table 2.1).

Table 2.1 The world's 20 most populous countries, 2007 and 2050.

2007		2050	
Country	**Population (m)**	**Country**	**Population (m)**
China	1,329	India	1,658
India	1,169	China	1,409
USA	306	USA	402
Indonesia	232	Indonesia	297
Brazil	192	Pakistan	292
Pakistan	164	Nigeria	289
Bangladesh	159	Bangladesh	254
Nigeria	148	Brazil	254
Russia	142	DRC	187
Japan	128	Ethiopia	183
Mexico	107	Philippines	140
Philippines	88	Mexico	132
Vietnam	87	Egypt	121
Ethiopia	83	Venezuela	120
Germany	83	Russia	108
Egypt	75	Japan	103
Turkey	75	Iran	100
Iran	71	Turkey	99
Thailand	64	Uganda	92
DRC	63	Kenya	85

Source: UN Department of Economic and Social Affairs (2006).

Population growth over the past century has been accompanied by enormous increases in food production [30]. But today's new investments are having much less effect on productivity. With steeply rising energy and fertilizer prices, some analysts now doubt that future production can keep pace if based on the same energy-hungry production model. There are two competing theories about the impact of population growth on natural resource degradation and agricultural productivity. The traditional Malthusian argument assumes that technological advance in agriculture is limited, hence growth in population leads to expansion of the cropped area into ever more marginal lands.

The result is a decline in labor productivity and per capita output. This process should go on until per capita output reaches subsistence levels, below which population pressure is unsustainable [31]. Also considering resource degradation, the vision of this theory is further exasperate into "downward spirals" that accelerate the process of impoverishment [32]. In contrast, Boserup [33] has offered a much more optimistic view assessing that population pressure makes labor become cheaper relative to land. Then a process of "induced innovation" can take place whereby communities invest in agricultural intensification and in improving their natural resources. The induced innovation model predicts increases in agricultural output per unit of land, although it does not necessarily predict that output per worker (or average labor productivity) will also increase, or that investments will be made in technologies that improve the long-term sustainability of resources. This will depend on the application characteristics of the induced technological change. If average output per worker continues to decline, then the induced innovation model can also lead to the same state of impoverishment as the Malthusian model, but over a longer time horizon. However, if technological change can raise labor productivity then, even as more workers are absorbed into the system, per capita incomes will rise on average, and a sustained process of economic development may be launched.

Another aspect related to food security and human pressure is that the world's population is becoming increasigly urbanized. This phenomenon has erupted dramatically in many developing countries in recent years as a result of both natural increase and rural-urban migration. In 2008, the world reached an invisible but momentous milestone: for the first time in history, more than half its population, 3.3 billion people, lived in urban areas. By 2030, this is expected to swell to almost 5 billion. Considering that over the last 15 to 20 years the absolute number of urban poor and undernourished people has increased at an extremely rapid rate, it is possible to forecast that many of the new urbanites will be poor, with a direct impact on food security [34]. A growing and more urban population will be accompanied by increases in income levels and changing food preferences as the three fundamental components of food security availability, access, and utilization differ in urban and rural contexts and across urban socio-economic groups [35]. A greater diversity of both local and imported food products are available in cities although most of the food is not produced within city boundaries. Similarly, much of the available food is processed either locally or imported in a processed form. In fact, urban dietary requirements are met to a considerable extent by relatively expensive processed and prepared foods, and access to food in urban areas is generally dependent on cash exchange, with few exceptions, where urban food production contributes directly to household intake. It follows that urban areas can provide at the same time a clear potential for food security and an increased risk [36, 37]. Urban diets can be more varied and balanced than rural ones once access to diversified food is achieved. However, cities and towns, in comparison with rural areas, are more cash-intensive and people often have to pay for goods and services which are non-food essentials. This means that urban dwellers must stretch their incomes across a wider range of goods such as housing, energy, transportation, household items, education, health care and personal items, in addition to food. Moreover, although a wider variety of food is available, the food consumed in urban areas is not necessarily of superior nutritional quality, and food safety is a growing concern in many urban environments [38].

2.2.1.3 *Access to Land, Security of Tenure and Gender*

Inadequate land tenure is still one of the main obstacles to ensuring sustainable agriculture and rural development [39]. The growth in large-scale and export-oriented production can exacerbate the marginalization of subsistence farmers and also encourage the further displacement of indigenous peoples by the process of urban migration. About half of the world's food is sourced from 400 million small farms of less than two hectares, producing both for household subsistence and surplus for market. This model has been unable to achieve self-sufficiency and economic growth and three-quarters of global hunger is located amongst the people who manage and work on these farms [40]. One barrier to prosperity is insecure tenure, a fact of life for the majority of poor farmers in many parts of the developing world. This impedes investment and lowers resistance to eviction by state and corporate interests for mining or property developments. Weak tenure has become more acute with the feminization of agriculture as men migrate for urban work. Although men can be key workers in the agricultural sector, women remain the dominant producers of food in subsistence agriculture for developing countries and they are considered part of the agricultural labor force [7]. Women work in agriculture as farmers on their own account, as unpaid workers on family farms and as paid or unpaid laborers on other farms and agricultural enterprises. They are involved in both crop and livestock production at subsistence and commercial levels. They produce food and cash crops and manage mixed agricultural operations often involving crops, livestock and fish farming.

Women make essential contributions to agriculture in developing countries, but their roles differ significantly by region and are changing rapidly in some areas. Women comprise, on average, 43 percent of the agricultural labor force in developing countries, ranging from 20 percent in Latin America to 50 percent in Eastern Asia and sub-Saharan Africa [7]. Their contribution to agricultural work varies even more widely depending on the specific crop and activity (Figure 2.4).

Women can play different roles in agriculture but almost everywhere they face more severe constraints than men in accessing

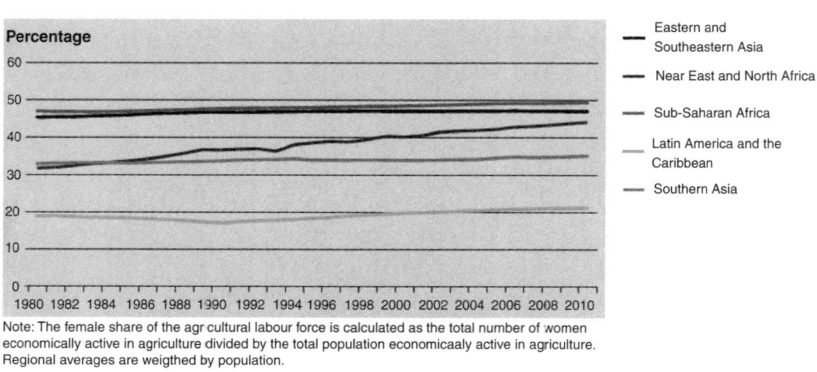

Figure 2.4 Female share of the agricultural labour force. Source: FAO.

productive resources, markets and services. This "gender gap" hinders their productivity and reduces their contributions to the agriculture sector and to the achievement of broader economic and social development goals. Closing the gender gap in agriculture would produce significant gains for society by increasing agricultural productivity, reducing poverty and hunger, and promoting economic growth.

2.2.1.4 Food Insecurity and Conflicts

The nature of conflicts has changed markedly in the late part of the twentieth century, and the proportion of civilian fatalities has increased markedly. Nowadays the state-against-state model is becoming the exception, and while the first half of the century was dominated by warfare between rich states, most contemporary conflicts take place overwhelmingly in the world's poorer countries, with Africa and Asia accounting for the greatest number of internal conflicts in the past decade. Studies on the relations between war and food security assess that hunger is either a cause or a consequence of a conflict. This is due both to the complexity of the evidence of causation and also to the changing conceptualization of conflict. During the Cold War, scholars and politicians focused on the struggle for land and access to subsistence underlying peasant wars of the 20th century [41]. After the Cold War, concern shifted from "war studies" to "peace studies," which analyze the causes of conflict and its prevention, management, and transformation. Some focused on perceived environmental scarcities and their consequences, including food insecurity, as either underlying or trigger causes [42], whereas others stressed political-cultural identities [43–45]. The economic correlates of war have also found conflict associated with factors closely related to food insecurity, such as high infant mortality, extreme poverty, inequality, declining per capita incomes, and intergroup competition over land and water [42, 46–48].

The causes and consequences of conflicts are often a complex mix of interlinked economic, environmental, political, cultural and religious factors, all having a negative impact on access to food by poor people. Gross Domestic Product (GDP) per capita is estimated to decline by about 2.2% per year during conflict, with sectors which have high transaction costs hit more severely. Although the agricultural sector is typically less affected than industry, per capita agricultural production falls by about 1.5% per year in periods of conflict.

There is a well-established correlation between the exposure of countries to external or internal conflicts, and the deterioration or long-term stagnation in their food security. Most conflicts, and especially the internal conflicts that have now become the dominant model of mass violence, mainly affect rural areas and their populations. They disrupt food production through physical destruction and plundering of crops and livestock, harvests and food reserves; they prevent and discourage farming; they interrupt the lines of transportation through which food exchanges and even humanitarian relief, take place; they destroy farm capital, conscript young and able-bodied males, taking them away from farm work and suppress income earning occupations [49]. The impact of conflicts on food security often lasts long after the violence has subsided, because assets have been destroyed, people killed or maimed, populations displaced, the environment damaged, and health, education and social services shattered; still more awesome are the landmines which litter agricultural land, kill and cripple people and deter them from farming for years after all violence has ceased The destruction of rural infrastructure, the loss of livestock, deforestation, the widespread use of land-mines as well as the population movements lead to long-term food security problems, particularly when these factors interact with natural disasters. Subsistence farming, crop diversification, divestment and migration are some of the survival strategies that people resort to. Agricultural sector recovery depends on successful demobilization of soldiers, land de-mining and the reconstruction of rural infrastructure, in particular roads and irrigation [50].

2.2.2 Economic Issues

2.2.2.1 *Finance Aid*

Among economic issues related with food insecurity, neglect of agriculture and world trade rules are the most severe. Despite the evidence that investment in agriculture results in growth and poverty reduction, spending on agriculture as a share of total public spending in developing countries fell by half between 1980 and 2004 [51]. The consequence of the prolonged lack of investment of foreign aid allocated to agriculture (from 18% in 1979 to 4.5% in 2008) is an inadequate infrastructure for rural economies. The situation is especially severe in sub-Saharan Africa, a region heavily reliant on agriculture for overall growth, where public spending for agriculture accounts for only 4 percent of total government spending and the sector is still taxed at relatively high levels [52]. In many African countries, spending on agriculture relative to GDP is well below the target set by the 2003 Maputo Declaration of Heads of State and Government of the African Union, which established that 10 percent of budgetary allocations should go to agriculture and rural development by 2008. Deregulation of the financial sector in many countries led to the closure of rural bank branches. This exacerbated the urban bias in loan allocation enabling rural savings to finance urban credit, thereby adversely impacting financing for agriculture [53]. In several countries, failure to adhere to IMF and World Bank (WB) conditionalities triggered temporary (and sometimes permanent) postponements of cash releases and changes in commitments from other donors. These externally imposed conditionalities prevented developing countries, especially African nations, from making much needed investments in agriculture. National government funding of agricultural research fell by 27 percent in sub-Saharan Africa between 1981 and 2000, with many governments currently allocating less than 1 percent of their national budgets to the sector (except Rwanda and Zambia). Many countries have reduced and even eliminated support for farm credit, crop distribution, and reserve programs. Elimination of seed and fertilizer subsidies, a keystone of World Bank austerity policies, resulted in African farmers abandoning higher-yield seeds with resulting decline in crop yields and production. When Zambia eliminated its corn seed and fertilizer programs, corn acreage and fertilizer application both declined sharply [54].

At the same time, multilateral investment in agricultural projects in poor countries and agricultural research by the governments of rich nations and institutions such as the World Bank have steadily declined [55]. USAID, the United States development agency, cut agricultural aid by 75 percent in the past two decades. Just 4 percent of current development aid to Africa goes to agriculture, and agricultural research grants were cut by more than half—from \$6 billion a year to \$2.8 billion—between 1980 and 2006, with the United States alone decreasing its contribution from \$2.3 billion to \$624 million [55]. In addition, the World Bank decreased its lending for agriculture from \$7.7 billion in 1980 to \$2 billion in 2004 [55].

Underinvestment in agriculture by national governments and international donors and the conditionalities they imposed have prevented the poorest developing countries from developing viable farm sectors, thereby eroding their ability to maintain agricultural production and only increasing their reliance on imported food [56].

2.2.2.2 *Trade*

By 2050 it is estimated that the world will need to increase food production by 70 percent to feed a larger, more urban, and, it is hoped, wealthier population [57, 58]. It will have to accomplish this in the context of shrinking availability of arable land and water and other environmental constraints. Self-sufficiency in food production is not a viable solution for most countries, as it is neither economically nor environmentally sustainable. With daunting challenges on the horizon, countries will need to rely more heavily on trade to be food secure [59]. Usually less emphasized but equally crucial for boosting productivity and availability of food is the existence of markets. Markets and trade also contribute to achieving global food security by increasing access to food. Improved access to agricultural input markets—such as seed and fertilizer—is crucial for productivity growth. Moreover, farmers will only increase production if they have access to viable markets for their agricultural outputs. At the simplest level, trade allows food to flow from areas of surplus to areas of deficit—in local, regional, and global markets. Well-functioning markets transmit price signals, which allow changes in demand to be met by supply. When demand is greater than supply, producers increase production in response to price signals, and this increased production, in turn, helps to stabilize prices. By transmitting information in this way, markets help to reduce price volatility. International agricultural trade has increased 10-fold since the 1960s owing to more open trade policies, market liberalization in many developing countries, and advances in communications and transport systems [60]. Some important consequences have been:

- more intense competition in export and domestic markets for nearly all major agricultural commodities,
- more integrated global and regional markets that are dominated by a few large international trading companies,
- increasing demand for higher quality and safer foods, and

- increasing amounts of food travel longer distances with growing concerns about the energy used in "food miles" and the transmission of pests and diseases to humans, plants and animals.

Nevertheless controversies rage about the effects of trade rules. Agricultural trade historically has failed to play a constructive role in addressing food security, safety and sustainability concerns [61]. It seems clear that "free trade," offered as a panacea by the powerful food exporters and their mainstream economists, is seriously flawed. Trade-distorting measures and restrictions can adversely affect the distribution of food, and border measures can destabilize world food markets and be detrimental to food security. The free trade promoters do not practice free trade in food. Determined to support the dominant profile of small family farms in the aftermath of the Second World War, the European Common Agricultural Policy and the US Farm Bill have protected their farming systems using domestic supports, import protections, and export/consumption subsidies to achieve food security within national borders, treating the rest of the world as a residual market. These policies proved successful, generating colossal internal food surpluses, although they depressed prices of basic food staples on international markets in surplus periods and amplified price spikes and supply unreliability in periods of tight supplies [62].

Ambitions of the poorer countries of the modern world to copy this approach remain unfulfilled, largely because they are bound by the system of open market rules adopted by the World Trade Organization in 1995 [63]. Moreover, many poor developing countries have taxed or ignored their agricultural systems, and international financial institutions often have abetted this by neglecting agriculture within their lending programs. Public policies in developing countries also harm poor farmers and producers who often lack the basic conditions for prosperity: health, education, land, capital, information, and the marketing infrastructure needed to take advantage of export opportunities. Developing-country governments can and must change domestic policies on markets, land tenure, research and extension, and credit to enable smallholder farmers to compete [64]. These policies have led to low productivity and degraded resources in many poor countries [65, 66]. Rich countries demand that poor countries accept trade barriers and under-priced imports (with serious damage to local farmers) and they urge these countries to switch to specialty crops for export. Developing countries often rely on exportable products for foreign exchange earnings, which are vulnerable to unstable commodity prices [67]. Economies that are largely dependent on their agricultural or fishing industries are even more vulnerable to shifts in global prices and markets, with impacts right down the production chain, e.g., farm/fleet jobs, processing, distribution and supply. Some governments, including India, Pakistan, Argentina, Russia and China, have recently taken steps to block exports of food, to protect their own "food sovereignty." Mainstream economists are strongly opposed to such trade barriers, pointing out that they harm poor food-importing countries and contribute to price rises on international markets [68].

Alternatively a number of other countries are dependent on food imports and subject to the fluctuations in the markets. Loss of confidence by net food-importing countries in global markets has reinforced self-sufficiency impulses and, most recently, led to purchasing of foreign agricultural land as a means to ensure supplies [69]. Food-short countries with large cash balances like Saudi Arabia, Japan, South Korea, and China are trying to secure future food supplies by buying up land in poor countries like Indonesia, the Philippines, and even Mongolia, promising to invest and bring prosperity to poor regions. Vast tracts have already been purchased amid controversy from citizens in the areas concerned. Such a rush to lock in food supplies is creating further trade distortions, privileging those with the most money and setting off multiple environmental problems, as mega-investors cut forests, drain wetlands and seek maximum production on an unsustainable basis [70].

Development assistance, food aid and trade preferences or exceptions for the benefit of poor, developing countries have been used to soften the external effects of such self-protecting initiatives. But these efforts have generally been too modest to offset the concerns of food-importing countries, and, in any case, do not represent a cost-effective long-term solution to food security, safety and sustainability concerns [71]. Moreover, food aid has been sometimes part of the trade problem since the rich countries often dump their surpluses as "aid for the hungry," undercutting local producers and even driving them out of business. Credits offered to poor countries for agricultural imports cause problems too. They boost indebtedness and often create import dependency. In addition, both net-food-importing and net-food-exporting countries could be broadly vulnerable because food security is also critically tied to ownership and exchange, which are exacerbated in contexts of high levels of poverty and inequality as well as economic crises and volatility.

The trade sector has many further problems. The rising cost of transportation from market to final consumer (due to soaring energy costs) is destabilizing the trade system and adding pressure to locate production closer to consumers The carbon emissions due to food shipping—especially air transport of perishables—are also forcing a rethinking of long-distance trade [72].

2.2.3 Environmental Issues

2.2.3.1 Climate Change and Natural Disasters

Mean global temperatures have been increasing since about 1850, mainly owing to the accumulation of greenhouse gases in the atmosphere. The process of global warming shows no signs of abating and is expected to bring about long-term changes in weather conditions. The main causes are the burning of fossil fuels (coal, oil and gas) to meet increasing energy demand, and the spread of intensive agriculture to meet increasing food demand, which is often accompanied by deforestation [73]. Intensive agricultural practices are, in particular, a major emitter of greenhouse gases. Depending on how emissions are counted (whether deforestation for agriculture is included, for example), global food and agriculture contributes between 17% and 32% of total global greenhouse gas emissions (comparable to emissions from the transport sector), with a particularly large share of nitrous oxide (owing to fertilizer use) and methane (particularly from livestock) [74, 12].

Climate change affects all dimensions of food security: food availability, food accessibility, food utilization, and food systems stability. It has an impact on human health, livelihood assets, food production and distribution channels, as well as changing purchasing power and market flows. Its impacts could be both short term, resulting from more frequent and more intense extreme weather events, and long term, caused by changing temperatures and precipitation patterns (Figure 2.5).

Rising sea levels and increasing incidence of extreme events pose new risks for the assets of people living in affected zones, threatening livelihoods and increasing vulnerability to future food insecurity in all parts of the globe. Such changes could result in a

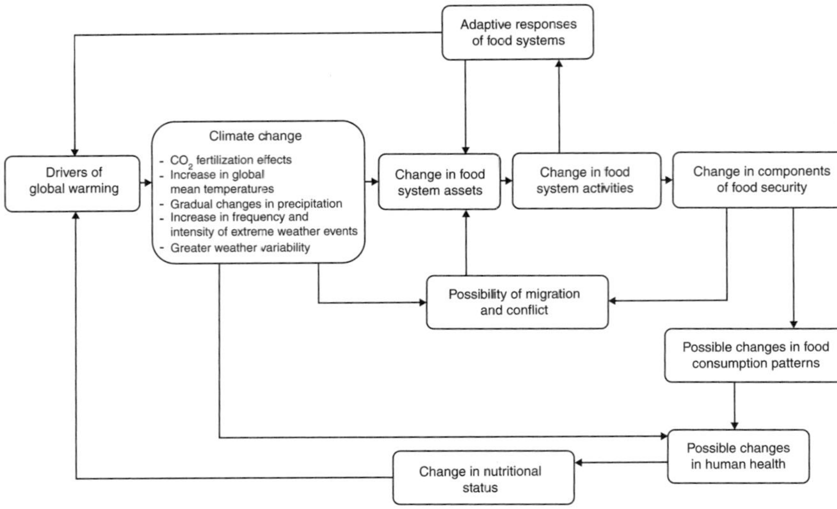

Figure 2.5 Climate change and food security.

geographic redistribution of vulnerability and a relocalization of responsibility for food security.

In this sense, these prospects need to be considered in the formulation of adaptation strategies for people who are currently vulnerable or could become so within the foreseeable future [75].

Intensive agricultural practices are one of the causes of global warming. On the other hand, agriculture, forestry and fisheries are all sensitive to climate change. Arable land and water constraints, combined with the likely impacts of climate change (more severe weather events, an increase in pests, and longer-term changes to agricultural production due to increasing temperatures) pose severe challenges to feeding a larger population. When a potential contribution of CO_2 fertilization is discounted, most crop yields are projected to decline signifcantly by 2050 as a result of climate change [76]. In general, impacts are expected to be positive in temperate regions and negative in tropical ones, but there is still uncertainly about how projected changes will play out at the local level. The food security implications of changes in agricultural production patterns and performance are of two kinds [77]:

- Impacts on the production of food will affect food supply at the global and local levels. Globally, higher yields in temperate regions could offset lower yields in tropical regions. However, in many low-income countries with limited financial capacity to trade and high dependence on their own production to cover food requirements, it may not be possible to offset declines in local supply without increasing reliance on food aid.

- Impacts on all forms of agricultural production will affect livelihoods and access to food. Producer groups that are less able to deal with climate change, such as the rural poor in developing countries, risk having their safety and welfare compromised.

Moreover it should be considered that other food system processes, such as food processing, distribution, acquisition, preparation and consumption, are as important for food security as food and agricultural production are [78]. They all can be in turn affected by climate change. Technological advances and the development of long-distance marketing chains that move produce and packaged foods throughout the world at high speed and relatively low cost have made overall food system performance far less dependent on climate than it was 200 years ago. However, as the frequency and intensity of severe weather increase, there is a growing risk of storm damage to transport and distribution infrastructure, with consequent disruption of food supply chains [79, 80].

Also, natural disasters such as earthquakes, floods or tsunamis can drastically impact on food production, especially in agriculture-intensive countries. An average of 500 weather-related disasters are now taking place each year, compared with 120 in the 1980s; the number of floods has increased sixfold over the same period [81]. Population increases, especially in coastal areas where most of the world's population now lives, mean that more and more people will be affected by catastrophic weather events. Evidence indicates that more frequent and more intense extreme weather events (droughts, heat and cold waves, heavy storms, floods), rising sea levels and increasing irregularities in seasonal rainfall patterns (including flooding) are already having immediate impacts on not only food production, but also food distribution infrastructure, incidence of food emergencies, livelihood assets, and human health in both rural and urban areas. In addition, less immediate impacts are expected to result from gradual changes in mean temperatures and rainfall. These will affect the suitability of land for different types of crop sand pasture; the health and productivity of forests; the distribution, productivity and community composition of marine resources; the incidence and vectors of different types of pests and diseases; the biodiversity and ecosystem functioning of natural habitats; and the availability of good-quality water for crop, livestock, and inland fish production. Arable land is likely to be lost owing to increased aridity (and associated salinity), groundwater depletion and sea-level rise. Food systems will be affected by internal and international migration resource-based conflicts and civil unrest triggered by climate change [12].

2.2.3.2 Soil and Forest Degradation

Degradation of agricultural land and declining soil fertility continue to be major threats to food security and sustainable development [82]. Nearly 40% of the world's agricultural land is seriously degraded. An estimated 500 million hectares of land has been affected by soil degradation since 1950, including as much as 65% of agricultural land. Land degradation is most severe in "hot spot" areas such as the foothills of the Himalayas, sloping areas in southern China, Southeast Asia and the Andes, the forest margins of East Asia and the Amazon, range-lands in Africa and West and Central Asia, and the Sahel [83, 84]. Farming in areas of fragile soils, poor management of crop, soil and water interaction, and unsustainable exploitation of soil nutrients are some of the major causes of land degradation [85]. Only some 16% of croplands globally are inherently free of soil constraints [86], and that figure is as low as 6–7% in Southeast Asia and sub-Saharan Africa. Modern ploughing, overgrazing, and fertilizer and pesticide use also result in the steady depletion of worldwide topsoils. Loss of tree cover leads to poorer water retention and storage and seasonal flooding, and soil erosion silts up reservoirs and irrigation and drainage structures downstream. In dry land areas, cropland encroachment into pastoral areas aggravates soil erosion problems and overstocking of the remaining grazing areas. Flooding and heavy rainfalls due to climate change worsen the process and an estimated 25 billion tons of topsoil are lost to erosion each year. All these aspects directly impact on the quantity and quality of food that can be produced in the long term and has lasting environmental implications. Modern agricultural production systems favor large farms, crop monocultures and mechanization, often at the expense of ecological principles. Intensive agriculture requires higher inputs of pesticides and herbicides to guarantee against crop failure [87]. Intensive farming reduces the amount of organic matter returned to the soil, decreasing productivity over time, whilst the leaching of nutrients creates a vicious circle demanding more and more pesticide and fertilizer application. On the other hand, soil nutrient mining is endemic in low-input farming systems, especially in areas with poor infrastructure and marketing institutions, where use of inorganic fertilizers is uneconomic [88]. This produces, in the absence of adequate levels of other forms of nutrient replenishment, soil nutrient depletion in unsustainable ways [89], often with harsh implications for rural lives and livelihoods [90, 91].

The economic costs of land degradation are difficult to assess and few of the available estimates are based on reliable data [92]. However, improved understanding of the role of processes such as silt deposition within catchments [93] and meta-analyses of empirical observations [94, 95], have recently provided more conservative assessments of long-term soil degradation. Nonetheless, costs to poor farmers in terms of lower yields are often very real and have important implications for their food security and income earning opportunities [96].

As far as forests are concerned, every year approximately 13 Mha of forest are lost or degraded in developing countries, equivalent to just over 1% of the current tropical forest reserves [97, 98]. More than 60% of deforestation has been attributed to subsistence farming in hillside areas, where declining yields force poor people to rely on shifting cultivation [97]. Developing countries have now lost about one-fifth of their total forest since 1960, with Asia losing 30%, and Africa and Latin America 18% [99]. Conversion or degradation of forests leads to loss of forest products, many of which (especially fuel wood, poles and non-timber forest products) are particularly important to the poor. Deforestation also gives rise to loss of important environmental services, especially watershed protection, maintenance of biodiversity, and carbon sequestration [97, 100].

2.2.3.3 *Water Resources*

Population growth and overuse of water resources is exacerbating hydrological poverty and water scarcity which are the significant limiting factors on agricultural production capacity during the 21st century. Only a tiny fraction of the world's water is available for human use. Just 2.5% of the world's water is fresh, and two-thirds of this is inaccessible (locked away instead as glaciers, snow, ice and permafrost). Of the remainder, the vast majority is groundwater, so that just 0.4% of the world's total freshwater is available at the surface as lakes, soil moisture, air humidity, marshes, wetlands, rivers, and in biomass [101].

During the 20th century, the world's demand for water rose sharply while in 2000, half a billion people lived in countries that were chronically short of water, out of a global population of around six billion. By 2050, however, the number of people living in such conditions is projected to grow to four billion, out of a global population of around nine billion [102]. Overall, the problem is simply a larger world population consuming more water per capita even as freshwater availability remains constant or declines. Moreover, land degradation and urbanization are considered important issues to be considered as well as agriculture which consumes 70% of the freshwater withdrawn annually by humans. But a number of changes in the food and agriculture sector are highly significant too. Water quality is affected by agricultural activities, fertilizer and pesticide runoff, salinization and alkalinization, and through other toxic substances which bio-accumulate affecting human health. Growing affluence is driving consumer demand, especially in urbanized areas of developing and developed countries, for more water-intensive fruit and vegetable crops. Many coastal habitats are also being degraded and polluted as a result of urbanization and run off from intensive agricultural practices, which in turn is impacting entire marine food chains.

Irrigated agriculture is associated with wasteful water use in many countries as well as unsustainable mining of ground water and aquifers [103, 104, 86]. As demand for water has grown, especially in the non-agricultural sectors, countries have increasingly faced water scarcities, and farmers are having to learn to produce more with less water. Increasing water scarcity has the potential to seriously worsen food balances in hot spot areas, perhaps even globally if timely and judicious action is not taken [105]. The impacts of unsustainable water use are already becoming clear in many parts of the world. One obvious impact is on surface water, for instance, rivers that run dry before they reach the sea. Another less visible impact is on the world's groundwater stocks—both aquifers and water tables—many of which are being depleted rapidly. With river water now close to being fully exploited in many of the world's key farming regions, groundwater is the default source of additional supply.

Salinization and waterlogging are two significant consequences of poor irrigation management and inadequate drainage and bring about decreased productivity and shifting ecological conditions [106]. If irrigated fields are not properly drained they can become waterlogged, allowing salts to build up in the soil which reduce its fertility. The problem of salinization has affected around 30% of all irrigated land. Globally, some 1.5 Mha of irrigated land per year are lost to production [83], and approximately US$11 billion is lost annually from reduced productivity [104], representing approximately 1% of the global totals of irrigated area and annual value of production, respectively [86]. As with land scarcity, water scarcity is likely to affect poor people most; equity in sharing water is frequently a highly contentious issue in irrigation management, corruption is widespread, and farmers without political power or money for bribes often find that they lose out.

2.2.3.4 *Biodiversity and Genetic Resources*

Biological diversity exists in terms of ecosystems, species, and genetic variety. The complex web of interactions between different life forms is increasingly being threatened by human-induced activities and pressures. Plant genetic resources are essential to sustain agriculture and food security for humanity now and in the future. FAO estimates that humans have used 10,000 species for food throughout history. Yet today, no more than 120 cultivated species provide around 90% of our food. From an agro-biodiversity perspective, there has been serious loss of traditional food crop species, and, even for the crop species that are grown, large areas are planted with a few modern varieties. This concentration of consumption has impacted the genetic viability of these cultivated species and in some cases has led to their extinction. Agriculture has large and well-documented adverse impacts on biodiversity in a number of ways. The first and most apparent impact has been a locally extensive, if globally declining, conversion of natural ecosystems for agricultural purposes. Second is the management of agricultural landscapes in ways that can limit the existence of natural biodiversity within them. Third is the use of production practices such as the application of pesticides and use of other agrochemicals that further constrain the viability of natural biodiversity, e.g., bees, bird populations and soil biodiversity. Since these animals and organisms can often perform beneficial economic services from a production perspective, these losses impact human well-being both directly and indirectly [107].

In this context, genetic modification (GM) technology should also be taken into account as GMOs could impact on genetic diversity. The increased competitiveness of GMOs could damage biologically-rich ecosystems as transgenic crops could encourage biodiversity loss through the establishment of monoculture agriculture which replaces traditional crops and other established varieties. The introduction of a transgene into a recipient organism is not a precisely controlled process and can result in a variety of outcomes with regard to integration, expression and stability of the transgene in the host [108]. The risks associated with modifying the genetic structure of crops are not well understood and there is little agreement on either the severity or likelihood of potential risks. It has been reported [109] that the future of sustainable agriculture may be irreversibly jeopardized by contamination of *in situ* preserved genetic resources (gene pollution) threatening a strategic resource for the world's food security. Because GM crops are truly biological novelties, their release into the environment poses concerns about the unpredictable ecological and evolutionary responses that GM species themselves and the interacting biota may express in the medium and long term. On the other hand, proponents of GM crops suggest that transgenic crops may be able to help preserve uncultivated habitats by increasing yields on land already under cultivation, reducing the need for conversion.

Also, from the economic point of view there are both potentials and constraints in introducing GM technology in relation to improving the agricultural outcome for small-scale subsistence farmers in developing countries. One potential is that GM technology enables the development of new crop varieties, which have beneficial characteristics for farming. This could be resistance to drought, pests or diseases. In situations of unstable food security due to bad harvests caused by climate or crop-diseases, GM crops present opportunities that can stabilize and ensure food supply for poor subsistence farmers [110]. Another potential is that some types of GM crops can reduce the use of chemical pesticides and fertilizers because of their pest resistance with transgenic pesticides. Some crops are made resistant to stress from drought, salt and low pH. This is an important consideration because chemical inputs are often not available for the subsistence farmers, as they often cannot afford any of these inputs [110]. GM allows crops to be bred by selectively inserting one or more gene into a plant to confer specific advantages. Plants that are resistant to pests and diseases can be produced this way, thereby reducing the amount of required insecticide. Nevertheless, there are some problems and constraints with the GM technology. One constraint is that the technology might not reach the poor farmers because of the privatization of the rights for implementing and using the technologies. The worldwide intellectual property right regime has already been extended to cover plants and animals, including their genes, making the technology expensive, and thus inaccessible for the subsistence farmers who already have limited opportunities for using the GM technology [110]. Furthermore, many developing countries do not have the capacity required to undertake the needed assessments and control on whether they would benefit from the GM crops and whether they can comply with the safety regulations. Finally, the GM technology may require adequate education and training as well. The farmers, especially in the developing countries, have to be willing to adopt the technique of GM crops. The GM technology thus has great potential in securing food supply for small-scale subsistence farmers, however, the technology cannot be transferred to the farmers without carefully considering the above-mentioned aspects [111].

It follows that if for one side GM technology may be considered a valuable tool to ensure food security considering the increasing world population and the limited amount of arable land, to the other, there are many environmental and economic concerns about the possibility of introducing this technology in developing countries [112].

2.2.3.5 *Pests and Pesticide Impacts*

Varietal specialization has occasionally led to widespread crop losses due to outbreaks of diseases and pests to which widely-planted varieties had no resistance. The experience of the Green Revolution gives considerable grounds for caution on this front; as early as 1993, excessive application of new insecticides and herbicides meant that 700 pests, 200 pathogens, and 30 weeds had already developed resistance to agrichemicals. In this regard, there is also the risk of pest and weeds emerging that will be resistant to GM technologies. The constant evolution of pest and diseases so as to overcome inbred resistance has required that larger shares of agricultural research expenditures be allocated to "maintenance" research and germplasm conservation programs [113].

The Green Revolution, and "industrialized" agriculture more generally, has often been associated with problems of environmental degradation and pollution [114]. Up to 70% of fertilizer applied to crops can be lost, rather than taken up by crops, polluting both groundwater sources and rivers, lakes and coastal zones (where fertilizers can stimulate algae or phytoplankton that then starve water, and the species that inhabit it, of oxygen). Today, significant areas of the world's oceans are classified as "dead zones" because of this problem, primarily related to agriculture in developed countries, but also around developing countries including Brazil, Mexico and China. The spread of emergent diseases and invasive species has increased dramatically in recent years—assisted by the rapid rise in global trade and movements of people. It highlights the need for international action on transboundary pests and diseases, especially where there are significant implications for food security. Control and management requires cooperation between countries. Pest-induced losses are more than 50% of attainable crop output. Factors affecting a country's ability to combat a disease include: globalization; conflict/civil unrest making it harder to enforce quarantine, unregulated movement of people, increased smuggling, and deregulation of animal and health services. International legislation, such as the Persistent Organic Pollutants (POPs) Convention, seek to increase regulation and reduce transportation of hazardous and polluting substances in agriculture [115].

2.3 The Food Insecurity Dimension

2.3.1 Current Situation at Global Level

The number of undernourished people in the world reached about one billion people in 2009 [116]. As can be seen in Figure 2.6, the trend during past decades shows a slow decline from 1970–71 to 1995–97 while the following years saw a gradual increase in the global number of undernourished people.

The upward trend accelerated sharply in 2008 during the food price crisis, and erupted in 2009 as a result of the financial crisis associated with the persistence of high food prices in the domestic markets of many countries in developing regions. In this sense, poor people were exposed to additional stress besides the decline of real wages and household incomes, the loss of jobs, and credit cuts, as the global recession also increased uncertainty about the levels of future aid and funds for social protection, both essential for avoiding hunger and starvation among the most vulnerable

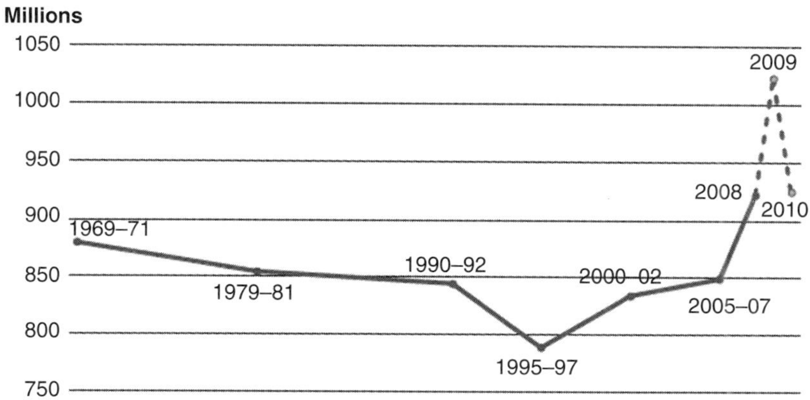

Note: Figures for 2009 and 2010 are estimated by FAO with input from the United States Department of Agriculture, Economic Research Service. Full details of the methodology are provided in the technical background notes (available at www.fao.org/publication/sofi/en/).

Figure 2.6 Number of undernourished people in the world, 1969–71 to 2010. Source: FAO.

people. This is of particular concern, because the crisis is still affecting large population segments living either in urban or in rural areas where they are both consumers and producers of food [38, 52]. Because they spend the majority of their disposable income on food and have minimal savings, they are particularly vulnerable to agricultural price spikes. In many cases, those who are the most affected by this situation, already reached, or came very close, to the limit of their ability to cope. The urban poor are likely to be particularly affected, as urban areas are linked more directly to world markets and may suffer more directly from declining export demand and reduced foreign direct investment. However, rural areas may also be affected by possible declines in agro-industrial activity and return migration. This widespread vulnerability persisting in both urban and rural environments, underscores the general principle that poverty, not geography, is mainly responsible for food insecurity [34].

Nevertheless, a decline of food insecurity was recorded in 2010 for the first time since 1995 as several indicators of food security—the number of food-insecure people, the food gap to meet the average nutritional requirement (nutritional gap), and the food gap associated with unequal purchasing power or food access (distribution gap)—all pointed to improvement between 2009 and 2010 [6]. This trend is largely attributable to increased economic growth, particularly in developing countries, and the fall in international food prices since 2008. The difference in the estimated number of food-insecure people from 2009 to 2010 highlights the fact that large portions of the populations in lower income countries consume just barely more than the nutritional target. This implies that their food security is precarious; even a brief economic slowdown or food production shock can result in millions of additional people being subjected to food insecurity. Conversely, a slight improvement in economic conditions can propel people past the nutritional target. However, a total of 925 million people are still estimated to be undernourished in 2010, representing almost 16 percent of the population of developing countries. The fact that nearly a billion people remain hungry even after the peaks of the recent food and financial crises have passed, indicates a deeper structural problem that gravely threatens the ability to achieve internationally agreed goals on hunger reduction: the first MDG and the 1996 World Food Summit goal. While the World Food Summit goal is to reduce by half the number of people who are undernourished, MDG 1 seeks to reduce by half the proportion of these people. Because the world's population is still increasing (albeit more slowly than in recent decades), a given number of hungry people represents a declining proportion of people who are hungry. In fact, developing countries as a group have seen an overall setback in terms of the World Food Summit goal (from 827 million in 1990–92 to 906 million in 2010), while some progress has been made towards MDG 1 (with the prevalence of hunger declining from 20 percent undernourished in 1990–92 to 16 percent in 2010) [7]. Developing countries account for 98 percent of the world's undernourished people and have a prevalence of undernourishment of 16 percent (Figure 2.7). This value is lower than 18 percent in 2009 but still well above the target set by MDG 1.

Most of the world's hungry people (62 percent of the total) live in Asia and the Pacifc, the world's most populous region, followed by sub-Saharan Africa, home to 26 percent of the world's undernourished population (Figure 2.8). Two-thirds of these 925 million people live in just seven countries (Bangladesh, China, the Democratic Republic of the Congo, Ethiopia, India, Indonesia and Pakistan) and over 40 percent live in China and India alone.

The highest proportion of undernourished people is found in sub-Saharan Africa, where in 2005–07 (the latest period with complete information by country) 30 percent of the total population were estimated to be undernourished; this value is lower in Asia

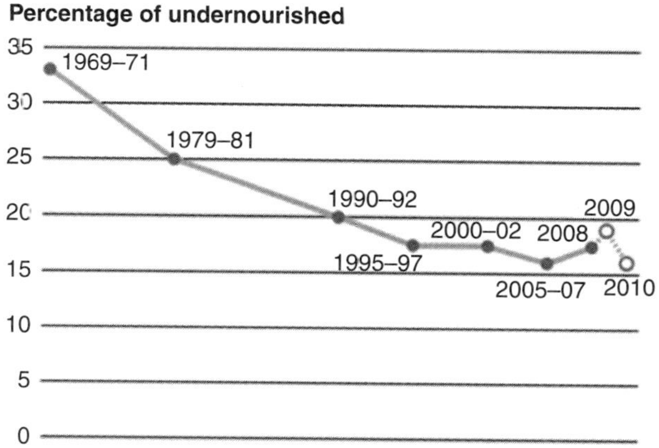

Figure 2.7 Proportion of undernourished people in developing countries, 1969–71 to 2010. Source: FAO.

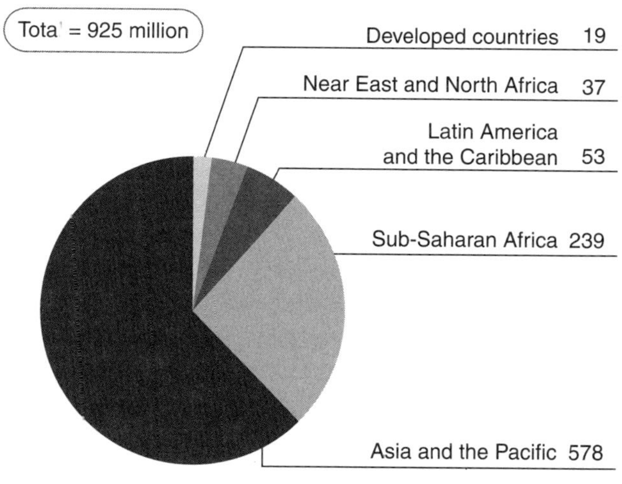

Figure 2.8 Undernourishment in 2010, by region (millions). Source: FAO.

and the Pacifc (16%), Latin America and the Caribbean (9%), and the Near East and North Africa (7%) (Figure 2.9).

However, large variations occur among subregions and by country; in fact, while a number of countries are currently on track achieving MDG 1, this target remains a challenge for many others. For example, Congo, Ghana, Mali and Nigeria had already achieved MDG 1 and Ethiopia and others were close to achieving it. Also, Asia, Armenia, Myanmar and Vietnam had achieved MDG 1 and China and others were close to doing so, while in Latin America and the Caribbean, Guyana, Jamaica, and Nicaragua had

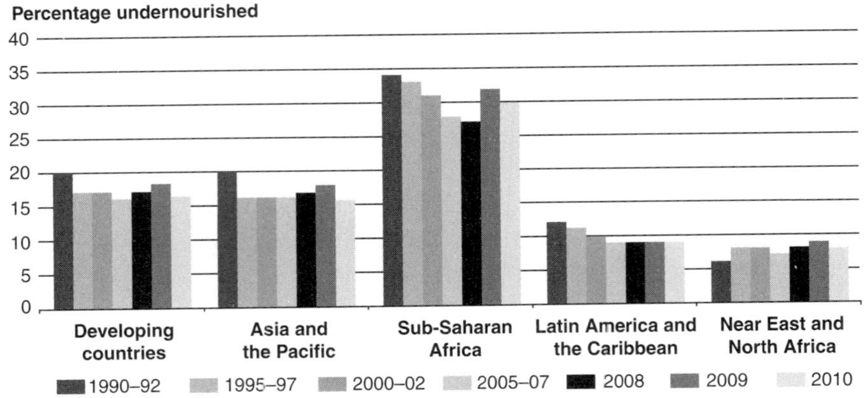

Figure 2.9 Regional trends in the proportion of undernourished, from 1990–92 to 2010. Source: FAO.

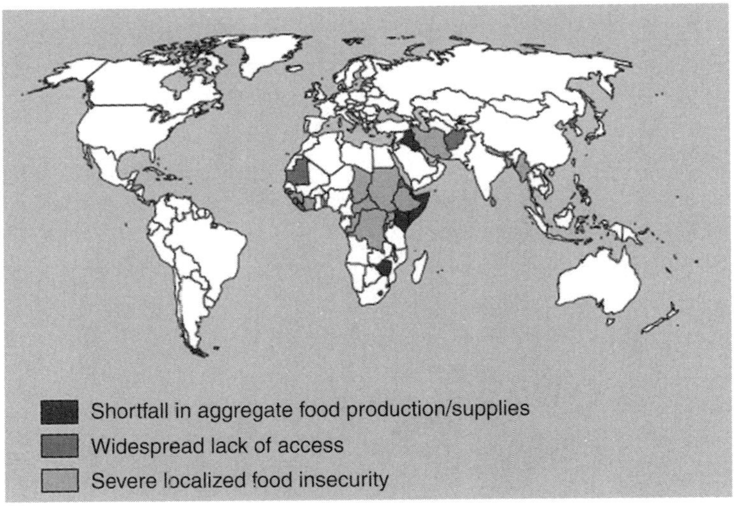

Figure 2.10 Food emergencies in the world. Source: FAO.

achieved MDG 1 and Brazil and others were approaching the target reduction [7].

When analyzing the current food insecurity situation it also should be considered that many countries are currently considered in situations of protracted crisis, characterized by recurrent natural disasters and/or conflict, longevity of food crises, breakdown of livelihoods, and insufficient institutional capacity to react to the crises (Figure 2.10).

In this regard, food crises affecting individual countries shock and destabilize the food security status of part of or the entire population (the newly food insecure) and worsen it for those who were already food insecure prior to the emergency (the chronically food insecure). Countries in protracted crisis face a particularly difficult situation as food security is significantly worse in this group of countries than in the rest of the developing countries in four out of the six key food security indicators: proportion undernourished (FAO); proportion stunted; mortality rate of children under five years old; and the Global Hunger Index (International Food Policy Research Institute). Countries in protracted crisis thus need to be considered as a special category with special requirements in terms of interventions by the development community. From 1981–2009, the region with the largest number of countries experiencing emergencies was Africa, followed by Asia, Latin America and the Caribbean, Eastern Europe, Commonwealth of Independent States and Oceania. According to *The State of Food Insecurity in the World 2010* [6], 22 countries are currently considered to be in a state of protracted crisis. All the countries have suffered some kind of human-induced emergency—a conflict or political crisis of some kind. Sixteen of them have also experienced some kind of natural disaster at some point, either as a stand-alone crisis or combined with a human-induced emergency, while 15 have experienced at least one occurrence of combined natural and human-induced emergency. These are countries that are expected to lack the resources to deal with reported critical problems of food insecurity and for the purposes of response planning, it is important to establish whether the nature of the food crises is predominantly related to lack of food availability, limited access to food, or severe but localized problems.

2.3.2 The Food, Financial and Economic Crisis and Their Implications on Food Security

Patterns in global food prices are indicators of trends in the availability of food, at least for those who can afford it and have access to world markets. Over the past century, food prices have generally fallen, leveling off in the past three decades but punctuated by price spikes such as that caused by the 1970s oil crisis (Figure 2.11).

In recent years, three successive crises have hit the world economy, albeit very unevenly. The episode of "soaring food prices," in fact, was followed in rapid succession by the most severe global

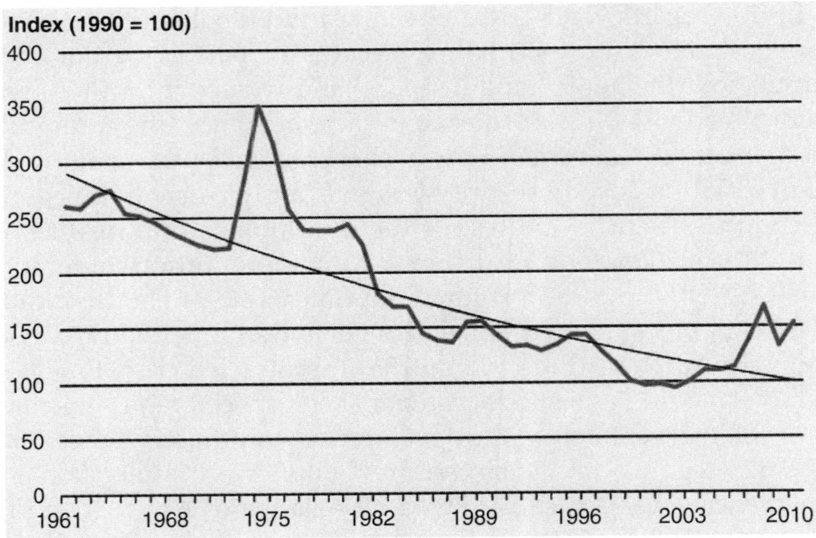

Note: Calculated using international prices for cereals, oilseeds, meats, dairy products and sugar. The FAO Food Price Index is calculated from 1990 to the present on a regular basis; in this figure it has been extended back to 1961 using proxy price information. The index measures movements in international prices and not necessarily domestic prices. The United States GDP deflator is used to express the Food Price Index in real rather than nominaòl terms.

Figure 2.11 FAO Food Price Index in real terms, 1961–2010. Source: FAO.

financial crisis and the deepest economic recession witnessed in the last 70 years.

From 2003 to their peak in mid-2008 world prices (in dollars) of the four commodities of primary interest (wheat, rice, maize, and petroleum) roughly tripled in real terms; they then fell to about 1.5 times their 2005 level during the last half of 2008 before again leveling off in 2009 and 2010 (Figure 2.12).

Just when food and energy prices started declining, around May 2008, it was becoming increasingly evident that a financial crisis of historic proportions was sweeping through the United States, western and eastern Europe, and Japan. By the end of 2008, it was also clear that the financial crisis was creeping into other sectors, notably trade, and that developing economies would also be hard hit. Civil unrest flared up in locations all over the world; over thirty countries introduced export restrictions on food, even as many importing countries attempted to tackle the issue through subsidies and price controls.

Despite early signs of a global recovery, scattered evidence suggests that many developing countries may have lost years of previous growth and poverty reduction. In fact, the food and fuel crisis

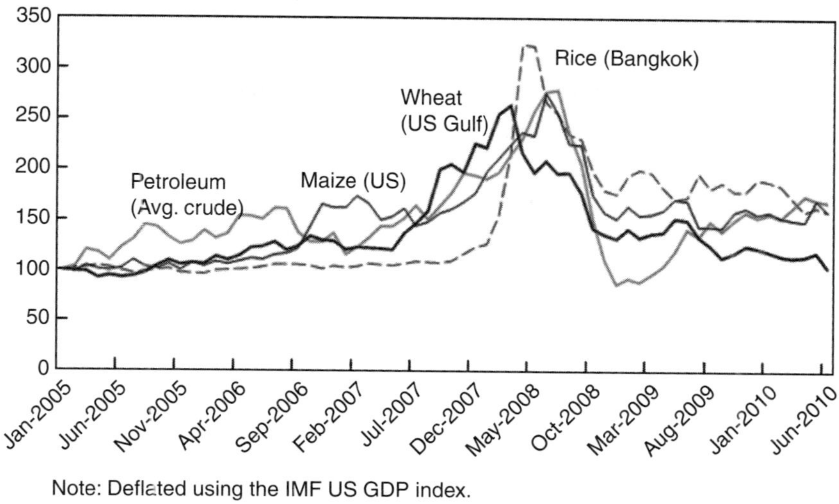

Figure 2.12 Real commodity price indexes, January 2005–June 2010. (Index, January 2005=100). Source: IMF International Financial Statistics, http://www.imfstatistics.org.

of 2007–08 led to rising inflation, deteriorating current-account balances and increasing government deficits in many countries. Since June 2010, an additional 44 million people fell below the 1.25 USD poverty line as a result of higher food prices and simulations showed that a further 10% increase in the Food Price Index could lead to 10 million people falling into poverty, and a 30% increase could increase poverty by 34 million people [117].

Although there is broad agreement on the main channels through which the food, fuel and financial crises affect developing countries [118–121], the developmental impact of each of these crises and how these impacts might have affected each other is not well understood. In addition, impacts are likely to differ widely between countries due to large differences in fiscal trade, and economic and household structure.

It has been pointed out that the drivers of food prices have become more complex, extending beyond traditional factors [122] consisting of fundamentals such as long-term demand (population expansion, income growth, and changing diets), supply (resource use and technology), and carryover stocks [123]. On the contrary, short-term variations in prices are influenced by weather variability, trade policies, more volatile oil prices (including through demand for biofuels based on agriculture feedstock), macroeconomic policy, and financial investments. Moreover, the presence of two of the main transmission mechanisms contributed in making the crisis "global," i.e., the trade in food (e.g., maize, rice, wheat, dairy products) or inputs to produce food (e.g., oil, fertilizers), and the effects of climate change on agricultural productivity. Another potential factor related to the food crisis has been the behavior of financial investors inside the financial and commodity markets. For many developing countries facing heightened food insecurity, the origins of soaring food prices were largely external, related mostly to the continuing surge in biofuels, major changes in policies, macroeconomic conditions and financial markets in rich countries, as well as the global recession. These factors compounded the problems of low crop productivity and increased reliance on food imports, and aggravated other internal causes of instability conflict, weak institutions, and inadequate infrastructure that typically plague the world's poorest countries [124].

Considering the factors that contributed to increased food prices in 2008, it is now uncontroversial that the oil-biofuels nexus was the driving force. Oil prices rose before cereal prices in relation to cereal production and trade costs, which might have raised US cereal production costs by 20–30 percent [125]. Once oil prices hit $50–$60 per barrel making biofuels production more economic when subsidies are included (Figure 2.13). Corn consumption for biofuels rose sharply as oil prices rose to the point where the biofuels sector consumed almost 30 percent of US corn production in 2008.

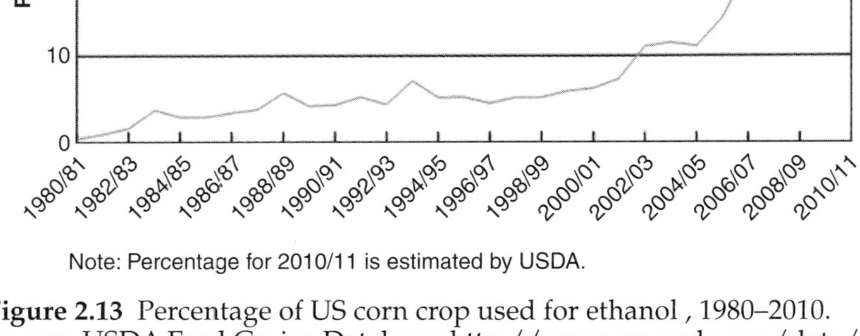

Figure 2.13 Percentage of US corn crop used for ethanol , 1980–2010. Source: USDA Feed Grains Database; http://www.ers.usda.gov/data/feedgrains/FeedYearbook.aspx#Usacre.

The decline in growth of agricultural production was considered another cause of the crisis, although it has been recently stated that the widely cited decline in cereal yields [126–128] was largely driven by the slowing down of Asia's Green Revolution. Timmer [129], Abbott [130], and Piesse [131] have all argued that the long period of low real food prices in the 1980s and 1990s led to under-investment in agricultural production. Consistent with this hypothesis, global food demand outstripped production for a number of years prior to the food crisis. Because of the buffer provided by the depletion of stocks, however, prices did not rise and farmers failed to increase production. However, Headey [132] rejected the notion that there was any crisis in global grain production. Authors examined trends in global production and trade and found that although per capita cereal production at a global level declined in recent decades, most of this slowdown was due to declines in the former Communist countries (FCM) (e.g., Russia, Ukraine, and Kazakhstan). However, FCM countries have actually increased their exports since the fall of the Berlin Wall, so authors concluded that the production decline was not a compelling explanation for rising international prices. The decline in global grain stocks, considered as a driving factor of the crisis as well, should also be treated cautiously as droughts and poor harvests in Australia, India, and Ukraine may have tightened wheat markets and added 50 percent to international prices, all else being equal [132]. But all else was not really equal because these poor harvests were compensated by strong harvests elsewhere, so that the global reduction in stocks was not large by historical standards.

Another common hypothesis in explanation of the crisis, i.e., changing diets in fast-growing Asian countries such as China, India, and Indonesia, has been recently rejected. Asia food and feed demand account for 25 and 15 percent, respectively, of wheat and coarse grain demand growth over 2005–2007. Neither change is much above trend, and China, India, and Indonesia account for only 8 percent of the increase in global demand over that period. Yet even this 8 percent grossly overstates the impact on prices because China and India are essentially self-sufficient in cereals (typically they are exporters), and Indonesia has actually substantially reduced its cereal imports in the last five years. Moreover, the change in diets in these countries is away from cereals toward meat, dairy, and seafood. Coarse grains are obviously a component of meat and dairy production, but the growth in meat demand is hardly large enough to have induced the crisis, and meat prices have not risen anywhere near as much as cereal prices. All these factors can therefore only be thought of as auxiliary factors. However, other channels seem to have influenced the cereal market, because for a number of years now China and India have significantly contributed to the surging demand for energy and metals [133]. At the same time, they substantially decreased their grain stocks, largely because of policy choices rather than surging demand and imposed export restrictions, all these aspects having significant impacts on grain markets. A more general Asian-led commodities boom could also have spilled over into agricultural commodities through other means, such as exchange rate movements and financial speculation [134].

Trade and financial factors have also been considered as a driving force in food crisis. Although fundamental factors were clearly responsible for shifting the world to a higher food price equilibrium in the years leading up the 2008 food crisis, there is little doubt that when food prices peaked in June of 2008, they soared well above the new equilibrium price. By March 2009, prices of staple grains had fallen by 30 percent from their peak in May 2008, while energy prices fell by around 50 percent, before stabilizing and then increasing again. This fact was indicative of a bubble (or "overshooting"), which supports the idea of exacerbating factors that turned tight markets into crisis markets. Macroeconomic imbalances (financial speculation, depreciation of the US dollar, low interest rates) have long been regarded as a significant channel of overshooting in commodity markets. Low real interest rates and crises in the housing and stock markets, especially in the United States, could have caused money to flow out of interest-bearing instruments and into foreign currencies, emerging market stocks, and other securities and commodity futures markets. The depreciation of the US dollar could have significantly boosted US agricultural exports, leading to higher prices in the United States and lower price increases elsewhere (all else being equal). Comparing the recent spike in food prices with historical episodes, Abbott [130] argued that the weak dollar accounted for closer to 50% of the recent spike. However, the econometric evidence regarding the impact of dollar movements on commodity prices has so far failed to provide a consensus on the importance of exchange rate movements [131, 135]. The impact of macroeconomic imbalances on commodity prices via futures market activity is even more controversial. Gilbert [134] argued that that futures market activity can only affect agricultural prices via inventory levels or stocks. If the futures price is driven above its market clearing level, stocks should accumulate. However, in the short run, stocks are largely predetermined by the carryover level from previous harvest, suggesting that increased demand may be accommodated by increased prices rather than stock accumulation. Empirically, Robles [136] and Gilbert [134] found time series evidence that futures market activity might have led to rising spot prices. Yet Irwin [137] found contradictory pieces of evidence, while Sanders [138] and Headey [133] observe that commodities with less speculative capital often experienced greater price increases than commodities with large speculative capital.

Speculation could have taken other forms, of course. In the case of rice, Timmer [129] argued that the large number of small producers and traders meant that the information available on the true level of stocks was unreliable, thus encouraging speculation, hoarding and panic purchases. Indeed, nearly all the most prominent reviews of this issue have identified export restrictions as significant determinants of price overshooting in late 2007 and 2008, especially in the relatively thin international rice market. Headey, in 2011 [139], explored the broader hypothesis that trade shocks (export restrictions and import surges) were a larger and more pervasive factor in the food crisis. While the case of rice is well known, author evaluated the importance of export restrictions in the wheat and maize markets by systematically tracking monthly export volumes in the world's largest grain markets: the United States for maize, wheat, and soybeans (for which Brazilian exports were also tracked) and Thailand, Vietnam, and India for rice. The analysis suggested that trade events were pervasively important in all of the major grain markets (with knock-on effects on soybeans) and arguably provide the most tangible explanation for the overshooting dynamics apparent in price series data.

At the moment global food prices remain high partly due to increasing fuel prices, and the World Bank's Food Price Index is around its 2008 peak. However, the current global food price situation seems to possess both similarities and differences with 2008 [122]. It is similar in four respects. First, global grain stocks are low driven by lower production. Second, higher oil prices have impacted agricultural commodity prices, and the recent events in the Middle East and North Africa add to the current uncertainty. Energy prices, in particular crude oil (which experienced a large price spike in 2008), are rising again. Crude oil prices underpin production costs of agricultural products relying on fertilizers and petroleum, in particular in developed and emerging economies, and transport costs in many developing countries. Third, depreciation of the dollar in 2008 against most currencies led to the perception of a larger increase of US dollar-denominated food prices compared to prices in other major currencies. Fourth, financial investment in agricultural commodities remains high. Much of the recent increase in commodity financial transactions has occurred in the futures markets, including for maize and wheat.

However the current situation differs in several critical respects. First, recent international price increases are more widespread across agricultural commodities than in 2008. Since June 2010, agricultural price increases have been broad-based, including increases in sugar, edible oils, beverages, animal products, and raw materials such as cotton. In contrast, 2008 price increases were predominantly driven by major grains—rice, wheat, and maize. Broad agricultural price increases, rather than just grain prices, provide less incentive for farmers to shift to the production of grains and away from the production of other agricultural commodities. Second, weather-induced production shortfalls are also more of a factor now as the number of reported droughts, floods and extreme temperatures seems to be increasing. Third, policy responses have further raised the amplitude of the grain price spikes in 2011, but not nearly as much as in 2008 when policy greatly exacerbated shortages. Export bans and tactical reductions in import duties were used by many countries in 2008 and accounted for an estimated 45 percent of the world price increase for rice and 29 percent of the increase for wheat. These impacts were compounded in 2008 by governments aggressively building up grain stocks in the face of high and escalating prices. Although these policy responses could be pragmatic answers to the food price spike in many low income countries, both instruments insulate domestic economies and shift the adjustment cost to the rest of the world, with their impact depending on the size of the economy. While a single individual food tariff reduction can serve to lower the domestic price of imported food for that country, if the same tariff reduction is pursued by a larger number of importing countries it would put upward pressure on global prices and off-set the tariff reduction. Insulating policies reduce the role that trade between nations can play in bringing stability to the world's food markets.

Latest data about food price trends show that in March 2011, the food index remained 36% above its level a year earlier, despite a small recent drop (Figure 2.14) [7].

Key staples that remain significantly higher than what they were at this point last year include maize (74%), wheat (69%), soybeans (36%), and sugar (21%); importantly, rice prices have been stable.

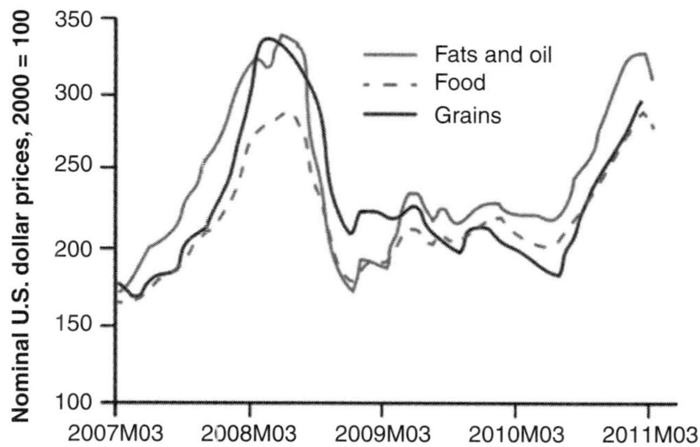

Figure 2.14 World Bank Global Price Indices (nominal U.S. dollar prices, 2000=100). Source: DECPG.

FAO reports that in the last quarter of 2010, among other agricultural commodities that are not part of the Food Price Index, international fruit prices moved closely together with those of the Food Price Index (i.e., cereals, oils, dairy, meat, and sugar), exhibiting a spike during the food price crisis and a decline during the subsequent financial crisis, while the price of beverage products moved less closely to prices of commodities contained in the Food Price Index. Raw material prices were generally not affected by the rise in other commodity prices during the food price crisis but decreased significantly in response to the economic downturn in 2009 before moving upwards again in response to economic recovery, reflecting the high income elasticity of demand for this group of commodities.

A comparison of average prices for the first quarter of 2011 with the last quarter of 2010 (Table 2.2) shows that prices have risen for a broad spectrum of food commodities, and all major agricultural outlooks [10, 140, 141] forecast that at least until 2019 international food prices will remain above the prices in the previous decade, influenced by a complex interplay of different factors, including higher production costs, increased demand by emerging and developing countries, and growing production of biofuels from agricultural feedstocks. Food price increases in 2011 are mostly linked to energy price increases; crude oil prices surged by 10.3% in March 2011 and are 36% higher than a year earlier, affecting the price of food through multiple channels.

First, higher crude oil prices encourage greater use of food products such as corn, vegetable oil, and sugar in the production of

Table 2.2 Specific food commodity price changes.

Commodity	Change in average price	
	1st quarter 2011/ 1st quarter 2010 (%)	1st quarter 2011/ 4th quarter 2010 (%)
Wheat (US, HRW)	69.1	16.9
Maize (No. 2, yellow	73.8	17.1
Rice (25%, Thai	−2.4	−1.3
Soybeans (U.S., cif, Rotterdam)	35.6	8.3
Soybeans meal (cif, Rotterdam)	18.3	3.1
Palm oil (Malaysia, 5% bulk)	54.9	12.9
Sugar (World)	21.0	8.1
Bananas (Central/South American)	23.4	21.1
Beef (Australia/New Zealand)	30.3	16.0

Source: DECPG. The price changes are for average prices of the reported commodities over the relevant quarters. For example, the first column reports the change in average prices in the January-March period in 2011 compared to average prices in January-March of 2010.

biofuels. A second channel of impact is that higher energy prices feed into the cost of food production through higher fertilizer prices, the cost of irrigation, and other farm inputs. The extent of energy price impact varies significantly depending on the type of crop and level of mechanization. A third channel of energy price impact is through increases in the costs of crop transportation to destination markets, which leads to larger price variations within countries and increases costs for importing countries.

The macro impacts of these increases in food prices feed into inflationary expectations. In East Asia, higher food price inflation is taking place in the context of higher than average credit growth in most countries, which has contributed to overall inflationary pressures. In Eastern Europe and Central Asia, several countries are making a gradual recovery from the financial crisis and any monetary tightening will need to take the state of the financial sector and growth into account. On the external front, net importers of food, fuel, and other commodities are the most vulnerable, especially those with large current account deficits and/or low reserve cover. Data from 46 countries for 2007–10 suggest that low- and low-middle-income countries have experienced higher levels of food price inflation compared to upper-middle- and high-income countries, particularly when international prices spike. One explanation is that food marketing channels in poorer countries are unable to absorb large fluctuations in commodity prices, whereas larger retailers in wealthier countries have larger margins partly because food commodity prices constitute a small share of the price of processed foods. Another explanation is that governments in poorer countries have a limited ability to cushion domestic consumers from price increases in international markets.

After the food price crisis, domestic commodity prices in many countries were slow in moving downwards, despite the rapid fall in international prices, suggesting a slow or low degree of transmission to domestic consumers. This phenomenon created a double threat to the food security of poor consumers, as domestic food prices remained high while income growth slowed or turned negative. Analyzing food prices at a country level, it has been reported that price spikes, and therefore poverty impacts, can be highly zone-dependent [142]. Localized shocks and emergencies have affected food security in specific countries as well as at the sub-national level. These differences relate to conflict and supply disruptions, as well as the fact that poor infrastructure limits the smoothing of prices within a country. Reversing the relationship, there is some evidence that historically higher food prices and the associated greater food insecurity have been contributing factors in social unrest.

2.3.3 The Last Concern: Food Prices Volatility

Price volatility can be difficult to define and still harder to measure. Broadly, price volatility is the movement of a price up or down over a given time period. That movement can be close to zero (low volatility) or some degree of magnitude larger (tending to high volatility). On the other hand, implied volatility represents the market's expectation of how much the price of a commodity is likely to fluctuate in the future. It is derived from the prices of derivative contracts, namely options, which are priced on the basis of the market's estimates of future prices as well as the uncertainty surrounding these estimates. The more divergent are traders' expectations about future prices, the higher the underlying uncertainty and thus the implied volatility. It has been reported that expectations—often faulty—played a key role in the price spike of 2008. They were most visible in the panic hoarding of rice in 2008, but they influenced fertilizer and feed markets as well. Uncertainty surrounding exchange rates and macro policies added to price misperceptions, as did flurries of speculative activity in organized futures markets. Events since 2005—including the most recent period of price variability in 2010—underscore the point that uncertainty and expectations can be as important as or even more important than actual changes in grain demand and supply in driving price variability.

Several authors have used a variety of methods to assess if food prices are becoming more volatile over time or not [143–146]. They almost unanimously conclude that there is no tendency towards increased price volatility over the past fifty years (1960 – now). However, they also notice that volatility in international agricultural commodity markets is currently higher than it was in the 1990s and 2000s but not higher than it was in the 1970s. A more pragmatic approach was applied by Naylor and Falcon [147] consisting of decomposing volatility into price trends, "normal" variability about those trends, and price spikes, all of which contribute to measured variation in prices. If all three components are deemed important in the variability calculation, then the coefficient of variation (cv)—the standard deviation divided by the mean—provides a useful standardized statistic for comparing variation across time. However, if the primary concern is about variations around trends, there are "exceptional" price movements (spikes or bubbles) which typically involve elements of misguided expectations. To provide the variability measurements, a simple breakdown of monthly data by decade is generally used. No time interval is perfect for all purposes, but monthly data by decade seems an appropriate compromise for the decision making and welfare impacts.

Obtained data confirm once again that price volatility since the turn of the century has not been unprecedented. Table 2.3 shows the most straightforward comparison of total price volatility by decade using coefficients of variation. Among the grains, rice prices were the most variable through time.

Table 2.3 Monthly variations, by decade, for selected real commodity prices.

	Coefficient of variation, in percent[a]			
	1970–79	**1980–89**	**1990–99**	**2000–09**
Wheat	36	24	21	32
Maize	25	27	20	29
Rice	41	44	43	49
Petroleum	69	41	25	46

[a]Standard deviation of each price series by decade, divided by its mean. Source: IMF International Financial Statistics.

This result is not surprising given the multiple end uses for maize and wheat and the well-functioning futures markets that exist for them, but not for rice. Perhaps more importantly, cvs for the grains during the post-2000 period were approximately the same as those that characterized the very volatile 1970s, although the relative impact of volatility on global food security was probably lower in the late 2000s than in the 1970s, mainly because of the phenomenal per capita income growth experienced in Asia since that time. This fact is small consolation, however, in a world in which almost 15 percent of the total population is still suffering from hunger.

The extreme variability of prices of basic food commodities over the most recent period has caused considerable concern as episodes of price volatility are detrimental to food security as the high uncertainty associated with food price affects producer viability and may lead to reduced agricultural investments. When prices move along well-established trends and seasonal patterns, producers, traders and consumers can adapt to them and in many cases profit from them. Steady, predictable, and high agricultural prices could even be good for poor net producers, in the short to medium term, as they would induce resource inflows into more profitable agriculturally-linked enterprises. However, volatile and unpredictable food prices increase economic risks for producers and traders, and lead to fundamental food security risks for consumers and governments, and thus can discourage needed investment in agriculture for development.

Three different but complementary interpretations of recent food price volatility in international markets have been proposed [148]. The first considers prices volatility as a natural and permanent problem of agricultural markets, related to low elasticity of demand and climate shocks affecting supply. In addition to the inherent "normal" level of volatility in agricultural markets, there is "excess" volatility, such as has characterized much of the period since 2007. The second interpretation points to the existence of periodic international food crises signal (1950s, 1970s, now) and says these can be explained by the cyclical nature of investments in agriculture, particularly the rise and fall of public investment. The third interpretation sees in the current price increases the early coming and lasting scarcities on agricultural markets as the volatility is linked to the lack of equilibrium in supply and demand when a new context emerges. This interpretation emphasizes the increasing pressures placed on natural resources, either directly linked to agricultural production (water, soil, biodiversity) or indirectly linked (oil, climate change). In this sense, new sources of demand, possibly coupled with diminishing productivity growth in agriculture, seem to affect supply and demand bringing them too close together for stable prices to be a likely outcome. Each of these three characterizations of price volatility is related to different temporal horizons: short-, medium- and long-term. Each also highlights different problems of economic efficiency and equity at the international level.

Although price volatility is considered an intrinsic characteristic of agricultural commodity markets it has increased markedly over the last six years. International grain price variability around its mean price doubled during the period between 2005 and 2010 relative to the period between 1990 and 2005, sugar price variability tripled, and rice price variability is four times higher (Figure 2.15).

Numerous causes are discussed in literature to explain food price volatility and its recent increase, and despite comparable episodes in the past, the current price environment has several unique features particularly referring to new linkages between agriculture–energy and agriculture–finance markets. In particular, the main factors connected with food volatility regards food demand, agricultural supply, trade policies, and speculation. The first aspect is mainly related to food price inelasticity, demand shocks, and the possible substitution between commodities.

For the poor consumers living in a less developed country (LDC), agricultural commodity prices represent a large proportion

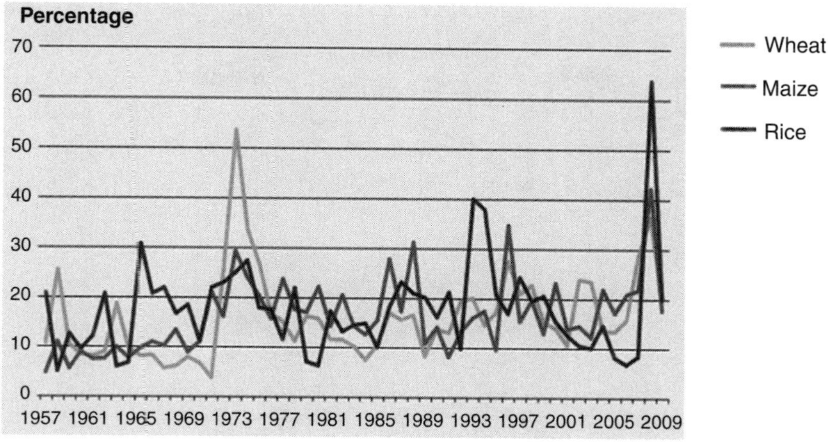

Note: Some price variability can be predicted (e.g. seasonal variation, business cycles or trending behaviour). The figure shows the coefficient of variation of prices after the predictable component has been removed from the observed values(for explanation, see OECD–FAO, 2010, p.57, footnote 5). Values close to zero indicate low volatility, higher values denote greater volatility.

Figure 2.15 Historic annualized volatility of international grain prices. Source: OECD-FAO.

of the final price they pay mostly for unprocessed food and food expenditures that are a large part of their household expenditures, making poorer countries very responsive to changes in food prices [149]. On the contrary, for the rich consumers of Organisation for Economic Cooperation and Development (OECD) countries, agricultural prices represent a small share of the overall value of the highly processed foods they eat and food expenditures are just a small part of their total budget.

Demand shocks is another aspect affecting food demand and is mostly related to the expanding production of biofuels generating a major shock on demand in cereal and vegetable oils markets. Moreover, substitutability between different commodities, and not only between agricultural commodities which always existed, has made the price of food affected also by the increasing use of agricultural commodities for the production of biofuels. This is based on agricultural feedstocks, which could tighten the link between prices of agricultural commodities, especially maize, and developments and conditions in international energy markets, implying an increased transmission of fluctuations in energy prices onto markets for agricultural and food commodities.

Higher and more volatile agricultural commodity prices are likely to persist in the foreseeable future largely due to continuing

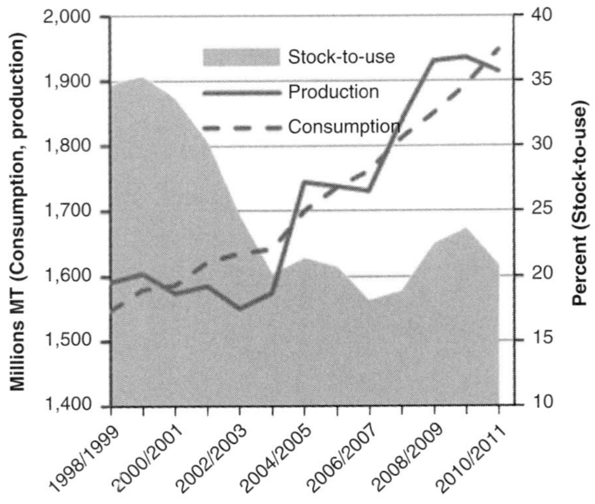

Figure 2.16 Higher world grain consumption, variable supply, and stock draw downs have contributed to the consecutive grain price spikes. Source: World Bank.

uncertainty on the supply side, against projected rising demand. Supply side uncertainty is reflected in the current price spike for cereals which was driven by a series of weather shocks in developed countries that ended up lowering their grain production in 2010 by an estimated 8 percent (Figure 2.16).

Good weather in the next growing season could lead to higher production, but long-term trends in tightening land and water constraints and climate change add to supply side uncertainty. These factors are likely to persist in the short to medium term suggesting that future volatility may be higher than that experienced in the 1980s and 1990s. Furthermore, a growing share of grain exports is being produced in Eastern Europe and Central Asia and Latin America, where weather outcomes and farm practices are less uniform than in the traditional grain exporting zones.

The difference between supply and demand is further amplified by low levels of grain stocks; estimated global grain stocks decreased significantly from the end of the 1990s, after a long period of hovering between 30–35 percent of use in the 1980s and 1990s, to about 20 percent after 2003. A change in producer income support mechanisms that induced stock holdings beyond food security concerns, associated with the reduction of stocks in Asia supported the overall global grain stock declines.

Trade policy aspects particularly related with food price volatility principally relate to stabilization policies and trade shocks.

Domestic price stabilization policies always include measures that aim to isolate domestic markets from international price fluctuations. In so doing, countries reduce the number of consumers and producers participating in the quantitative adjustment between supply and demand, which in turn imposes a bigger adjustment for the rest of the world, and therefore, a bigger international price variation. The larger the world market, the smaller the price variations that are supposed to be necessary to balance supply and demand, as was intended by the liberalization policies and the WTO trade negotiations. In one unified world market big enough "to absorb," with limited price variations, any localized supply or demand shock, the role of trade is considered as a vital mechanism to smooth prices. However, very significant income disparities between countries and among different population segments within countries imply very unequal adjustments between those who spend half or more or their income on agricultural commodities and those who spend less than 10 percent of their income on food, of which an even smaller share is spent on raw commodities. It follows that uncoordinated national policy responses to increasing food prices based exclusively on concerns about domestic food security, with little regard for their effects on trading partners, may exacerbate international market volatility and jeopardize global food security. A world market comprised of about two hundred countries provides a mechanism for individual countries to diversify risk, especially to weather shocks. However, policy actions inducing volatility, such as through price insulation, reduce the effectiveness of the world market in diversifying away these shocks supporting the idea that trade shocks are considered one of "the great uncertainties" underlying the most recent volatility in food prices [133]. Moreover, it is important to note that local price volatility in many developing countries is still higher than volatility in world markets, pointing to huge benefits from better integration of domestic markets with world markets and impacts of higher and more volatile food prices that vary by region, depending on their net trade position among other factors. Regions with large net importers of food—such as the Middle East, North Africa, and West Africa—face higher import bills, reduced fiscal space and greater transmission of world prices to local prices for imported goods such as rice and wheat. On the contrary, those countries with large net exports in Latin America and Eastern Europe stand to benefit from higher export revenues and farmer incomes, but may also face higher internal pressure to impose export bans when domestic food prices spike.

As already stated, the synchronicity of price movements during the soaring of food prices suggests that, beyond the specific fundamental situation of each commodity, some common factors were present. Speculation could be one of them. Speculation is an intrinsic part of how the futures market works and speculators provide a market for hedgers. Hedgers need risk insurance—farmers want to lock into prices in case prices are low at harvest time; processors want to lock into prices in case prices rise. Because speculators buy when the price is low and sell when the price is high, they even out price extremes. However, if unregulated, speculators can also do significant harm to the market. In particular, the volume of activity on future markets leads many commentators to believe that increased speculation is an important, if not the leading, cause of increasing volatility of food prices. The phenomenon is described as the "financialization" of the commodity markets [150], or, as UNCTAD described it, the "growing presence of financial investors in future commodity exchanges" [151]. In this context, the deregulation of markets and the breakdown of the regulatory walls that once separated banks from insurance firms, the mobility of capital in the global economy, and the enlarged mix of interests among those trading contracts, have probably complicated the role played by commodity speculators.

With the 2008 price spike over, the outlook for food price variability still remains tenuous. The climate shocks in Russia and Eastern Europe in the summer of 2010, coupled with floods in Pakistan, the declining estimates of maize stocks in the United States and uncertainties about global GDP growth, have captured the attention of many analysts and policymakers; but what will happen to prices in terms of spikes, trends, and variations during 2011–13 and beyond is unclear. The main conclusion is that food price variability, particularly price spikes, deserves much more attention in order to improve food security globally as such variability has profound effects on poor consumers and also is a major impediment to improved food and trade policy in developing countries.

2.3.4 The Food Sector Numbers: Trends in Global Food Production and Trade

According to estimates based on FAO production index numbers [116] and OECD-FAO [140] data, after two years of performance below the trend growth for the decade of about 2.2 percent, global agricultural production grew in 2008 by 3.9 percent as a number

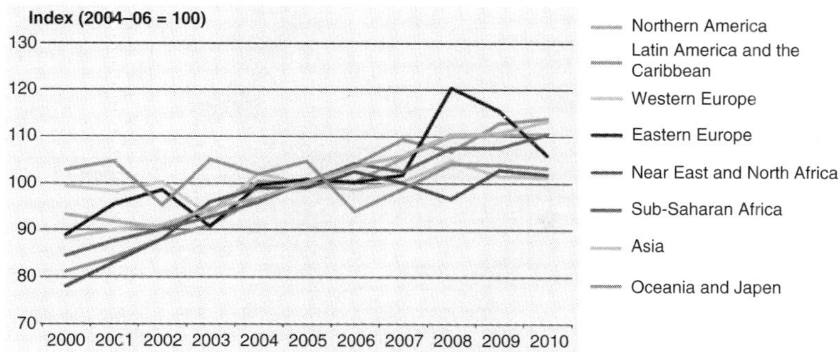

Note: Net of feed and seedstock. Estimates are in constant US dollars (2004–2006 basis). Data for 2010 are projected; those for 2009 are provisional estimates.

Figure 2.17 Indices of food production by region, 2000–10. Source: FAO.

of countries expanded production in response to the higher prices of 2007 and even better price prospects for 2008. Moreover, positive price prospects boost plantings in both the southern and northern hemispheres. This aspect, combined with good weather, have already resulted in larger outputs in the southern hemisphere for grains as well as for soybeans.

The strongest growth in food production over the last decade has been recorded by Eastern Europe and Latin America and the Caribbean (Figure 2.17).

The Eastern European countries, after recording bumper crops in 2008, were unable to sustain potential growth in the subsequent years, and the 2010 drought led to substantially reduced levels of crop production in the region. On the contrary, Latin America and the Caribbean suffered weather-related production shortfalls in 2008 but recovered in 2009 and 2010. In Asia, growth in food production remained strong throughout the last decade, generally in the range of 2–4 percent per year, although they faced a slowdown in 2009 and 2010. Production failed to grow in 2009 in sub-Saharan Africa, which had seen growth in the range of 3–4 percent per year over the previous decade, while the region registering the slowest growth in food production in recent years is Western Europe. Production did increase in 2007 and 2008 under the effect of high prices and reduced set-aside requirements in the European Union, but declined by around 2 percent in 2009 as a result of lower prices and unfavorable weather conditions. In this regard, the prospect for an expansion in grain production in 2011 is particularly related to the expectation of a return to regular climatic conditions firstly in the Russian Federation, after last year's devastating dryness.

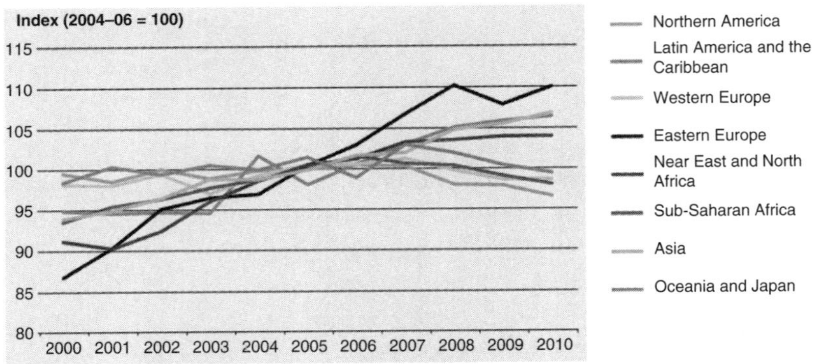

Note: Estimates are in constant US dollars (2004–2006 basis). Data for 2010 are projected; those for 2009 are provisional estimates.

Figure 2.18 Indices of per capita food consumption by geographic region, 2000–10. Source: FAO.

Encouragingly, the country has announced the lifting of its export ban from July 2011 and weather permitting, excellent crops are also anticipated in Ukraine. However, other important producing regions (Europe and North America) are now facing difficult weather situations which eventually may hamper yields.

Global food consumption, which increased at over 2 percent per year fell marginally in per capita terms during the economic recession in 2009. The most rapid growth in per capita consumption of basic foods in recent years has been recorded in Eastern Europe, followed by Latin America and the Caribbean, then Asia and the Near East and North Africa (Figure 2.18), where consumption generally continued to rise even during the recession.

An exception was Eastern Europe, which saw a decline of some 2 percent in 2009, when the region was particularly hard hit by the economic crisis. Food consumption per capita has remained stagnant-to-falling in the developed regions of North America, Western Europe and Oceania, while in sub-Saharan Africa, it rose between 2000 and 2007, but is estimated to have fallen somewhat on a per capita basis since then.

Food exports by nearly all regions, fell or stagnated in 2009 during the economic crisis (Figure 2.19). From 2000 to 2008, Eastern Europe saw cumulative export growth of around 350 percent; however, exports declined the following year even more significantly as a result of drought in 2010. Food exports from Western Europe declined, possibly as a result of the rise in the value of the euro as well as of successive policy reforms, including the reform of the EU Common Agricultural Policy.

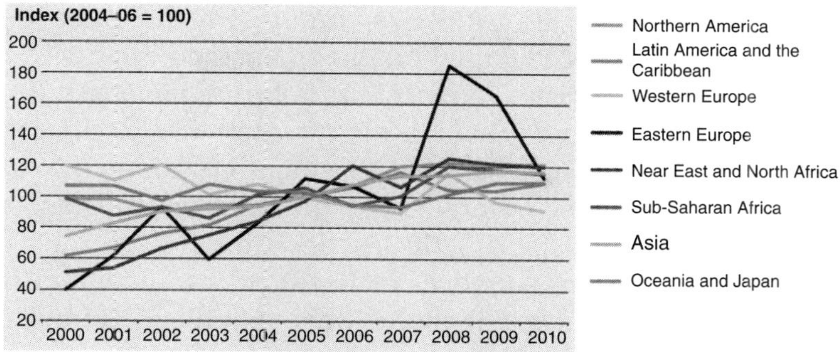

Note: Estimates are in constant US dollars (2004–2006 basis). Data for 2010 are projected; those for 2009 are provisional estimates.

Figure 2.19 Indices of food export volumes by geographic region, 2000–10. Source: FAO.

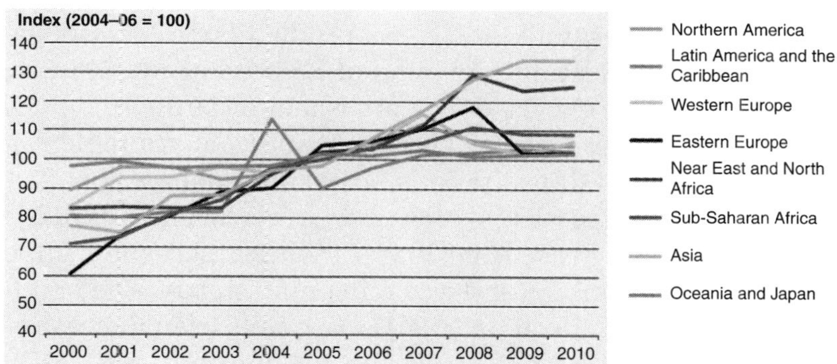

Note: Estimates are in constant US dollars (2004–2006 basis). Data for 2010 are projected; those for 2009 are provisional estimates.

Figure 2.20 Indices of food import volumes by geographic region, 2000–10. Source: FAO.

Strong export performances by countries in Latin America and the Caribbean, for which food exports nearly doubled over the decade, have made this region an increasingly important supplier of food to global markets. Export volumes from North America grew by 24 percent over the decade, but growth may have been dampened by the rising use of domestic grains for biofuel production.

Food imports have been rising more rapidly in Asia than in any other region (Figure 2.20), increasing in volume terms by almost 75 percent between 2000 and 2010, and they continued to grow during the food price crisis and the recession as the region succeeded in sustaining relatively high rates of income growth.

Food imports by countries in the Near East and North Africa have also grown, financed by growing oil revenues, but were considerably reduced during the recession. Imports by all other regions also grew significantly over time, with the exception of North America and Oceania, where they remained relatively stagnant. Sub-Saharan Africa's food import volumes increased during the first half of the decade, but the higher international prices during the food price crisis and the subsequent economic downturn translated into a decline in import volumes in 2008 and stagnating levels in 2009 and 2010. During the last decade, net food imports by sub-Saharan Africa, measured in constant prices, increased more than 60 percent, implying a further widening of the food trade deficit faced by this region over the past several decades, as population growth has outstripped growth in food production.

Analyzing the global food production and trade by commodity, an increase in world cereal production in 2011 is expected (Table 2.4) [141, 152].

FAO's first forecast for world cereal production in 2011 points to a record amount, indicating a rebound of 3.5 percent after a 1 percent decline in 2010. The expected increase is mainly supported by yield recoveries and larger plantings yet is not sufficient for replenishing stocks as the stocks-to-use ratio is hovering around a low 21 percent. FAO's first forecast of world trade in cereals in 2011/12 [152] indicates a slight increase from 2010/11 with larger wheat imports, a decline in coarse grains and rice remaining steady. The first forecast for total cereal utilization in 2011/12 points to an increase of 1.4 percent from 2010/11, compared with a 2 percent rise in 2010/11, as a result of a slowdown in the rate of increase of industrial use of cereals for production of biofuels. With total cereal production barely meeting consumption, international prices are likely to stay high, especially in the wheat and coarse grain markets. Although the removal of the Russian Federation export ban could help put some downward pressure on prices, due to the uncertain crop prospects in the United States and leading producers in the EU, international cereal prices are expected to remain volatile.

Also production of coarse grains is set to increase in 2011 exceeding the 2008 record. FAO's first forecast for world production [152] stands at 1,165 million tonnes, a record level that is 3.9 percent up from last year and some 23 million tonnes above the previous high in 2008 (Table 2.5).

The bulk of the increase is expected in the United States, the world's largest producer, where a record maize crop is forecast, as well as in the Russian Federation where production of coarse grains is set to recover sharply after last year's drought-reduced harvest. In

Table 2.4 World cereal market at a glance[1]

	2009/10	2010/11 (estim.)	2011/12 (f'cast)	Change 2011/12 over 2010/11
	Million tonnes			%
WORLD BALANCE				
Production	**2262.7**	**2237.6**	**2314.9**	**3.5**
Trade[2]	**276.1**	**274.8**	**276.0**	**0.4**
Total utilization	**2234.4**	**2279.1**	**2311.3**	**1.4**
Food	1037.3	1054.2	1069.2	1.4
Feed	767.2	774.3	785.8	1.5
Other uses	430.0	450.7	456.3	1.2
Ending stocks	**533.6**	**490.0**	**493.9**	**0.8**
SUPPLY AND DEMAND INDICATORS Per caput food consumption:				
World (Kg/year)	151.9	152.4	152.9	0.3
LIFDC (Kg/year)[3]	156.9	158.0	158.9	0.6
World stock-to-use ratio (%)	**23.4**	**21.2**	**21.0**	
Major exportes' stock-to-disappearance ratio (%)	**18.6**	**15.3**	**15.4**	
FAO CEREAL PRICE INDEX (2002–2004 = 100)	**2009**	**2010**	**Jan–May 2011**	**Change : Jan–May 2011 over Jan–May 2010 (%)**
	174	183	256	59.8

[1]Rice in milled equivalent.
[2]Trade data refer to exports based on a July/June marketing season for wheat and coarse grains and on a January/December marketing season for rice.
[3]Low-Income Food-Deficit Countries.
Source: World Bank.

Table 2.5 World coarse grain market at a glance.

	2009/10	2010/11 (estim.)	2011/12 (f'cast)	Change 2011/12 over 2010/11
	Million tonnes			%
WORLD BALANCE				
Production	**1122.3**	**1121.3**	**1165.4**	**3.9**
Trade[1]	**115.0**	**120.0**	**119.0**	**–0.8**
Total utilization	**1127.0**	**1149.3**	**1164.9**	**1.4**
Food	191.2	196.9	199.5	1.4
Feed	634.4	636.9	646.1	1.4
Other uses	301.4	315.4	319.2	1.2
Ending stocks	**194.4**	**165.5**	**167.7**	**1.3**
SUPPLY AND DEMAND INDICATORS Per caput food consumption:				
World (Kg/year)	28.0	28.5	28.5	0.2
LIFDC (Kg/year)	37.2	38.4	38.2	–0.4
World stock-to-use ratio (%)	**16.9**	**14.2**	**13.9**	
Major exportes' stock-to-disappearance ratio (%)[2]	**14.7**	**8.4**	**8.5**	
FAO CEREAL PRICE INDEX (2002–2004 = 100)	**2009**	**2010**	**Jan–May 2011**	**Change : Jan–May 2011 over Jan–May 2010 (%)**
	157	176	279	82.4

[1]Trade data refer to exports based on a July/June marketing season.
[2]Major exports include Argentina, Australia, Canada, EU and the United States.
Source: World Bank.

southern Africa, prospects for the current main coarse grains season are mixed. In South Africa, the largest producer in the subregion, a 14 percent reduction in output to 11.5 million tonnes is forecast, due to less area planted in response to low maize prices in 2010. Elsewhere in the subregion, Malawi, Mozambique, Zambia and Zimbabwe are expecting similar or higher maize harvests compared with 2010, but reductions are forecast for Botswana, Lesotho and Namibia due to floods in January and a February dry spell. The expected output in coarse grains production may be just sufficient to meet anticipated utilization in 2011/12. Feed and industrial usages of coarse grains in 2011/12 are likely to increase, although not as fast as in 2010/11, leading to an increase of about 1.4 percent in total utilization. Against these expectations for production and utilization, world stocks are likely to recover slightly from the anticipated heavy drawdown in 2011, but the build-up may prove marginal at 1.3 percent, to 167.7 million tonnes. As a result, the stocks-to-use ratio will remain near historic lows. World trade, which expanded sharply in 2010/11, is expected to decline slightly to 119 million tonnes.

However, with coarse grain harvests in the northern hemisphere many months away and prevailing weather uncertainty, this forecast is very tentative. Elevated prices are certainly an important factor behind this contraction, but good crop prospects in several importing countries are also expected to keep imports in check. International prices have been expressing the tightening of coarse grain markets for many months, with quotations exceeding by 50 to more than 100 percent of their corresponding 2010 levels.

Following a sharp drop in world wheat production in 2010, global output is forecast to increase by 3.2 percent to nearly 674 million tonnes in 2011 [152], mostly reflecting improved yield prospects in the Russian Federation (Table 2.6).

A sharp rebound in FSU-12 production, combined with larger expected crops in India, North Africa, Canada, and EU-27 account for most of the increase in world wheat output for 2011/12. World production will not be sufficient to meet the expected demand, in spite of demand not rising as fast as in the previous season. World wheat utilization is forecast to increase by 1 percent, to 677 million tonnes, in 2011/12. The growth in feed use is likely to slow in the new season, largely in anticipation of a recovery of coarse grains supplies in the Commonwealth of Independent States (CIS). World wheat inventory, which is forecast to end in 2011 well below the 2010 level, is anticipated to drop further by the close of the 2012

Table 2.6 World wheat market at a glance.

	2009/10	2010/11 (estim.)	2011/12 (f'cast)	Change 2011/12 over 2010/11
	Million tonnes			%
WORLD BALANCE				
Production	**684.7**	**652.6**	**673.6**	**3.2**
Trade[1]	**129.8**	**123.0**	**125.0**	**1.6**
Total utilization	**658.6**	**670.3**	**677.0**	**1.0**
Food	463.3	468.1	472.0	0.8
Feed	121.0	125.3	127.5	1.8
Other uses	74.3	76.9	77.5	0.8
Ending stocks	**209.6**	**187.8**	**182.9**	**–2.6**
SUPPLY AND DEMAND INDICATORS Per caput food consumption:				
World (Kg/year)	67.8	67.7	67.5	–0.3
LIFDC (Kg/year)	54.4	54.0	53.9	–0.1
World stock-to-use ratio (%)	**30.9**	**27.7**	**27.1**	
Major exportes' stock-to-disappearance ratio (%)[2]	**21.8**	**18.9**	**17.9**	
FAO CEREAL PRICE INDEX (2002–2004 = 100)	**2009**	**2010**	**Jan–May 2011**	**Change : Jan–May 2011 over Jan–May 2010 (%)**
	154	169	242	72.2

[1]Trade data refer to exports based on a July/June marketing season.
[2]Major exports include Argentina, Australia, Canada, EU and the United States.
Source: World Bank.

season, to 183 million tonnes. At this level, the global stocks-to-use ratio in the new season (2011/12) could drift slightly lower, to around 27 percent, which would still be above the low 22.6 percent of 2007/08.

Initial indications suggest a small rebound in world wheat trade after a plunge in 2010/11 [152]. At 125 million tonnes, world trade in 2011/12 will be 2 million tonnes higher than in 2010/11, mostly driven by larger imports by several countries in Asia and the EU. Increased supplies in Russia, Ukraine, and Kazakhstan and a return to exporting are expected to increase competition for EU-27 and U.S. wheat. A recovery in production and improved wheat quality in Canada is also expected to increase export competition. A sharp decline in wheat exports from the United States is forecast to be more than offset by larger deliveries from the CIS. In May 2011, international wheat prices have reacted to weather concerns and uncertain production prospects. Prices remain below their February highs but with the United States wheat futures some 75 percent above the corresponding period last year, a return to more normal price levels is unlikely, at least during the first half of the new season (July–December).

Despite a season fraught with problems, which have resulted in lower crop performance than originally envisaged in November, global rice production is estimated to have risen by 1.8 percent to a new record in 2010. Global 2010/11 rice production is projected at a record 463.8 million tons, up 1.8 percent from 2009/10 (Table 2.7) [152]. Large crops are projected for most of Asia including record or near-record crops in Bangladesh, Burma, Cambodia, Indonesia, the Philippines, Thailand, and Vietnam. In contrast, rice crops in many Western Hemisphere nations including Argentina, Brazil, Peru, the United States, and Uruguay are forecast lower than the previous year. Trade in rice is forecast to increase by 1.4 percent in 2011, to a level approaching the 2007 record, sustained by increased deliveries to countries in Africa, North America and Europe. Among exporters, Thailand and Vietnam are likely to cover much of the expansion, while Egypt, Pakistan and the United States are foreseen to ship less than last year. Global exports in 2011/12 are projected at a marketing-year record 32.2 million tons, up 0.8 million from 2010/11 with increases expected for India, Pakistan, and Vietnam, while exports from the U.S., Cambodia, and Brazil are expected to decline. Larger imports are projected for Middle Eastern, Sub-Saharan Africa, and Western Hemisphere markets, although the expected increases are slight.

Table 2.7 World rice market at a glance.

	2009/10	2010/11 (estim.)	2011/12 (f'cast)	Change 2011/12 over 2010/11
	Million tonnes			%
WORLD BALANCE				
Production	**458.5**	**455.6**	**463.8**	**1.8**
Trade[1]	**29.6**	**31.4**	**31.8**	**1.4**
Total utilization	**444.5**	**448.9**	**677.0**	**2.4**
Food	379.6	382.8	389.2	1.7
Ending stocks	**126.6**	**132.3**	**137.6**	**3.3**
SUPPLY AND DEMAND INDICATORS **Per caput food consumption:**				
World (Kg/year)	56.3	56.1	56.4	0.5
LIFDC (Kg/year)	68.5	68.0	68.2	0.3
World stock-to-use ratio (%)	**28.8**	**28.8**	**29.1**	**1.2**
Major exportes' stock-to-disappearance ratio (%)[2]	**21.7**	**19.4**	**18.6**	**–2.1**
FAO CEREAL PRICE INDEX (2002–2004=100)	**2009**	**2010**	**Jan–May 2011**	**Change : Jan–May 2011 over Jan–May 2010 (%)**
	253	229	249	11.7

[1]Trade data refer to exports based on a July/June marketing season.
[2]Major exports include Argentina, Australia, Canada, EU and the United States.
Source: World Bank.

Global rice utilization is predicted to increase by 2 percent in 2011. With global production outpacing consumption, world rice stocks in 2011 are forecast to reach their highest level since 2002. Global ending stocks are expected to decline 0.9 million tons from 2010/11 to 96.2 million. The stocks-to-use ratio for 2011/12 is calculated at 21.0 percent, down from last year's 21.6 percent.

After last season's extraordinary rise, only a modest increase in world oilcrop production is expected in 2010/11 (Table 2.8) [152]. Estimated at 465 million tonnes, production should exceed last season's all-time record by no more than 2 percent. Growth will be mainly area-driven as average yield levels should remain close to those of last season. Looking at individual oilcrops, a sizeable drop is reported for rapeseed and copra. Global soybean, cottonseed, groundnut and palm kernel production are forecast to increase. Global oilseed production for 2011/12 is projected with an only marginal rise from 2010/11 due particularly to increased competition for arable land between oilseeds and grains. Global soybean production is projected to increase less than 1 percent to 263.3 million tons. The Argentina crop is projected at 53 million tons, up 3.5 million from 2010/11 crop based on a higher harvested area and yields. The Brazil soybean crop is projected at 72.5 million tons, down 0.5 million from the projected record 2010/11 crop. A 3 percent increase in harvested area is more than offset by a return to trend yields. China soybean production is projected at 14.8 million tons, down 0.4 million from 2010/11 due to lower area and yields. Higher rapeseed production for Canada, Australia, China, and Ukraine more than offsets lower production for EU-27. For sunflowerseed, production gains for Russia, Ukraine, and EU-27 more than offset reduced production in Argentina.

Expansion in global oil/fat demand is expected to proceed in 2010/11. However, with an anticipated rise of 3 percent, consumption growth would be below the rate recorded in past years. Persistently firm oils/fats prices are contributing strongly to this slowdown. In numerous developing countries, growth in demand is expected to decelerate. The exception is China, where oils/fats consumption is accelerating while in India and Indonesia, Asia's second and third largest oil users, year-on-year rises should fall well behind past rates. Slowdowns are also expected among developed nations, notably the EU and the United States, where consumption expansion is constrained by thin domestic availabilities.

Table 2.8 World oilseed and product market at a glance.

	2009/10	2010/11 (estim.)	2011/12 (f'cast)	Change 2011/12 over 2010/11
	Million tonnes			%
TOTAL OILSEEDS				
Production	458.5	455.6	463.8	1.8
OILS AND FATS				
Production	161.2	172.2	175.2	1.7
Supply	184.5	195.6	201.0	2.8
Utilization	161.7	170.1	175.1	3.0
Trade	86.3	89.1	91.2	2.3
Stoke-to-utilization ratio (%)	14.5	15.2	14.7	
MEALS AND CAKES				
Production	98.2	113.8	116.1	2.0
Supply	116	127.7	135.0	5.7
Utilization	102.9	107.6	116.1	7.9
Trade	62.3	67.2	71.2	6.0
Stoke-to-utilization ratio (%)	13.6	17.6	16.2	
FAO PRICE INDEX (2002–2004=100)	**2009**	**2010**	**Jan–May 2011**	**Change: Jan–May 2011 over Jan–May 2010 (%)**
Oilseeds	161	172	221	40.8
Meals/cakes	194	217	231	6.5
Oils/fats	150	193	267	56.1

Source: World Bank.

As opposed to last season, when the global oils/fats output exceeded demand, production in 2010/11 is anticipated to just match consumption. Consequently, total inventories (measured as oil/fat stocks, plus the oil contained in stored oilseeds) are expected to remain about unchanged compared with last season. When related to the projected world consumption, current stock forecasts indicate a global stock-to-use ratio of 14.7 percent, down from last season's 15.2 percent and close to the low levels recorded during and immediately after the 2007/08 crisis.

In 2010/11, global trade in oils/fats (including the oil contained in traded oilseeds) is forecast at 91 million tonnes, which amounts to a year-on-year increase of 2.3 percent – well below the average rise of previous seasons. Trade expansion is anticipated to rely primarily on soybean and palm oil. Among main soy oil suppliers, only Brazil can expect a strong expansion in exports (following the country's abundant harvest). In Argentina and the United States, poor domestic output and additional demand from biodiesel industries should constrain export growth. While Indonesia should be able to raise palm oil shipments by 1.4 million tonnes (or about 8 percent), in Malaysia, below-record production may lead to an unprecedented contraction in the volume of shipments. Interestingly, Canada is set to expand exports of rapeseed oil despite this season's poor harvest.

Based on the latest 2010/11 crop estimates, global meals/cakes production (measured in protein equivalent) should exceed last season's all-time record by a small margin of 2 percent [152]. World supplies of meals/cakes in 2010/11, which comprise 2010/11 production plus 2009/10 ending stocks, are anticipated to expand by almost 6 percent. Supplies are set to surpass previous records in Brazil, Canada, China and India, owing to ample opening stocks, abundant crops or a combination of the two. Although domestic availabilities in Argentina and the United States have improved marginally, they are estimated to fall short of historic records. By contrast, the EU's combination of low carry-in stocks and poor harvests should result in an unusual drop in supplies. In spite of historically high prices, global consumption of meals/cakes (measured in protein equivalent) is estimated to expand by about 8 percent in 2010/11, well above the average rate of recent years. The expansion in demand will be primarily on account of soybean meal, the consumption of which should increase strongly. About two thirds of the global consumption rise is expected to occur in

Asia, with China alone responsible for over half of global growth. Last season's abundance of meal production over consumption proved short-lived and 2010/11 global output is expected to just match demand. As a result, the overall stock-to-use ratio is anticipated to fall again, thus departing from last season's comfortable level. Last season's strong rise in global meal/cake transactions is expected to be followed by another robust increase in 2010/11. World trade is forecast to expand by 6 percent, Headed by Brazil, South American suppliers are anticipated to supply the bulk of increased world meal exports, thanks to good harvests and/or ample opening stocks. Other exporters, such as Canada, Paraguay and Ukraine, are set to drive up their exports to take advantage of favorable international prices. India should enjoy a strong recovery in soymeal shipments following this season's ample crop.

The upward trend in world prices for oilseeds and oilseed products that started in 2009 continued into the current 2010/11 marketing year and, in February 2011, quotations for several oilseeds and derived products came close to the 2008 peaks. The renewed surge in prices mainly reflects a progressive tightening in global supplies combined with steady demand growth and robust buying interest by major importing countries. At this point, this means that supplies in the coming season may not be sufficient to satisfy the steadily expanding oil and meal demand, which would imply further reductions in global inventories as well as in stock-to-use ratios. As a consequence, firmness in prices for oilcrops and oilcrop products is expected to continue in the months to come.

According to the latest FAO estimate, world sugar production is expected to reach 165.7 million tonnes in 2010/11, an increase of 5.8 percent over the 2009/10 season (Table 2.9) [152].

This is largely attributed to bumper crops in Brazil and Thailand and a recovery in India. For the first time since 2007/08, global production will surpass consumption, but the surplus is not expected to be large enough to bring global sugar inventories back to normal levels. Production increases were prompted by strong overall international sugar prices that prevailed in the past two seasons. Although world sugar consumption is set to recover from a slowdown in 2009/10, amid buoyant economic growth in 2010/11, relatively high domestic sugar prices will contain the expansion. As a result, little growth in average per capita sugar intake is currently anticipated. World trade is expected to decline by 3.6 percent as a result of reduced export availabilities in several major exporting

Table 2.9 World sugar market at a glance.

	2009/10	**2010/11 (estim.)**	**2011/12 (f'cast)**	**Change 2011/12 over 2010/11**
	Million tonnes			**%**
WORLD BALANCE				
Production	151.0	156.6	165.7	5.8
Trade	47.5	53.2	51.3	–3.6
Utilization	160.7	162.5	165.1	1.5
Ending stocks	60.8	54.8	55.3	1.0
SUPPLY AND DEMAND INDICATORS				
Per caput food consumption:				
World (Kg/year)	23.8	23.8	23.9	0.4
LIFDC (Kg/year)	16.2	16.3	16.1	–1.3
World stock-to-use ratio (%)	**37.8**	**33.7**	**33.5**	
ISI DAILY PRICE AVERAGE (US Cents/lb)	**2009**	**2010**	**Jan–May 2011**	**Change : Jan–May 2011 over Jan–May 2010 (%)**
	18.1	21.2	26.3	28.9

Source: World Bank.

countries. Under expectation of a return to normal weather patterns, early estimates for the new 2011/12 season indicate the likelihood of a large production surplus, reflecting expansion in planted areas. If confirmed, international sugar prices are likely to decline from the peaks of early 2011. However, given the relatively low inventory levels, any unexpected weather events in major producing regions could again trigger sudden and sharp rises in international sugar prices.

High feed prices, disease outbreaks, and depleted animal inventories are forecast to limit the expansion of global meat production to only 1 percent in 2011, to 294 million tonnes (Table 2.10) [152].

The increase is anticipated to be driven by gains in the poultry and pig meat sectors, while world bovine and ovine meat outputs are expected to be constrained by a retention of animals for herd rebuilding. Strong demand for imports, especially in Asia where a number of countries are facing tight supplies and high domestic prices, is expected to foster a 2.4 percent growth in world meat trade, bringing it to 26.8 million tonnes. Much of the expansion would stem from increased flows of pig meat, and to a lower extent, poultry and bovine meats. On the other hand, trade in ovine meat may stagnate, limited by short availabilities in traditional exporting countries. Relatively high retail prices are foreseen to keep per capita meat consumption in 2011 stalling around 41.9 kg. In the developing countries, steady economic growth may foster a minimal increase to 32.0 kg, while per capita consumption in the developed countries is expected to remain at 78.4 kg. International meat prices have maintained steady increases since January 2011, progressing by 5 percent over the first quarter, mainly sustained by a 10 percent increase in pig meat prices. In the short-term, the combination of strong world import demand and limited export availabilities points toward a further firming of world meat prices in the next few months.

FAO is currently forecasting world dairy production in 2011 to grow by 14 million tonnes or 2 percent, to 724 million tonnes (Table 2.11) [152].

Much of the increase would be accounted for by developing countries, especially Argentina, Brazil, China and India, but the sector is also expected to advance in the developed countries, driven by the EU, New Zealand and the United States. World import demand is anticipated to boost trade in dairy products by 5 percent, reaching 48.3 million tonnes in liquid milk equivalent. The

Table 2.10 World cereal market at a glance.

	2009/10	2010/11 (estim.)	2011/12 (f'cast)	Change 2011/12 over 2010/11
	Million tonnes			%
WORLD BALANCE				
Production	**283.2**	**290.6**	**294.0**	**1.1**
Bovine meat	64.9	64.9	65.0	0.2
Poultry meat	93.6	98.0	100.2	2.3
Pig meat	106.3	109.2	110.0	0.7
Ovine meat	12.9	13.0	13.1	0.5
Trade	**25.2**	**26.2**	**26.8**	**2.4**
Bovine meat	7.2	7.5	7.7	1.9
Poultry meat	11.1	11.5	11.7	1.6
Pig meat	5.8	6.1	6.4	5.0
Ovine meat	0.9	0.8	0.8	0.8
SUPPLY AND DEMAND INDICATORS Per caput food consumption:				
World (Kg/year)	41.3	41.3	41.8	0.1
Developed (Kg/year)	78.0	78.4	78.4	0.0
Developing (Kg/year)	31.1	31.8	32.0	0.5
FAO MEAT PRICE INDEX (2002–2004 = 100)	**2009**	**2010**	**Jan–May 2011**	**Change: Jan–May 2011 over Jan–May 2010 (%)**
	133	152	175	19.9

Source: World Bank.

Table 2.11 World dairy market at a glance.

	2009/10	2010/11 (estim.)	2011/12 (f'cast)	Change 2011/12 over 2010/11
	Million tonnes milk equivalent			%
WORLD BALANCE				
Total milk Production	**698.5**	**710.0**	**723.8**	**1.9**
Total milk Trade	**44.0**	**46.0**	**48.3**	**4.5**
SUPPLY AND DEMAND INDICATORS				
Per caput food consumption:				
World (Kg/year)	101.3	101.8	102.6	0.8
Developed countries (Kg/year)	235.7	235.0	235.2	0.1
Developing countries (Kg/year)	65.7	66.9	68.2	1.9
Trade – share of prod. (%)	6.3	6.5	6.7	
FAO MEAT PRICE INDEX (2002–2004 = 100)	**2009**	**2010**	**Jan–May 2011**	**Change: Jan–May 2011 over Jan–May 2010 (%)**
	142	200	229	14.5

Source: World Bank.

positive environment should foster growth in all major internationally traded dairy products, especially skim milk powder (SMP), whole milk powder (WMP) and cheese. The expansion in trade is expected to rely mainly on increased exports from Argentina, Belarus, the EU, New Zealand, and the United States. Sluggish production growth in a number of exporting countries led to a drawing down of public and private stocks to meet rising import demand. As such inventories are now at minimal levels, the availability of supplies for trade in 2011 is increasingly dependent on production performance. As a result, international dairy quotations will be particularly sensitive to climatic conditions for the rest of the year, both in relation to pasture growth and the availability and price of fodder and feed.

Dairy prices surged during the first quarter of the year propelled by strong import demand in Asia and limited supplies in traditional exporting countries. During April, prices fell but bounced back in May as many countries in Northern Europe experienced lower than average rainfall. With the peak season in the region ending soon, international dairy prices during the remainder of the year will be highly dependent on weather conditions in the southern hemisphere.

World production of fish and fishery products is set to reach a new record in 2011, at around 149 million tonnes (Table 2.12) [152].

This is due to both the growth in aquaculture production and the comeback of small pelagic catches in South America after a weak 2010. Increased catches are also forecast for other important species, such as Atlantic cod, Alaska pollack and Atlantic mackerel. Higher fishing quotas and an increased supply of wild species indicate that the fisheries management measures implemented by many countries are having a positive long-term effect on the sector's sustainability. The FAO Fish Price Index reached its highest level ever in April 2011. This means that the crisis experienced in late 2008 and throughout 2009, which depressed prices, margins and volumes of trade, is now a matter of the past for most operators. Demand is strong in developing countries and is rebounding in developed markets. Supply is increasing, but costs, especially of feed, labor and energy are also up, which means consumers are likely to face rising fish prices throughout 2011. Trade volumes and prices both increased in 2011 sustained by a dynamic demand, in particular, from emerging economies. The price surges mainly reflect lagging supply, which, despite solid growth in overall aquaculture

Table 2.12 World fish market at a glance.

	2009/10	2010/11 (estim.)	2011/12 (f'cast)	Change 2011/12 over 2010/11
	Million tonnes			%
WORLD BALANCE				
Production	**144.6**	**145.1**	**149.0**	**2.7**
Captures fisheries	89.9	87.0	88.5	1.8
Aquaculture	55.7	58.1	60.4	4.0
Trade value (export USD billion)	**99.4**	**104.9**	**108.4**	**3.4**
Trade volume (live weight)	**54.9**	**55.2**	**55.4**	**0.4**
Total utilization				
Food	117.8	120.0	121.7	1.4
Feed	20.0	17.7	20.3	14.4
Other uses	68.0	7.3	7.0	–4.8
SUPPLY AND DEMAND INDICATORS **Per caput food consumption:**				
Food fish (Kg/year)	**17.2**	**17.3**	**17.4**	**0.3**
From capture fisheries (Kg/year)	9.1	8.9	8.8	–2.1
From aquaculture (Kg/year)	8.2	8.4	8.6	2.8
FAO FISH PRICE INDEX (2005 = 100)	**2009**	**2010**	**Jan-May 2011**	**Change: Jan-May 2011 over Jan-May 2010 (%)**
	128	117	127	8.5

Source: Norwegian Seafood Export Council

production, remains short of demand for a number of farmed species, including Atlantic salmon, trout, seabass and seabream, tilapia, and Vietnamese catfish. In addition, growing domestic consumption of local fish products, especially in Asia and South America, is constraining export availability.

2.4 Conclusions

Unfortunately, increasing hunger is a global problelm today and no part of the world is immune as the global food system now faces substantial challenges. It must help eliminate the chronic hunger crisis and nutritional deficiencies while smoothing the transition of developing countries from agricultural to industrial societies and increasing security and opportunity for the world's poor. It must move food through longer, more integrated supply chains while meeting consumers' rising expectations for safer, healthier products. The challenge that lies ahead is to secure the food security of these one billion hungry people, and also to double food production, in order to feed a population projected to reach 9.2 billion by 2050. Arable land and water constraints, combined with the likely impacts of climate change pose additional challenges to agricultural and food production to meet the demand of an always increasing population.

The challenge can be seen on two levels. Firstly, to achieve subsistence or basic food security requires provision of the main dietary requirements to a population. Food security should aim to safeguard the rights and interests of local communities, allowing each individual the basic human right to have access to food. Secondly, achieving food security must also contribute to sustainable agriculture, rural development, and the achievement of sustainable production and consumption. Achieving these outcomes requires both a much more open global food system and institutional and resource support to make that system more equitable and trustworthy. Urgent action is necessary and will require both short- and long-term measures as well as policy measures that help to address the food crisis and ensure the food sovereignty of developing nations. It will require a package of ambitious reform commitments, institutional innovations in managing food security, safety and sustainability risks, as well as sufficient resources to ensure food and nutrition for the hungry, safety and value for the well-nourished, and sustainability for all.

The already grave situation for the fate of the world's hundreds of millions of poor and hungry people has currently worsened as the world is going through a financial turbulence that has led to a serious economic setback. The recent food crisis and the associated spike in commodity prices has heightened concerns about global access to safe and stable food supplies, and the sharpness of the price increases and their persistence has left many developing countries struggling to cope with the consequences. The impact has been particularly severe owing to the overlap with the food crisis of 2006–08, which had pushed basic food prices beyond the reach of millions of poor people. The events of the past few years have highlighted the vulnerability of global food security to major shocks—both in the global agricultural markets and in the world economy. The food price crisis and the ensuing economic crisis reduced the purchasing power of large segments of the population in many developing countries, severely curtailing their access to food and thus undermining their food security. In a remarkable turn of events, earlier prospects for more comfortable supply situations and stable prices gave way to increasingly worrisome outlooks and to an escalation of international prices to levels not seen in decades, and the prospects for an early reversal of food price rises are not promising due to strong fundamental factors that will continue to push food prices upwards. On the demand side, these include population growth and recovering per capita income growth, especially in Asia. On the supply side, agricultural expansion will continue to be impeded by high oil prices, which are keeping production and distribution costs high and continuing to divert maize crops to ethanol production. Moreover, price volatility in international markets is of particular concern as it influences food policy and price stability in national markets, both aspects being key issues for food security. Although the precise impact of all these factors is uncertain, it will probably be most severe for countries already affected by protracted food-related crises and/or dysfunctional politics.

While unfavorable weather was the main culprit, a host of other unpredictable factors negatively impacted stability in the food markets, including the catastrophe in Japan, an unprecedented wave of political unrest engulfing many countries in North Africa and the Near East, another strong increase in oil prices, and prolonged uncertainty in financial markets and the global economy. In the cereal market, barley, maize and wheat are being, for the most part, influenced by production problems and depleting inventories.

Maize stocks have fallen to a critical low in the United States, the world's largest maize producer and exporter. Rice is an exception thanks to a record world output and large opening stocks. In addition, generally good cereal production in importing countries, as opposed to exporting countries, also dampened the impact of high international prices this time around as compared with 2007/08. In the oilseeds sector, prices have also risen sharply, supported by a tightening supply and demand balance. Quotations for dairy and meat have not been spared, as prices have been propelled (to record levels in the case of meat) by climbing costs of production, low animal inventories and virtually exhausted product stockpiles. On the back of dwindling export supplies, sugar markets also experienced a sharp price surge before retreating in recent months. Against this backdrop, food import bills are projected to soar to an all time high of almost USD 1.3 trillion.

References

1. FAO. *National programmes for food security: FAO's vision of a world without hunger*. Rome, Italy: FAO. 2007.
2. FAO. *Rome declaration and world food summit plan of action*. Rome, Italy: FAO. 1996.
3. E. Clay. Food security: Concepts and measurement. In *Trade reforms and food security: Conceptualising the linkages*. Rome: Food and Agriculture Organization of the United Nations (FAO). 2002.
4. FAO. *Guidelines for national FIVIMS: Background and principles*. Rome, Italy: FAO. 2000.
5. S. Maxwell, R. Slater. Food policy old and new. *Devel. Pol. Rev.* 21:531–553, 2003.
6. FAO. *The state of food insecurity in the world. Addressing food insecurity in protracted crises*. Rome, Italy: FAO. 2010.
7. FAO. *The state of food agriculture. Women in agriculture. Closing the gender gap for development*. Rome, Italy: FAO. 2010.
8. A. Thomsen, M. Metz. *Implications of economic policy for food security: A training manual*. Rome. FAO and the German Agency for Technical Cooperation (GTZ). 1998.
9. GECAFS Online. About GECAFS. Available at: ww.gecafs.org/glossary/index.html#foodsystems.
10. USDA – US: Department of Agriculture. Agricultural projections to 2019. Washington, DC: USDA. 2010.
11. FAO. Land resource potential and constraints at regional and country levels. World Soil Resources Report 90. Rome, Italy: FAO. 2000.
12. FAO. *Climate change and food security: A framework document*. Rome, Italy: FAO. 2008.

13. World Bank. *World development indicators*. Washington, DC: World Bank. 2008.
14. MSF-H. Food security assessments in emergencies. Report of an Inter-agency Workshop. Amsterdam. 1997.
15. UNHCR/WFP/ENN. Food security assessments, self-reliance and phasing out in on-going refugee situations. Summary Report of an Inter-Agency Workshop. Rome, Italy: UNHCR. 2000.
16. T. Boudreau. *The food economy approach: A framework for understanding rural livelihoods*. Network Paper 26. London, UK: Relief and Rehabilitation Network. 1998.
17. IFPRI. *Toward a typology of food security in developing countries*. Development Strategy and Governance Division. Discussion Paper 00945. 2010.
18. A. Sen. *Poverty and famines: An essay on entitlement and deprivation*. Oxford: Clarendon Press. 1981.
19. WHO – World Health Organization. *Globalization, diets and non-communicable diseases*. Geneva, Switzerland: WHO. 2002.
20. WHO. *Diet, nutrition and the prevention of chronic diseases*. WHO Technical Report Series 916. Geneva, Switzerland: WHO. 2003.
21. T.A. Reardon, S.A. Vosti. Links between rural poverty and environment in developing countries: Asset categories and "investment poverty." *World Devel*. 23:1495–1506, 1995.
22. J. von Braun, M.W. Rosegrant, R. Pandya-Lorch, M.J. Cohen, S.A. Cline, M. Ashby, M. Brown, M.S. Bos. *New risks and opportunities for food security: Scenario analyses for 2015 and 2050*. 2020 Discussion Paper No. 39. Washington, D.C: IFPRI. 2005.
23. L.C. Smith, A. Subandoro. *Measuring food security using household expenditure surveys*. Washington, D.C: IFPRI. 2007.
24. J. Dixon, A. Gulliver, D. Gibbon. *Farming systems and poverty: Improving farmers' livelihoods in a changing world*. Rome: FAO; Washington, DC: World Bank. 2001.
25. A. Dorward, S. Fan, J. Kydd, H. Lofgren, J. Morrison, C. Poulton, N. Rao, L. Smith, H. Tchale, S. Thorat, I. Urey, P.I. Wobst. Institutions and economic policies for pro-poor agricultural growth. Discussion Paper No. 15. Washington, DC: Development Strategy and Governance Division, International Food Policy Research Institute (IFPRI). 2004.
26. S.D. Mink. Poverty, population and the environment. World Bank Discussion Paper No. 189. Washington, D.C: The World Bank. 1993.
27. IAASTD – International assessment of agricultural knowledge, science and technology for development. Agriculture at a crossroads, synthesis report. Washington, DC: Island Press. 2009.
28. J. von Braun, D.G. Johnson. *The world food situation: An overview*. Washington, D.C.: IFPRI. 2005.
29. FAO. Assessment of the world food security and nutrition situation. Committee on World Food Security, 34th Session. Rome, Italy: FAO. 2009.
30. L.T. Evans. *Feeding the ten billion: Plans and population growth*. Cambridge, UK: Cambridge University Press. 1998.
31. T. Malthus. *An essay on the principle of population*. Oxford, UK: Oxford World's Classics, Oxford University Press. (First published in 1798.) 1993.

32. K. Cleaver, G. Schrieber. *Reversing the spiral: The population agriculture, and environment nexus in sub-Saharan Africa*. Washington, DC: World Bank. 1994.
33. E. Boserup. *The conditions of agricultural growth*. London, UK: Allen and Unwin. 1965.
34. M. Ruel. Are the urban poor particularly vulnerable? *Mitigating the Nutritional Impacts of the Global Food Price Crisis: Workshop Summary*. Washington, DC: The National Academies Press. 2010.
35. D. Bezemer, D.D. Headey. Agriculture, development and urban bias. *World Devel.*, 36:1342–64, 2008.
36. D.E. Sahn, D.C. Stifel. Urban-rural inequality in living standards in Africa. *J. Afr. Econ.* 12:564–597, 2003.
37. FAO. Globalization, urbanization and changing food systems in developing countries. In *The state of food insecurity in the world 2004*. Rome, Italy: FAO. 2004.
38. M. Ravallion, S. Chen, P. Sangraula. New evidence on the urbanization of global poverty. Washington, D.C: World Bank. 2007.
39. F. Place, P.B.R. Hazell. Productivity effects of indigenous land tenure systems in sub-Saharan Africa. *Am. J. Agricult. Econ.* 75:10–19, 1993.
40. M. Lipton. The family farm in a globalizing world: The role of crop science in alleviating poverty. Discussion Paper No. 40. Washington, DC: IFPRI. 2005.
41. E. Wolf. *Peasant wars of the twentieth century*. New York: Harper and Row. 1969.
42. T. Homer-Dixon. *Environment, scarcity, and violence*. Princeton, NJ, USA: Princeton University Press. 1999.
43. K. Rupesinghe. Strategies for conflict resolution: The case of South Asia. In K. Rupesinghe and K. Mumtaz, *Internal conflicts in South Asia*. London, UK: Sage. 1996.
44. R. Paarlberg. The weak link between world food markets and world food security. *Food Pol.* 25:317–335, 2000.
45. T.R. Gurr, B. Harff. *Ethnic conflict in world politics*. 2nd edition. Boulder, CO, USA: Westview. 2000.
46. J. Markakis. *Resource conflict in the Horn of Africa*. Thousand Oaks, CA, USA.: Sage Publications for the International Peace Research Institute (PRIO), Oslo. 1998.
47. P. Collier. On the economic consequences of civil war. *Oxford Econom. Pap.* 51:168–183, 1999.
48. M. Eriksson, P. Wallensteen, M. Sollenberg. Armed conflict, 1989–2002. *J. Peace Res.* 40:593–607, 2003.
49. D. Keen. *The economic functions of violence in civil wars*. Adelphi Paper 320. Oxford, UK: Oxford University Press for the International Institute for Strategic Studies. 1998.
50. J. Macrae, A. Zwi. *War and hunger: Rethinking international responses to complex emergencies*. London, UK: Zed Books. 1994
51. H. Jiang. *Rising agricultural commodity prices: How we got here and where do we go*. Office of Global Analysis. Foreign Agricultural Service. Washington, DC: USDA. 2008.
52. World Bank. World development report 2008: Agriculture for development. Washington, DC: World Bank. 2007.

53. A. Chowdhury. Politics, society, and financial sector reform in Bangladesh. *Int. J. Social Econom.* 29:963–988, 2002.
54. World Bank. Implementation completion report on a credit in the amount of SDR 41.2 to the Republic of Zambia for an agricultural sector investment program. Report No. 24444. 30 June. Washington, DC: World Bank. 2002.
55. K.S. Jomo. Washington rediscovers agriculture: The political economy of the agrarian turn. Keynote address. Vancouver, Canada: Wall Summer Institute, University of British Columbia. 2008.
56. S. Fan, N. Rao. Public spending in developing countries: Trends, determination, and impact. Environment, Production and Technology Division Discussion Paper No. 99. Washington, DC: IFPRI. 2003.
57. X. Irz, L. Lin, C. Thirtle, S. Wiggins. Agricultural productivity growth and poverty alleviation. *Devel. Pol. Rev.* 19:449–466, 2001.
58. N. Majid. Reaching millennium goals: How well does agricultural productivity growth reduce poverty? Employment Strategy Paper 2004 No. 12. Geneva, Switzerland: International Labor Organization. 2004.
59. E. Diaz-Bonilla, M. Thomas, S. Robinson, A. Cattaneo. Food security and trade negotiations in the World Trade Organization: A cluster analysis of country groups. Trade and Macroeconomics Division Discussion Paper 59. Washington, DC: IFPRI. 2000.
60. T. Hertel, P. Preckel, J. Cranfeld, I. Maros. The earnings effects of multilateral trade liberalization: Implications for poverty. *World Bank Econ. Rev.* 18:205–236, 2004.
61. C. Stevens, S. Devereux, J. Kennan. International trade, livelihoods and food security in developing countries. IDS Working Paper No. 215. Brighton, UK: Institute of Development Studies, 2003.
62. C.F. Runge, B. Senaur, P. Pardey, M.W. Rosegrant. *Ending hunger in our lifetime: Food security and globalization.* Baltimore, MD, USA: Johns Hopkins University Press, 2003.
63. M. Khor. *The impact of trade liberalization on agriculture in developing countries: The experience of Ghana.* Penang, Malaysia: Third World Network, 2008.
64. T. Dorsey, H. Tadesse, S. Singh, Z. Brixiova. The landscape of capital flows to low-income countries. IMF Working Paper and Subsequent Personal Communication, 2008
65. S. Narayanan, A. Gulati. Globalization and the smallholders: A review of issues, approaches and implications. MTID Discussion Paper No. 50. Washington, DC: IFPRI, 2003.
66. P.G. Pardey, N. Beintema, S. Dehmer, S. Wood. Agricultural research: A growing global divide? Food Policy Report. Agricultural Science and Technology Indicators Initiative. Washington, DC: IFPRI, 2006.
67. P. Warr. World food prices and poverty incidence in a food exporting country: A multihousehold general equilibrium analysis for Thailand. *Agric. Econ.* 39:525–37, 2008.
68. K. Dollive. The impact of export restraints on rising grain prices. Washington, D.C.: U.S. International Trade Commission, 2008.
69. F. Ng, M.A. Aksoy. Who are the net food importing countries? Policy Research Working Paper Series 4457. Washington, DC: World Bank, 2008.

70. IPC – International Food and Agricultural Trade Policy Council. Food security: The role of agricultural trade. International Food & Agricultural Trade Policy Council Discussion Paper, 2009.
71. A. Bulir, A.J. Hamann. Aid volatility: An empirical assessment. *IMF Staff Papers*, 50:64–89, 2003.
72. J. Rubin, B. Tal. Will soaring transport costs reverse globalization? *CIBC World Markets Strateg Econ Newsletter* 27 May, 2008.
73. W.F. Laurence, G.B. Williamson. Positive feedbacks among forest fragmentation, drought and climate change in the Amazon. *Conser. Biol.* 28:1529–1535, 2001.
74. G.J. Monteny, A. Bannink, D. Chadwick. Greenhouse gas abatement strategies for animal husbandry. *Agric. Ecosys. Environ.* 112:163–170, 2006.
75. M. Mendis, K. Openshaw. The clean development mechanism: Making it operational. *Environ. Devel. Sustain.* 6:183–211, 2004.
76. FAO. Adaptation to climate change in agriculture, forestry and fisheries: Perspective, framework and priorities. Report of the FAO Interdepartmental Working Group on Climate Change. Rome, Italy: FAO. 2007
77. K. Stamoulis, A. Zezza. Conceptual framework for national, agricultural, rural development, and food security strategies and policies. Rome: FAO, 2003.
78. FAO. The energy and agriculture nexus. Environment and Natural Resources Working Paper No. 4. Rome, Italy: FAO, 2000.
79. J.N. Pretty, A.S. Ball, T. Lang, J.I.L. Morrison. Farm costs and food miles: An assessment of the full cost of the UK weekly food basket. *Food Pol.* 30:1–19, 2005.
80. P.J. Ericksen. Conceptualising food systems for global environmental change (GEC) research. GECAFS Working Paper No. 2, 2006.
81. Oxfam. Weather disasters getting worse. Report cited in BBC Online. 2007.
82. R. Lal. Soil carbon impacts on global climate change and food security. *Science* 304:1623–1627, 2004.
83. H. Dregne, M. Kassa, B. Rzanov. A new assessment of the world status of desertification. *Desert. Contr. Bull.* 20:6–18, 1991.
84. S.J. Scherr, S. Yadav. Land degradation in the developing world, issues and policy options for 2020. Washington, DC: IFPRI, 1996.
85. R. Lal. Degradation and resilience of soils. *Phil. Trans. R. Soc. B* 352:997–1010, 1997.
86. S. Wood, K. Sebastian, S.J. Scherr. Pilot analysis of global ecosystems: Agroecosystems. A joint study by the International Food Policy Research Institute and the World Resources Institute, Washington, DC, 2000.
87. J.R. Porter, M.A. Semenov. Crop responses to climatic variation. *Phil. Trans. R. Soc. B* 360:2021–2035, 2005.
88. J. Pretty, ed. *The pesticide detox*. London, UK: Earthscan, 2005.
89. E.M.A. Smaling, J.J. Stoorvogel, P.N. Windmeijer. Calculating soil nutrient balances in Africa at different scales: District scale. *Fertilizer Res.* 35:237–250, 1993.
90. I. Scoones, ed. *Dynamics and diversity: Soil fertility and farming livelihoods in Africa*. London, UK: International Institute for Environment and Development, Earthscan, 2001.

91. P. Sanchez. Soil fertility and hunger in Africa. *Science* 295:2019–2020, 2002.
92. P.R. Crosson, J.R. Anderson. Resources and global food prospects: Supply and demand for cereals to 2030. World Bank Technical Paper No. 184. Washington, DC: World Bank, 1992.
93. S.W. Trimble. Decreased rates of alluvial sediment storage in the Coon Creek basin, Wisconsin, 1975–93. *Science* 285:1244–1246, 1999.
94. P.H. Lindert. *Shifting ground: The changing agricultural soils of China and Indonesia*. Cambridge, MA, USA: MIT Press, 2000.
95. D. Biggelaar, R. Lal, K. Wiebe, V. Breneman. Soil erosion impact on crop yields in North America. *Adv. Agron.* 72:1–52,2001.
96. S.J. Scherr. Soil degradation. 2020 Vision Briefs 58. Washington, DC: *IFPRI*, 1999.
97. FAO. Global forest resource assessment. Rome, Italy: FAO, 2005.
98. FAO. Global planted forests thematic study: Results and analyses. Planted Forest and Trees Working Paper No. FP/39. Rome, Italy: FAO, 2006.
99. D. Bryant, D. Nielsen, L. Tangley. The last frontier forests: Ecosystems and economies on the edge. Washington, DC: World Resources Institute, 1997.
100. Millennium Ecosystem Assessment. *Ecosystems and well-being*. Washington, DC: Island Press, 2005.
101. P. Hazell, S. Wood. Drivers of change in global agriculture. *Phil. Trans. R. Soc. B* 363:495–515, 2008.
102. L. Brown. *Outgrowing the earth: The food security challenge in an age of falling water tables and rising temperatures*. London, UK: Earthscan, 2005
103. S. Postel. *Last oasis: Facing water scarcity*. New York, NY, USA: W.W. Norton, 1997.
104. S. Postel. *Pillar of sand: Can the irrigation miracle last?* New York, NY, USA: W.W. Norton, 1999.
105. M.W. Rosegrant, X. Cai, S. Cline. World water and food to 2025: Dealing with scarcity. Colombo, Sri Lanka: IFPRI; Washington, DC: International Water Management Institute, 2002.
106. F. Ghassemi, A.J. Jakeman, H.A. Nix. *Salinisation of land and water resources: Human causes, extent, management, and case studies*. Wallingford, UK: CAB International, 1995.
107. T.H. Ricketts, G.C. Daily, P.R. Ehrlich, C.D. Michener. Economic value of tropical forest to coffee production. *Proc. Natl Acd. Sci. USA* 101:579–582, 2004
108. FAO, WHO. FAO/WHO Expert consultation on the safety assessment of foods derived from genetically modified animals, including fish. Rome, Italy: FAO, 2003.
109. M.A. Garcia. Transgenic crops: Implications for biodiversity and sustainable agriculture. *Bull. Sci. Technol. Soc.* 25:335–353, 2005.
110. H. Egelyng. Managing agriculture biotechnology for sustainable development: The case of Semi-Arid India. *Int. J. Biotechnol.* 2:343–354, 2000.
111. A.M. Closter, E. Embree, M. Petersen, S.H. Pedersen. Organic farming and genetically modified crops in relation to food security. *Henning Høgh Jensen Publication*, 2004.
112. H. Azadi, P. Ho. Genetically modified and organic crops in developing countries: A review of options for food security. *Biotechnol. Adv.* 28:160–168, 2010.

113. J. Anderson, P. Hazell, L. Evans. Variability in cereal yields: Sources of change and implications for agricultural research and policy. *Food Pol.* 12:199–212, 1987
114. P.L. Pingali, P.A. Roger, eds. *Impact of pesticides on farmer health and the rice environment*. Laguna, Philippines: IRRI, 1995.
115. J. Pretty. Agricultural sustainability: Concepts, principles and evidence. *Phil. Trans. R. Soc. B* 363:447–465, 2008.
116. FAO. State of Food Insecurity in the World 2009. Rome, Italy: FAO, 2009.
117. M. Plant. *Food security and the increase in global food prices*. Washington, DC: IMF, 2008.
118. World Bank. Double jeopardy: Responding to high food and fuel prices. Working Paper presented at G8 Hokkaido-Toyako Summit. Washington, DC: World Bank, 2008.
119. K. Collins. The role of bio-fuels and other factors in increasing farm and food prices. A review of recent developments with a focus on feed grain markets and market prospects. Kraft Foods Global, 2008.
120. M. Ivanic, W. Martin. Implications of higher global food prices for poverty in low- income countries. *Agric. Econom.* 39:405–416, 2009.
121. N. Jones, C. Harper, S. Pantuliano, S. Pavanello, K. Kyunghoon, S. Mitra, K. Chalcraft. Impact of the economic crisis and food and fuel price volatility on children and women in the MENA region. Working Paper 310. London and New York: Overseas Development Institute and UNICEF, 2009
122. World Bank. DC2011–0002. *Responding to global food price volatility and its impact on food security*. Development Committee. Washington, DC: World Bank, 2011.
123. R. Trostle. *Global agricultural supply and demand: Factors contributing to the recent increase in food commodity prices*. Washington, DC: USDA Economic Research Service, 2008.
124. M. Khor. *Rising world prices reinforce need for food security policies*. Penang, Malaysia: Third World Network, 2008.
125. D. Mitchell. A note on rising food prices. Policy Research Working Paper 4682. Washington, DC: World Bank, 2008.
126. ADB – Asian Development Bank. Soaring food prices: Response to the crisis. Manila, Philippines: ADB, 2008.
127. IRRI - International Rice Research Institute. The rice crisis: What needs to be done? A background paper. Manila, Philippines: IRRI, 2008.
128. J. von Braun, M. Torero. Physical and virtual global food reserves to protect the poor and prevent market failure. Policy Brief No. 004, Washington, DC: IFPRI, 2009.
129. C.P. Timmer. Did speculation affect world rice prices? ESA Working Paper No. 09–07, Agricultural Development Economics Division, Food and Agriculture Organization of the United Nations. Rome, Italy: FAO, 2009.
130. P.C. Abbott, C. Hurt, W.E. Tyner. What's driving food prices? March 2009 Update, Issue Report, Farm Foundation, 2009.
131. J. Piesse, C. Thirtle. Three bubbles and a panic: An explanatory review of recent food commodity price events. *Food Pol.* 34:119–129, 2009.
132. D. Headey, S. Fan. *Reflections on the global food crisis: How did it happen? How has it hurt? and How can we prevent the next one?* Washington, DC: IFPRI, 2010.

133. D. Headey, S. Fan. Anatomy of a crisis: The causes and consequences of surging food prices. *Agric. Econom.* 39:375–391, 2008.
134. C. Gilbert. How to understand high food prices. *J. Agric. Econom.* 61:398–425, 2010.
135. D. Orden, F. Cheng. *Currency policy and agriculture, toward a global food and agricultural policy for an open international economy in honor of G. Edward Schuh.* University of Minnesota, USA: Humphrey Institute, 2007.
136. M. Robles, B. Cooke. Recent food prices movements: A time series analysis. IFPRI Discussion Paper No. 00942. Washington, DC: IFPRI, 2009.
137. S.H. Irwin, D.R. Sanders, R.P. Merrin. Devil or angel? The role of speculation in the recent commodity boom (and bust). *J. Agric. Appl. Econom.* 41:393–402, 2009.
138. D.R. Sanders, S.H. Irwin. A speculative bubble in commodity futures prices? Cross-evidence. *Agric. Econom.* 41:25–32, 2010.
139. D. Headey. Rethinking the global food crisis: The role of trade shocks. *Food Pol.* 36:136–146, 2009.
140. OECD (Organisation for Economic Co-operation and Development) – FAO. 2009. OECD-FAO Agricultural Outlook 2009–2018. Geneva, Switzerland: OECD; Rome, Italy: FAO, 2009.
141. World Bank. *Global commodity markets: Review and price forecasts.* Development Prospects Group. Washington, DC: World Bank, 2010.
142. J. Compton, S. Wiggins, S. Keats. *Impact of the global food crisis on the poor: What is the evidence?* London, UK: Overseas Development Institute, 2010.
143. G. Calvo. Exploring commodity prices, lax monetary policy, and sovereign funds. London, UK: Vox: Research-based policy analysis and commentary from leading economist, 2008.
144. C. Gilbert, C. Moran. Food price volatility. *Phil. Trans. R. Soc. B* 365:3023–3034, 2010.
145. M. Huchet-Bourdon. *Developments in commodity prices volatility.* Paris, France: OECD, 51, 150.
146. P. Abbott. *Stabilisation policies in developing countries after the 2007–08 crisis.* Paris, France: OECD, 54, 2011.
147. R.L. Naylor, W.P. Falcon. Food security in an era of economic volatility. *Popul. Devel. Rev.* 36:693–723, 2011.
148. C. Gouel. Agricultural price instability: A survey of competing explanations and remedies. *J. Econom. Surv.* DOI: 10.1111/j.1467–6419.2010.00634.x, 2010
149. A. Regmi, M.S. Deepak, J.L. Seale, L. Bernstein. *Cross-country analysis of food consumption patterns.* In A. Regmi, *Changing Structure of Global Food Consumption and Trade,* 2001.
150. D. Domanski, A. Health. Financial investors and commodity markets. *BIS Quaterly Rev.* 53–67, 2007.
151. UNCTD – United Nations Conference on Trade and Development. Trade and Development Report 2009. Geneva, Switzerland: *UNCTAD* 218, 2009.
152. FAO. Food Outlook. Global Market Analysis. Global information and early warning system on food and agriculture. Rome, Italy: FAO, 2011.

3

Nanotechnology in Food Applications

Rui M. S. Cruz[1,3], Javiera F. Rubilar[2,3], Igor Khmelinskii[2,3] and Margarida C. Vieira[1,3]

[1]*Department of Food Engineering, Institute of Engineering, University of Algarve, Faro, Portugal*
[2]*Department of Chemistry and Pharmacy, Faculty of Science and Technology, University of Algarve, Faro, Portugal*
[3]*CIQA- Chemistry Research Centre of Algarve, Department of Chemistry and Pharmacy, Faculty of Science and Technology, University of Algarve, Faro, Portugal*

Abstract
The application of nanotechnology in the food industry has increased in the last 10 years. There are different definitions regarding the use of "nano." Different ingredients/nutrients can be delivered at nanoscale and change food formulations and contribute to the development of value added food products. On the other hand, food product shelf life can also be enhanced using different types of packaging designs, applying nanomaterials in their matrices. Nevertheless, commercialization and use of some nanomaterials may be compromised due to the lack of studies on their undesired effects on public health.

Keywords: Nanotechnology, food formulation, packaging, nanocapsules, nanocomposites, active packaging, intelligent packaging

3.1 What is Nanotechnology?

The concept of nanotechnology (nanometer, 10^{-9} m) was first introduced by Richard Feynman in 1959 at a meeting of the American Physical Society held at the California Institute of Technology [1]. It was only fifteen years later that the term "nanotechnology" was

Visakh P. M., Sabu Thomas, Laura B. Iturriaga, and Pablo Daniel Ribotta (eds.) Advances in Food Science and Technology, (103–122) © 2013 Scrivener Publishing LLC

used, when Professor Norio Taniguchi of Tokyo Science University referred to the ability to engineer materials at the nanoscale [2].

According to the Royal Society and Royal Academy of Engineering [3] in the UK, nanotechnologies are defined as: "the design, characterization, production and application of structures, devices and systems by controlling shape and size at the nanometer scale." In fact, nanotechnology is a very general term and there are several definitions proposed. The National Nanotechnology Initiative (NNI), which promotes nanoscale science activities among federal agencies in the United States, defines nanotechnology as "the understanding and control of matter at dimensions between approximately 1 and 100 nanometers, where unique phenomena enable novel applications" [4–5], while nanoscience is defined as "the study of phenomena and manipulation of materials at atomic, molecular and macromolecular scales, where properties differ significantly from those at a larger scale."

The US Environmental Protection Agency (EPA), which regulates many aspects of the field, defines nanotechnology as "research and technology development at the atomic, molecular, or macromolecular levels using a length scale of approximately 1 to 100 nanometers in any dimension; the creation and use of structures, devices and systems that have novel properties and functions because of their small size; and the ability to control or manipulate matter on an atomic scale" [5].

Nanotechnology is an important tool that is influencing a large number of industrial segments. The food industry is investing in mechanisms and procedures to use nanotechnology to improve production processes and produce food products with better and more convenient functionalities [6].

The global nanotechnology market is expected to grow around 19% during 2011–2013 according to the "Nanotechnology Market Forecast to 2013" report [7]. It is projected that the global market for nanotechnology-based manufactured goods will be worth US$ 1.6 trillion. This potential growth will be due to important investments of both governments and corporations worldwide into nanotechnology R&D and commercialization.

In 2006, about 400 companies around the world, included in the agricultural and food industry segment, actively invested in the research and development of nanotechnology and by 2015 this is expected to happen in more than 1,000 companies [8].

Nanotechnology offers several possibilities; this chapter will focus on the application of nanotechnology in food products' formulations and in food packaging.

3.2 Food Formulations

Food ingredients are formulated and processed into food products to perform several roles such as improvement of flavor or texture. Moreover, some ingredients have also physiological properties, including, among others, vitamins, mineral and proteins [9]. Systems that may allow the incorporation and delivery of these nutrients in food are being studied, and nanotechnology may be applied to these types of food systems [10].

One of the technologies used to deliver a range of food ingredients within small capsules is called encapsulation. This technique may be used when direct addition of a food ingredient compromises the quality of the manufactured food product. Capsules that are less than 100 nm in diameter have been classified as nanocapsules, whereas those on the order of microns are termed microcapsules. The use of encapsulation can improve the nutritional content of food since the core is protected from other components in the food and from the environment, and thus, taste, aroma and texture of food are not affected. Moreover, it also has the capability to mask off-flavors, extend the shelf life and stability of the ingredient and the final food product quality [11].

Currently, encapsulation techniques used in the food industry are based on biopolymer matrices composed of sugars, starches, proteins, synthetics, dextrins, alginates, and liposomes [12–14].

Liposomes are spherical bilayer vesicles obtained from the dispersion of polar lipids in aqueous solvents, having the ability to act as delivery vehicles by shielding reactive or sensitive compounds prior to release. These compounds are thereby made stable against a range of environmental and chemical changes, including enzymatic and chemical modification. In the food industry, liposomes have been used to deliver food flavors and nutrients in various food applications, and more recently, have been investigated for their controversial ability to incorporate food antimicrobials that could aid in the protection of food products against microorganisms [11].

Some current uses of nanomaterials in food formulations include: nutritional supplement with molecular cages 1–5 nm in diameter made of silica-mineral hydride complex from RBC Lifesciences, oat chocolate nutritional drink mix with 300 nm particles of iron from Toddler Health, meat products with 30 nm micelles to encapsulate active ingredients from Aquanova, nanotea with nanoparticles from Shenzhen Become Industry & Trading, and lemonade, fruit juices, cheese and margarine with nanoscale synthetic lycopene produced by the German multinational BASF.

The use of nanomaterials in food formulations has the potential to produce stronger flavorings, colorings, and nutritional additives, and on the other hand, improve production operations, lowering the costs of ingredients and processing [15]. Nevertheless, major companies such as Kraft Foods are still waiting for the confirmed benefits in terms of food safety, product quality, nutrition and sustainability of nanotechnology application in food products, and thus, are keeping their main interest and efforts focused on food packaging applications [16]. Moreover, Dr. Hilary Green, head of R&D communications at the food giant Nestlé, reported that they recognize the potential of nanotechnology to improve the properties of food and food packaging, however, the company declares no research in the field of nanotechnology [17]. A similar position was taken by Cargill at the British Parliament in 2009, when the company assured that they will not intentionally incorporate engineered nanomaterials into its products until health, safety, and environmental issues are overcome [18].

Thus, the application of nanotechnology in food formulations is still a controversial issue (Figure 3.1). On one hand, food companies believe and recognize the nanotechnology potential and

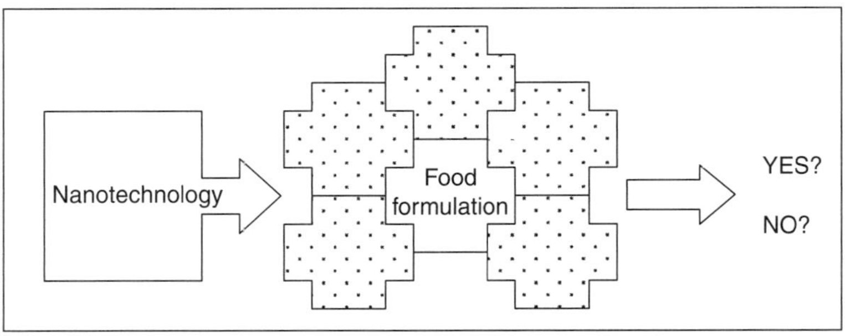

Figure 3.1 Controversial application of nanotechnology in food formulations.

opportunity to develop new valuable foods. On the other hand, they also believe that consumer health and safety risks, related to this type of application, were not yet circumvented.

3.3 Food Packaging

One of the functions of food packaging is to increase the shelf life of foods protecting it from microbial and chemical contamination and other factors, such as oxygen and light. The use of nanotechnology in food packaging is a promising application aimed at achieving longer shelf life of food products, rendering them safer [4]. New solutions can be provided for food packaging, through the modification of the permeability behavior of the packaging systems. Some of those include: enhanced barrier (mechanical, microbial and chemical), antimicrobial, and heat-resistance properties [19–20].

The Project on Emerging Nanotechnologies and the Grocery Manufacturers/Food Products Association (GMA/FPA) held a joint meeting in 2007 with several experts to begin discussing possible applications of engineered nanomaterials for use in packaging case studies. Three hypothetical applications were designed to be developed, illustrating the range of possible future uses of engineered nanomaterials in packaging [19].

Thus, enhanced barrier properties, active packaging, and intelligent packaging are the three basic categories of nanotechnology applications and functionalities that appear to be in development for food packaging applications.

3.3.1 Enhanced Barrier Properties

3.3.1.1 Clays and Silicates

3.3.1.1.1 Structure and Types of Composites

In the late 1980s, the concept of polymer-clay nanocomposites (PCN) was developed and first commercialized by Toyota [21], but only since the late 1990s have works been published on the development of PCN for food packaging [22]. There are different forms to improve the plastic materials' barrier properties. One of them is the incorporation of clays or silicates in the polymer matrix. These layered inorganic solids have drawn the attention of the packaging industry due to their availability, low cost, significant enhancements, and relatively simple processing [23]. The nanocomposites most commonly used are layered silicates consisting of two-dimensional layers around 1 nm in thickness, and several microns in extension, depending on the kind of silicate [23]. The presence of the layered silicates in polymer formulations increases the irregularity of the diffusive path for a penetrant molecule (Figure 3.2), providing excellent barrier properties against oxygen, water vapor, carbon dioxide, and aromas [19, 24–26].

In a tactoid structure, predominating in microcomposites (conventional composites), the polymer and the clay tactoids remain immiscible, resulting in agglomeration of the clay in the matrix and poor macroscopic properties of the material [27–28], while the interaction between layered silicates and polymer chains may produce two types of ideal nanoscale composites (Figure 3.3). One type are the intercalated nanocomposites obtained from the penetration of polymer chains into the interlayer region of the clay, resulting in an ordered multilayer structure with alternating polymer/inorganic layers at a repeated distance of a few nanometers [29]. The other types are the exfoliated nanocomposites which involve extensive polymer penetration, with the clay layers delaminated and randomly dispersed in the polymer matrix [28]. It has been reported that the exfoliated nanocomposites exhibit the best properties due to the optimal interaction between clay and polymer [27, 30].

One of the most studied clay fillers is Montmorillonite (MMT), a hydrated aluminosilicate layered clay consisting of an edge-shared octahedral sheet of aluminum hydroxide between two tetrahedral layers of silica [29]. The imbalance of the negative charges at the

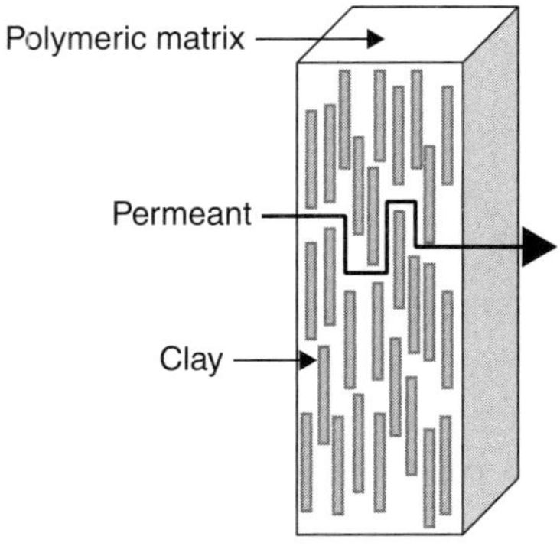

Figure 3.2 Tortuous path of a permeant in a clay nanocomposite. Adapted from de Azeredo, [23].

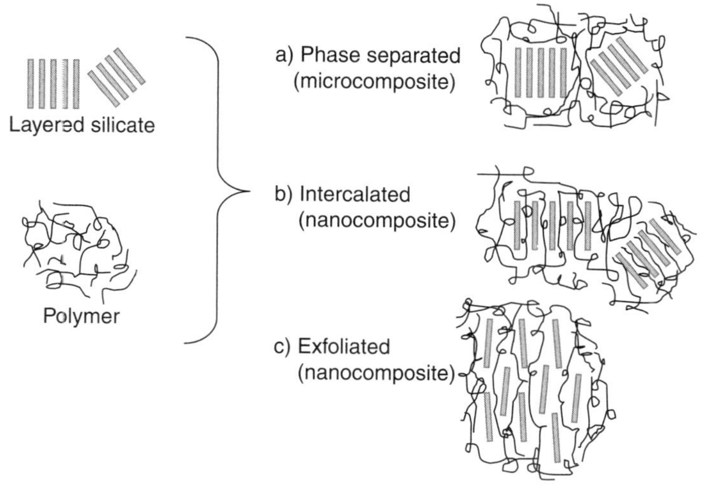

Figure 3.3 Types of composites derived from interaction between layered silicates and polymers: (a) phase-separated microcomposite; (b) intercalated nanocomposite and (c) exfoliated nanocomposite. Based on Alexandre and Dubois [27] and Weiss *et al.* [29].

surface is compensated by exchangeable cations (typically Na^+ and Ca^{2+}) [23]. The parallel layers are linked together by weak electrostatic forces [31–32]. This type of clay is characterized by a moderate negative surface charge (known as the cation exchange capacity, CEC, measured in meq/100 g), which is an important factor defining the equilibrium layer spacing [23]. The charge of a layer is not locally constant, varying from layer to layer, and thus an average value over the whole crystal should be considered instead [27]. MMT is an efficient reinforcing filler due to its high surface area and large aspect ratio (50–1000) [33].

3.3.1.1.2 Applications of Clay Nanocomposites

The introduction of nanoclays into polymer biostructures has been shown to greatly improve barrier properties, constituting a barrier to gas and water molecules and forcing them to follow a much longer path; the path length is increased by the aspect ratio of the clay nanoflakes times their relative fraction [34], reducing one of the main drawbacks of biopolymer films. Several studies have reported the effectiveness of nanoclays in reducing permeabilities to oxygen [24–25, 35–40] and water vapor [38, 41–42]. The mechanical strength of biopolymers can also be improved by the use of clays [29]. A thermoplastic starch (TPS)/clay nanocomposite with improved mechanical properties and decreased water vapor permeability was generated by Park *et al.* [43] using only 5% (w/w) clays. In a study reported by Petersson and Oksman [44], bentonite improved the strength and modulus of a polylactic acid (PLA) matrix, even though drastically decreasing elongation of the material. Lotti *et al.* [38] and Xu *et al.* [45] showed similar results for low-density polyethylene (LDPE) treated with organoclay and chitosan film with the incorporation of MMT, respectively. Alternatively, Marras *et al.* [46] showed that elongation of poly(ε-caprolactone) (PCL) was not impaired by MMT.

Nevertheless, improvement of mechanical properties of several polymers by the addition of nanoclays was observed by other authors [42, 47–51]. Other advantages, such as increased glass transition and thermal degradation temperatures, have been reported in the performance of a diversity of polymers as a result from adding clay nanoparticles [25, 44, 47, 51]. However, some decrease in transparency has also been observed [47].

3.3.1.2 Other Nanofillers

Laminar clays have been used in several applications of nanocomposites in bioplastics for packaging [52] along with carbon nanotubes [53] and nanoparticles of metals and oxides [54]. Biodegradable cellulose nanowhiskers (CNW) and nanostructures obtained by electrospinning, which are very promising in a number of application fields, are other types of reinforcing elements [55–57]. The generation of fully biobased formulations can be achieved by the use of biobased nanofillers to reinforce bioplastics [52]. These nanobiofillers (CNW and electrospun nanofibers), besides other properties, have very large surface to mass ratios (up to 10^3 higher than a microfiber), excellent mechanical strength (CNW and some reinforced electrospun fibers), flexibility, lightness, and, possible edibility when made of food hydrocolloids [58–60].

The properties of nanocomposites composed of cellulose fibers are strongly dependent on their dimensions and aspect ratio (shifting from micro- to nanosized fibers allows for improvements in optical and mechanical properties), as well as on their compatibility with the polymer matrix [61–63]. These nanomaterials have already been used for controlled release of bioactive substances in pharmaceutical and biomedical applications, and also as reinforcing fillers [53]. Controlled release of active and bioactive compounds in food packaging applications, and nanoencapsulation of functional added-value food additives are other possible applications [64–65].

3.3.1.2.1 Applications of Other Nanofillers

Helbert *et al.* [59] reported that a poly(styrene-co-butyl acrylate) latex film containing 30% of straw cellulose whiskers presented a modulus that was more than a thousand times higher than that of the bulk matrix. This effect is due to the geometry and stiffness of the whiskers, but also to the formation of a fibril network within the polymer matrix, the cellulose fibers probably being linked through hydrogen bonds. Zimmermann *et al.* [66] observed that fibril contents of up to 5% resulted in no strength or stiffness improvement of polyvinyl alcohol composites, and it was suggested that probably a minimum content of fibrils is required to induce intense interactions between fibrils and thus the formation of networks.

These cellulose fibers have been effective in improving strength and modulus of polymers, especially at temperatures above the glass transition temperature (T_g) of the matrix polymer [67–68]. The cellulose nanoreinforcements showed increased moisture barrier of polymer films [57, 69–70]. The lower permeability is thought to be related with the presence of crystalline fibers increasing the tortuosity in the materials leading to slower diffusion processes [57]. Fillers less permeable, with good dispersion in the matrix and a high aspect ratio, can improve the barrier properties [71]. Improved thermal properties of polymers have also been reported in studies with nanosized cellulose fibrils. In these studies the thermal stability of polymers in nanocomposites with cellulose whiskers was improved compared to the corresponding bulk polymers [59, 72–73]. Nevertheless, controversial results, such as T_g increasing effects on polymer films [74–75], and inconsistent or even negligible effect of cellulose nanoreinforcements on T_g have been reported [57, 76–77]. In a study with a sorbitol-plasticized starch nanocomposite with tunicin whiskers it was observed that the T_g first increased up to the whisker content around 10–15 wt.% and then decreased. The increase of T_g was attributed to the increase in the crystallinity of the starch matrix with tunicin content, the restricted mobility of amorphous amylopectin chains resulting from the physical crosslinks induced by the crystallization. On the other hand, a possible explanation for the T_g decrease, could be that sorbitol is probably not totally included into the crystalline domains during crystallization, which increases its concentration in the amorphous domains of the matrix [77].

Two studies proposed possible explanations of negligible variation of T_g values of polymers with the contents of cellulose nanoreinforcements in composites. One explanation is that the inclusion of cellulose nanofibrils results in a smaller portion of the matrix participating in the glass transition instead of a consistent increase in T_g [78]. Another mechanism was proposed by Azizi Samir *et al.* [76], whereby the presence of whiskers could influence the T_g values in different manners. First, the solid surface of cellulose whiskers could restrict mobility of polymer chains in the vicinity of the interfacial area, which would result in a global shift of T_g toward higher temperatures. On the other hand, in the presence of whiskers, the crosslinking density of the polymeric matrix decreased, indirectly decreasing the T_g.

3.3.2 Active Packaging

Conventional packaging is known as a passive barrier to and from the external environment [79]. On the other hand, a system which allows changes in the structure and condition of the package to improve the preservation of food properties, improve safety, enhance sensory quality and further extend shelf life is called active packaging (AP) [80]. AP is designed to deliberately incorporate components that would release or absorb substances into or from the packaged food environment surrounding the food [81]. The use of nanotechnology may allow the incorporation of active components to deliver functional attributes beyond those of conventional AP [19].

There have been developments for antimicrobial and oxygen scavenging packaging applications. Other main promising applications include ethylene removers and carbon dioxide absorbers/emitters.

3.3.2.1 Antimicrobial Nanocomposites

The incorporation of antimicrobial compounds into food packaging materials in AP is a promising technology, having received considerable attention since it may allow microbial inactivation and/or inhibition to enhance product safety and extend its shelf life [23]. An antimicrobial nanocomposite film is particularly desirable due to its acceptable structural integrity and barrier properties imparted by the nanocomposite matrix, and the antimicrobial properties contributed by the natural antimicrobial agents impregnated within [82].

Metal and metal oxide nanoparticles and carbon nanotubes are the nanoparticles most used for the development of active packaging with antimicrobial properties [52]. Silver is the most common nanoadditive used in antimicrobial packaging, with several advantages such as strong toxicity to a wide range of microorganisms, high temperature stability, and low volatility [23]. Several mechanisms were proposed to explain the antimicrobial properties of silver nanoparticles. The adhesion to the cell surface, degrading lipopolysaccharides and forming "pits" in the membranes, largely increasing permeability [83], penetration inside bacterial cell, damaging DNA [84], and releasing antimicrobial Ag^+ ions by Ag-nanoparticles dissolution [85] are some of the proposed hypotheses.

Titanium dioxide (TiO_2) has also been used to inactivate several food-related pathogenic bacteria [86–88]. A TiO_2 powder-coated packaging film was developed by Chawengkijwanich and Hayata [89] reducing *Escherichia coli* counts on food surfaces. In another study, TiO_2-coated films exposed to sunlight inactivated fecal coliforms in water [90]. Moreover, doping TiO_2 with silver greatly improved photocatalytic bacterial inactivation [91–92]. A nanocomposite with PVC and TiO_2/Ag^+ nanoparticles also showed good antibacterial properties [93]. Actually, attention is particularly focused on the photocatalytic activity of TiO_2 under ultraviolet radiation [94]. Oxygen scavenger films were successfully developed by adding titania nanoparticles to different polymers. The authors suggested their use for packaging of a wide variety of oxygen-sensitive products. Nevertheless, its major drawback is the requirement of UVA light [23, 95]. Carbon nanotubes (CNTs) have also been reported to have antibacterial properties. The long and thin CNTs perforate microbial cells causing irreversible damage [96]. Nevertheless, CNTs can be cytotoxic to human cells when in contact with skin and lungs [97–99]. Antibacterial activity of nanoscale chitosan has also been studied [100]. Its mechanism of action involves interactions between positively charged chitosan and negatively charged cell membranes, increasing membrane permeability and eventually causing rupture and leakage of intracellular material.

3.3.3 Intelligent Packaging

Systems that include an external or internal indicator providing the consumer information on the history of the product/or the quality of the food are called intelligent packaging [101]. These systems can detect and record changes in the product's external or internal environment and inform the customer on the consequences of these changes to the safety and quality of the food product [102–103].

3.3.3.1 Nano-based Sensors

Nanoparticles can be applied as reactive particles in packaging materials. These nanosensors are able to respond to environmental changes (e.g., temperature, humidity and levels of oxygen), degradation products or microbial contamination [104]. The food expiration date is estimated by the food industries, considering the distribution and storage conditions (mainly temperature) to which the food product is predicted to be exposed [23]. Nevertheless, special attention must be given to products requiring cold chain conditions since temperature abuses may occur. Moreover, sealing defects or micropores in packaging systems can contribute to an oxygen concentration increase leading to undesirable changes [23]. The incorporation of these nanosensors allows the detection of certain chemical compounds, pathogens and toxins in food, providing real-time status of food freshness and, consequently, eliminating the need for inaccurate expiration dates [105]. Moreover, tracking certain ingredients or products through the processing chain is already under development or has been commercialized [106].

Mahadevan Iyer, an expert from the Packaging Research Center of the Georgia Institute of Technology in Atlanta, pointed out several advantages of these sensors. These include: rapid and high-throughput detection, simplicity, cost effectiveness, reduced power requirements and easy recycling [107].

3.3.3.2 Detection of Gases Produced by Food Spoilage

Several types of gas sensors have been developed based on applied studies of the surface properties of materials. Conducting polymer nanocomposites (CPC) and metal oxide gas sensors are the most popular types of sensors due to their high sensitivity and stability [108]. Food spoilage is mainly caused by microorganisms, whose metabolism produces gases which can be quantified and/or identified by these types of sensors. CPC sensors are constituted by conducting particles embedded into an insulating polymer matrix. The emitted gases can be detected since the sensor resistance changes produce the corresponding pattern [108]. An "electronic tongue" device for inclusion in packaging is being developed by Kraft Foods and researchers at Rutgers University in the US. This equipment is composed of an array of nanosensors highly sensitive to gases released by food as it spoils, producing a color change indicating whether the food has deteriorated [23].

3.4 Regulation Issues and Consumer Perception

Nanotechnology can be applied in all aspects of the food chain, both for improving food safety and quality control, and to incorporate novel food ingredients or additives [81]. This application or utilization in foods is a matter of concern in terms of public health. Currently, there are no special regulations in the United States; however, in the European Union (EU) some recommendations for regulations have been made [52]. As a general recommendation, nanocomposites within the EU must comply with the European Food Safety Authority (EFSA) total migration limit of 10 mg/dm^2, with the functional barrier stringent migration level of 0.01 mg/kg of food or food simulant and/or with the specific migration levels for their constituents in case they comprise food-contact components (Commission Directive 2007/19/CE that modifies Directive 2002/72/CE) [51]. On the other hand, the US Food and Drug Administration (FDA) states that it regulates "products, not technologies," and anticipates that many products of nanotechnology will fall under the jurisdiction of multiple centers within the FDA and will therefore be regulated by the Office of Combination Products. FDA regulates on a product-by-product basis and stresses that many products that are currently regulated produce particles in the nano-size range. The FDA says that "particle size is not the issue" and stresses that new materials, regardless of the technology used to create them, will be subject to the standard battery of safety tests. Nevertheless, a recent report by the Institute of Food Science and Technology (IFST) in the United Kingdom stated that size matters and recommends that nanoparticles be treated as new, potentially harmful materials until testing proves their safety [29]. Thus, it is mandatory to know the eventual health effects of nanotechnology applications, since the risk of ingestion of particles incorporated into food packaging material must be taken into account because of the possibility of their migration to food.

The acceptance of new technologies by consumers, in particular nanotechnologies, depends on the consumer's perception and reaction to the information about those types of technology. Several reports showed that European consumer awareness of nanotechnology is progressively emerging and that they are positive about the opportunities of nanotechnology in several applications, however, there is still some skepticism regarding the use of nanoparticles in food. In the US, studies revealed that very few consumers heard about nanotechnology, nevertheless, they are expecting safer and better food with the application of nanotechnology [81].

Moreover, in 2006 the National Science Foundation (US) funded a survey and observed that US consumers are willing to use specific products with nanoparticles when the potential benefits are high, even if there are health and safety risks.

Acknowledgements

The author Rui M. S. Cruz would like to thank Fundação para a Ciência e Tecnologia (grant SFRH/BPD/70036/2010).

References

1. A. Khademhosseini, and R. Langer. Nanobiotechnology: Drug delivery and tissue engineering. *Chemical Engineering Process* 102(2), 38–42, 2006.
2. R. Sequeira, A. Genaidy, R. Shell, W. Karwowski, G. Weckman, and S. Salem. The nano enterprise: A survey of health and safety concerns, considerations, and proposed improvement strategies to reduce potential adverse effects. *Human Factors and Ergonomics in Manufacturing* 16(4), 343–368, 2006.
3. Royal Society, Royal Academy of Engineering. Nanoscience and nanotechnologies: Opportunities and uncertainties. http://www.nanotec.org.uk/finalReport, 2004.
4. S. Neethirajan, and D.S. Jayas. Nanotechnology for the food and bioprocessing industries. *Food and Bioprocess Technology* 4, 39–47, 2011.
5. K. Gibson, and D. Pula. Nanoparticles: Environmental risk and regulation environmental quality management, 2009.
6. M.C. Roco. Nanoscale science and engineering for agriculture and food systems. Washington: National Planning Workshop, 2002.
7. Nanotechnology market forecast to 2013. RNCOS E-Services Private Limited, 2011.

8. T. Joseph, and M. Morrison. Nanotechnology in agriculture and food: A nanoforum report. Institute of Nanotechnology, 2006.
9. R.E.C. Wildman. *Handbook of nutraceuticals and functional foods*. CRC Press, Boca Raton, FL, USA, 2001.
10. D.K. Bhatt. Nanotechnology: Changing dimensions of food processing. *International Journal of Food Science, Technology & Nutrition* 4(1), 31–39, 2010.
11. M.A. Augustin, and Y. Hemar. Nano- and micro-structured assemblies for encapsulation of food ingredients. *Chemical Society Reviews* 38, 902–912, 2009.
12. B.F. Gibbs, S. Kermasha, I. Alii, and C.N. Mulligan. Encapsulation in the food industry: a review. *International Journal of Food Science and Nutrition* 50, 213–224, 1999.
13. C. Kirby. Microencapsulation and controlled delivery of food ingredients. *Food Science and Technology Today* 5:74–78, 1991.
14. G. Reineccius. Liposomes for controlled release in the food industry. In S. Risch, and G. Reineccius, eds. *Encapsulation and Controlled Release of Food Ingredients*. Washington, DC: American Chemical Society, pp. 113-131, 1995.
15. G. Miller, and R. Senjen. Out of the laboratory and on to our plates. Nanotechnology in food and agriculture. Friends of the Earth Report, 2008.
16. Kraft foods, Nanotechnology, http://www.kraftfoodscompany.com/deliciousworld/food-safety-quality/nanotech.aspx, 2011.
17. C. Shaffer. Is food nanotech withering on the vine? *Food Quality* 2011.
18. Cargill, Nanotechnology in Cargill. ST/NF/74, British Parliament documents. http://www.parliament.uk/documents/lordscommittees/sciencetechnology/st174cargillev081409.pdf., 2009.
19. A.L. Brody. Case studies on nanotechnologies for food packaging. Packaging, *Food Technology* 102–107, 2007.
20. Q. Chaudhry, M. Scotter, J. Blackburn, B. Ross, A. Boxall, L. Castle, R. Aitken, and R. Watkins. Applications and implications of nanotechnologies for the food sector. *Food Additives and Contaminants* 25(3), 241–258, 2008.
21. J. Collister. Commercialization of polymer Nanocomposites. In R. Krishnamoorti, R.A. Vaia, eds. *Polymer nanocomposites: Synthesis, characterization and modeling*. Washington: American Chemical Society, 2002.
22. S. Ray, A. Easteal, S.Y. Quek, and X.D. Chen. The potential use of polymer-clay nanocomposites in food packaging. *International Journal of Food Engineering* 2(4), article.5, 2006.
23. H.M.C. de Azeredo. Nanocomposites for food packaging applications. *Food Research International* 42, 1240–1253, 2009.
24. R.K. Bharadwaj, A.R. Mehrabi, C. Hamilton, C. Trujillo, M. Murga, R. Fan, A. Chavira, and A.K. Thompson. Structure-property relationships in cross-linked polyester-clay nanocomposites. *Polymer* 43(13), 3699–3705, 2002.
25. L. Cabedo, E. Giménez, J.M. Lagaron, R. Gavara, and J.J. Saura. Development of EVOH-kaolinite nanocomposites. *Polymer* 45(15), 5233–5238, 2004.
26. A. Mirzadeh, and M. Kokabi. The effect of composition and draw-down ratio on morphology and oxygen permeability of polypropylene nanocomposites blown films. *European Polymer Journal* 43(9), 3757–3765, 2007.
27. M. Alexandre, and P. Dubois. Polymer-layered silicate nanocomposites: Preparation, properties and uses of a new class of materials. *Materials Science and Engineering* 28, 1–63, 2000.

28. L.N. Ludueña, V.A. Alvarez, and A. Vasquez. Processing and microstructure of PCL/clay nanocomposites. *Materials Science and Engineering*: A, 121–129, 2007.
29. J. Weiss, P. Takhistov, and D.J. McClements. Functional materials in food nanotechnology. *Journal of Food Science* 71(9), R107–R116, 2006.
30. M.A. Osman, J.E.P. Rupp, and U.W. Suter. Effect of non-ionic surfactants on the exfoliation and properties of polyethylene-layered silicate nanocomposites. *Polymer* 46, 8202–8209, 2005.
31. W. Tan, Y. Zhang, Y.S. Szeto, and L. Liao. A novel method to prepare chitosan/montmorillonite nanocomposites in the presence of hydroxyl-aluminum olygomeric cations. *Composites Science and Technology* 68(14), 2917–2921, 2008.
32. R.E. Grim, and N. Guven. *Bentonites: Geology, mineralogy, properties and uses.* Elsevier Scientific, Amsterdam, 1978.
33. H. Uyama, M. Kuwabara, T. Tsujimoto, M. Nakano, A. Usuki, and S. Kobayashi. Green nanocomposites from renewable resources: Plant oil-clay hybrid materials. *Chemistry of Materials* 15, 2492–2494, 2003.
34. D. Adame, and G.W. Beall. Direct measurement of the constrained polymer region in polyamide/clay nanocomposites and the implications for gas diffusion. *Applied Clay Science* 42, 545–552, 2009.
35. D. Cava, E. Giménez, R. Gavara, and J.M. Lagaron. Comparative performance and barrier properties of biodegradable thermoplastics and nanobiocomposites versus PET for food packaging applications. *Journal of Plastic Film and Sheeting* 22, 265–274, 2006.
36. H.C. Koh, J.S. Park, M.A. Jeong, H.Y. Hwang, Y.T. Hong, S.Y. Ha, and S.Y. Nam. Preparation and gas permeation properties of biodegradable polymer/layered silicate nanocomposite membranes. *Desalination* 233, 201–209, 2008.
37. J.M. Lagaron, L. Cabedo, D. Cava, J.L. Feijoo, R. Gavara, and E. Gimenez. Improving packaged food quality and safety part 2: Nanocomposites. *Food Additives and Contaminants* 22(100), 994–998, 2005.
38. C. Lotti, C.S. Isaac, M.C. Branciforti, R.M.V. Alves, S. Liberman, and R.E.S. Bretas. Rheological, mechanical and transport properties of blown films of high density polyethylene nanocomposites. *European Polymer Journal* 44, 1346–1357, 2008.
39. D.A. Pereira de Abreu, P. Paseiro-Losada, I. Angulo, and J.M. Cruz. Development of new polyolefin films with nanoclys for application in food packaging. *European Polymer Journal* 43, 2229–2243, 2007.
40. F.J. Rodríguez, M.J. Galotto, A. Guarda, and J.E. Bruna. Modification of cellulose acetate films using nanofillers based on organo-clays. *Journal of Food Engineering*. doi:10.1016/j.jfoodeng.2011.05.004, 2011.
41. R.K. Bharadwaj. Modeling the barrier properties of polymer-layered silicate nanocomposites. *Macromolecules* 34, 9189–9192, 2001.
42. P. Jawahar, and M. Balasubramanian. Preparation and properties of polyester-based nanocomposite gel coat system. *Journal of Nanomaterials* 4 [article ID 21656], 2006.
43. H.M. Park, W.K. Lee, C.Y. Park, W.J. Cho, and C.S. Ha. Environmentally friendly polymer hybrids: Part I. Mechanical, thermal, and barrier properties of the thermoplastic starch/clay nanocomposites. *Journal of Materials Science* 38, 909–915, 2003.

44. L. Petersson, and K. Oksman. Biopolymer based nanocomposites: Comparing layered silicates and microcrystalline cellulose as nanoreinforcement. *Composites Science and Tehcnology* 66, 2187–2196, 2006.
45. Y. Xu, X. Ren, and M.A. Hanna. Chitosan/clay nanocomposite film preparation and characterization. *Journal of Applied Polymer Science* 99(4), 1684–1691, 2006.
46. S.I. Marras, K.P. Kladi, I. Tsivintzelis, I. Zuburtikudis, and C. Panayiotou. Biodegradable polymer nanocomposites: The role of nanoclays on the thermomechanical characteristics and the electrospun fibrous structure. *Acta Biomaterialia* 4(3), 756–765, 2008.
47. Y.H. Yu, C.Y. Lin, J.M. Yeh, and W.H. Lin. Preparation and properties of poly(vinyl alcohol)-clay nanocomposite materials. *Polymer* 44(12), 3553–3560, 2003.
48. M. Avella, J.J. De Vlieger, M.E. Errico, S. Fischer, P. Vacca, and M.G. Volpe. Biodegradable starch/clay nanocomposite films for food packaging applications. *Food Chemistry* 93, 467–474, 2005.
49. B. Chen, and J.R.G. Evans. Thermoplastic starch-clay nanocomposites and their characteristics. *Carbohydrate Polymers* 61, 455–463, 2005.
50. G.M. Russo, V. Nicolais, L. Di Maio, S. Montesano, and L. Incarnato. Rheological and mechanical properties of nylon 6 nanocomposites submitted to reprocessing with single and twin-screw extruders. *Polymer Degradation and Stability* 92(10), 1925–1933, 2007.
51. V.P. Cyras, L.B. Manfredi, M.T. Ton-That, and A. Vázquez. Physical and mechanical properties of thermoplastic starch/montmorillonite nanocomposite films. *Carbohydrate Polymers* 73, 55–63, 2008.
52. J.M. Lagaron, and A. Lopez-Rubio. Nanotechnology for bioplastic: Opportunities challenges and strategies. *Trends in Food Science and Technology*. doi:10.1016/j.tifs.2011.01.007, 2011.
53. M.D. Sanchez-Garcia, and J.M. Lagaron. On the use of plant cellulose nanowhiskers to enhance the barrier properties of polylactic acid. *Cellulose* 17(5), 987–1004, 2010.
54. A. Travan, C. Pelillo, I. Donati, E. Marsich, M. Benincasa, T. Scarpa, S. Semeraro, G. Turco, R. Gennaro, and S. Paoletti. Non-cytotoxic silver nanoparticle-polysaccharide nanocomposites with antimicrobial activity. *Biomacromolecules* 10(6), 1429–1435, 2009.
55. Z.M. Huang, Y.Z. Zhang, M. Kotaki, and S. Ramakrishna. A review on polymer nanofibers by electrospinning and their applications in nanocomposites. *Composites Science and Technology*, 63(15), 2223–2253, 2003.
56. A. Lopez-Rubio, J.M. Lagaron, M. Ankerfors, T. Lindstrom, D. Nordqvist, A. Mattozzi, and M.S. Hedenqvist. Enhanced film forming and film properties of amylopectin using micro-fibrillated cellulose. *Carbohydrate Polymers* 68(4), 718–727, 2007.
57. M.D. Sanchez-Garcia, E. Gimenez, and J.M. Lagaron. Morphology and barrier properties of solvent cast composites of thermoplastic biopolymers and purified cellulose fibers. *Carbohydrate Polymers* 71(2), 235–244, 2008.
58. J.R. Capadona, K. Shanmuganathan, S. Trittschuh, S. Seidel, S.J. Rowan, and C. Weder. Polymer nanocomposites with nanowhiskers isolated from microcrystalline cellulose. *Biomacromolecules* 10(4), 712–716, 2009.

59. W. Helbert, C.Y. Cavaillé, and A. Dufresne. Thermoplastic nanocomposites filled with wheat straw cellulose whiskers. Part I: Processing and mechanical behaviour. *Polymer Composites* 17(4), 604–611, 1996.
60. O.J. Rojas, G.A. Montero, and Y. Habibi. Electrospun nanocomposites from polystyrene loaded with cellulose nanowhiskers. *Journal of Applied Polymer Science* 113(2), 927–935, 2009.
61. D. Dubief, E. Samain, and A. Dufresne. Polysaccharide microcrystals reinforced amorphous poly(b-hydroxyoctanoate) nanocomposite materials. *Macromolecules* 32(18), 5765–5771, 1999.
62. M.A. Hubbe, O.J. Rojas, L.A. Lucia, and M. Sain. Cellulosic nanocomposites: A review. *Bioresources* 3(3), 929–980, 2008.
63. G. Siaueira, J. Bras, and A. Dufresne. Cellulose whiskers versus microfibrils: Influence of the nature of the nanoparticle and its surface functionalization on the thermal and mechanical properties of nanocomposites. *Biomacromolecules* 10(2), 425–432, 2009.
64. A. Fernandez, S. Torres-Giner, and J.M. Lagaron. Novel route to stabilization of bioactive antioxidants by encapsulation in electrospun fibers of zein prolamine. *Food Hydrocolloids* 23(5), 1427–1432, 2009.
65. A. Lopez-Rubio, E. Sanchez, Y. Sanz, and J.M. Lagaron. Encapsulation of living bifidobacteria in ultrathin PVOH electrospun fibers. *Biomacromolecules* 10, 2823–2829, 2009.
66. T. Zimmermann, E. Pöhler, and T. Geiger. Cellulose fibrils for polymer reinforcement. *Advanced Engineering Materials* 6(9), 754–761, 2004.
67. A. Dufresne, and M.R. Vignon. Improvement of starch film performances using cellulose microfibrils. *Macromolecules* 31, 2693–2696, 1998.
68. A. Dufresne, D. Dupeyre, and M.R. Vignon. Cellulose microfibrils from potato tuber cells: Processing and characterization of starch–cellulose microfibril composites. *Journal of Applied Polymer Science* 76(14), 2080–2092, 2000.
69. S.A. Paralikar, J. Simonsen, and J. Lombardi. Poly(vinyl alcohol)/cellulose nanocrystal barrier membranes. *Journal of Membrane Science* 320(1-2), 248–258, 2008.
70. A.J. Svagan, M.S. Hedenqvist, and L. Berglund. Reduced water vapour sorption in cellulose nanocomposites with starch matrix. *Composites Science and Technology* 69(3-4), 500–506, 2009.
71. J.M. Lagaron, R. Catalá, and R. Gavara. Structural characteristics defining high barrier polymeric materials. *Materials Science and Technology* 20, 1–7, 2004.
72. K. Oksman, A.P. Mathew, D. Bondeson, and I. Kvien. Manufacturing process of cellulose whiskers/polylactic acid nanocomposites. *Composites Science and Technology* 66(15), 2776–2784, 2006.
73. L. Petersson, I. Kvien, and K. Oksman. Structure and thermal properties of poly(lactic acid)/cellulose whiskers nanocomposite materials. *Composites Science and Technology* 67, 2535–2544, 2007.
74. A. Alemdar, and M. Sain. Biocomposites from wheat straw nanofibers: Morphology, thermal and mechanical properties. *Composites Science and Technology* 68, 557–565, 2008.
75. M.N. Anglès, and A. Dufresne. Plasticized starch/tunicin whiskers nanocomposites. Structural analysis. *Macromolecules* 33, 8344–8353, 2000.

76. M.A.S. Azizi Samir, F. Alloin, and A. Dufresne. Review of recent research into cellulosic whiskers, their properties and their application in nanocomposite field. *Biomacromolecules* 6, 612–626, 2005.
77. A.P. Mathew, and A. Dufresne. Morphological investigation of nanocomposites from sorbitol plasticized starch and tunicin whiskers. *Biomacromolecules* 3(3), 609–617, 2002.
78. Q. Wu, M. Henriksson, X. Liu, and L.A. Berglund. A high strength nanocomposite based on microcrystalline cellulose and polyurethane. *Biomacromolecules* 8, 3687–3692, 2007.
79. E.L. Bradley, L. Castle, and Q. Chaudhry. Applications of nanomaterials in food packaging with a consideration of opportunities for developing countries. *Trends in Food Science & Technology*. In press, 2011.
80. P.N. Skandamis, and G.E. Nychas. Preservation of fresh meat with active and modified atmosphere packaging conditions. *International Journal of Food Microbiology* 79, 35–45, 2002.
81. C. Silvestre, D. Duraccio, and S. Cimmino. Food packaging based on polymer nanomaterials. *Progress in Polymer Science*. In press, 2011.
82. J.W. Rhim, and P.K.W. Ng. Natural biopolymer-based nanocomposite films for packaging applications. *Critical Reviews in Food Science and Nutrition* 47(4), 411–433, 2007.
83. I. Sondi, and B. Salopek-Sondi. Silver nanoparticles as antimicrobial agent: A case study on *E. coli* as a model for Gram-negative bacteria. *Journal of Colloid Interface Science* 275, 177–182, 2004.
84. Q. Li, S. Mahendra, D.Y. Lyon, L. Brunet, M.V. Liga, D. Li, and P.J.J. Alvarez. Antimicrobial nanomaterials for water disinfection and microbial control: Potential applications and implications. *Water Research* 42(18), 4591–4602, 2008.
85. J.R. Morones, J.L. Elechiguerra, A. Camacho, K. Holt, J.B. Kouri, J.T. Ramirez, and M.J. Yacaman. The bactericidal effect of silver nanoparticles. *Nanotechnology* 16(10), 2346–2353, 2005.
86. B. Kim, D. Kim, D. Cho, and S. Cho. Bactericidal effect of TiO_2 photocatalyst on selected food-borne pathogenic bacteria. *Chemosphere* 52(1), 277–281, 2003.
87. T.Y. Kim, Y.H. Lee, K.H. Park, S.J. Kim, and S.Y. Cho. A study of photocatalysis of TiO_2 coated onto chitosan beads and activated carbon. *Research on Chemical Intermediates* 31(4-6), 343–358, 2005.
88. J.M.C. Robertson, P.K.J. Robertson, and L.A. Lawton. A comparison of the effectiveness of TiO_2 photocatalysis and UVA photolysis for the destruction of three pathogenic micro-organisms. *Journal of Photochemistry and Photobiology A: Chemistry* 175(1), 51–56, 2005.
89. C. Chawengkijwanich, and Y. Hayata. Development of TiO_2 powder-coated food packaging film and its ability to inactivate *Escherichia coli* in vitro and in actual tests. *International Journal of Food Microbiology* 123(3), 288–292, 2008.
90. S. Gelover, L.A. Gómez, K. Reyes, and M.T. Leal. A practical demonstration of water disinfection using TiO_2 films and sunlight. *Water Research* 40, 3274–3280, 2006.
91. K. Page, R.G. Palgrave, I.P. Parkin, M. Wilson, S.L.P. Savin, and A.V. Chadwick. Titania and silver–titania composite films on glass-potent antimicrobial coatings. *Journal of Materials Chemistry* 17(1), 95–104, 2007.

92. M.P. Reddy, A. Venugopal, and M. Subrahmanyam. Hydroxyapatite-supported Ag-TiO_2 as *Escherichia coli* disinfection photocatalyst. *Water Research* 41, 379–386, 2007.
93. Q. Cheng, C. Li, V. Pavlinek, P. Saha, and H. Wang. Surface-modified antibacterial TiO_2 /Ag^+ nanoparticles: Preparation and properties. *Applied Surface Science* 252, 4154–4160, 2006.
94. L. Xiao-e, A.N.M. Green, S.A. Haque, A. Mills, and J.R. Durrant. Light-driven oxygen scavenging by titania/polymer nanocomposite films. *Journal of Photochemistry and Photobiology A: Chemistry* 162, 253–259, 2004.
95. A. Mills, G. Doyle, A.M. Peiro, and J. Durrant. Demonstration of a novel, flexible, photocatalytic oxygen-scavenging polymer film. *Journal of Photochemistry and Photobiology A: Chemistry* 177, 328–331, 2006.
96. S. Kang, M. Pinault, L.D. Pfefferle, and M. Elimelech. Single-walled carbon nanotubes exhibit strong antimicrobial activity. *Langmuir* 23, 8670–8673, 2007.
97. N.A. Monteiro-Riviere, R.J. Nemanich, A.O. Inman, Y.Y. Wang, and J.E. Riviere. Multi-walled carbon nanotube interactions with human epidermal keratinocytes. *Toxicology Letters* 155(13), 377–384, 2005.
98. A. Shvedova, V. Castranova, E. Kisin, D. Schwegler-Berry, A. Murray, V. Gandelsman, A. Maynard, and P. Baron. Exposure to carbon nanotube material: Assessment of nanotube cytotoxicity using human keratinocyte cells. *Journal of Toxicology and Environmental Health, Part A* 66(20), 1909–1926, 2003.
99. D.B. Warheit, B.R. Laurence, K.L. Reed, D.H. Roach, G.A.M. Reynolds, and T.R. Webb. Comparative pulmonary toxicity assessment of single-wall carbon nanotubes in rats. *Toxicological Sciences* 77, 117–125, 2004.
100. L.F. Qi, Z.R. Xu, X. Jiang, C. Hu, and X. Zou. Preparation and antibacterial activity of chitosan nanoparticles. *Carbohydrate Research* 339, 2693–2700, 2004.
101. G.L. Robertson, ed. *Food packaging – Principles and practice*. Second edition, CRC Press, Boca Raton, FL, USA, 2006.
102. K. Huff. Active and Intelligent packaging: Innovations for the future. Department of Food Science & Technology. Virginia Polytechnic Institute and State University, Blacksburg, Va, pp. 1–13, 2008.
103. N. de Kruijf, R. Rijk, and H.A. Jongbloed. Evaluating safety, effectiveness, economic-environmental impact and consumer acceptance of active and intelligent packaging. www.packaginglaw.com, 2002.
104. H. Bouwmeester, S. Dekkers, M.Y. Noordam, W.I. Hagens, A.S. Bulder, C. de Heer, S.E. ten Voorde, S.W. Wijnhoven, H.J. Marvin, and A.J. Sips. Review of health safety aspects of nanotechnologies in food production. *Regulatory Toxicology and Pharmacology* 53(1), 52–62, 2009.
105. F. Liao, C. Chen, and V. Subramanian. Organic TFTs as gas sensors for electronic nose applications. *Sensors and Actuators B: Chemical* 107(2), 849–855, 2005.
106. K. Nachay. Analyzing nanotechnology. *Food Technology* 61(1), 34–36, 2007.
107. A. Šetkus. Heterogeneous reaction rate based description of the response kinetics in metal oxide gas sensors. *Sensors and Actuators B* 87, 346–357, 2002.
108. K. Arshak, C. Adley, E. Moore, C. Cunniffe, M. Campion, and J. Harris. Characterisation of polymer nanocomposite sensors for quantification of bacterial cultures. *Sensors and Actuators B* 126, 226–231, 2007.

4

Frozen Food and Technology

Elisabete M.C. Alexandre, Teresa R.S. Brandão and Cristina L.M. Silva

Center of Biotechnology and Fine Chemistry, Superior School of Biotechnology, Catholic University of Portugal, Porto, Portugal

Abstract

Freezing has been successfully implemented worldwide for long-term preservation of an endless variety of food products. The low temperatures achieved in freezing processes change the physical state of water and, consequently, water becomes unavailable to support deteriorative processes. Freezing, when conveniently applied, may preserve some of the original attributes of a food, but overall quality is inevitably affected. Ice crystallization that occurs during freezing processes, and along frozen storage, may cause important physic and/or chemical changes in food products. So, it is important that products have high quality raw characteristics before the freezing stage. Freezing may reduce microbial loads and microbial activity, yet it cannot assure the safety of post-thawed products. To inactivate undesirable microorganisms and enzymes responsible for quality decay, adequate treatments are often applied before the freezing processes of foods.

The success of the freezing operation depends mainly on the composition, physical properties and shape of product to be frozen, the freezing method and conditions applied, the type of equipment used and packaging materials selected.

This chapter provides an overview of treatments pre-applied in freezing processes of meat, fish, fruits and vegetables products, freezing methods and equipment industrially used, and innovations in freezing processes. Main impacts of frozen technology on food properties are also highlighted.

Visakh P. M., Sabu Thomas, Laura B. Iturriaga, and Pablo Daniel Ribotta (eds.) Advances in Food Science and Technology, (123–150) © 2013 Scrivener Publishing LLC

Keywords: Frozen foods, pre-freezing treatments, freezing methods, freezing equipment, food quality, frozen food properties

4.1 Introduction

Freezing is the unit operation in which the temperature of a substance is reduced below its freezing point. Changes in the structure of the product occur due to the ice crystals formation when energy is removed. Freezing is one of the oldest and most frequently used processes for long-term food preservation. The use of ice and snow to cool and preserve food goes back to the Paleolithic and Neolithic periods. The use of mountain snows, pond and lake ice to form freezing baths, and ice manufacture by evaporative and radiative cooling of water on cloudless clear nights was a common practice.

Nowadays, the freezing process is strongly implemented worldwide, being one of the most common preservation methods used for all kinds of commercialized foods: fruits (whole, puréed or as juice concentrates) and vegetables; fish fillets and seafood, including prepared dishes; meats and meat products; baked goods (such as bread, cakes, pizzas); desserts and an endless number of precooked dishes [1].

Food preservation by freezing occurs through different mechanisms. When temperature is lowered below 0°C, there is a reduction in the microbial loads and microbial activity; therefore, deterioration rates of foods decrease. Freezing temperatures affects biological materials in various ways, depending on their chemical composition, microstructure and physical properties. The low temperatures also have a strong impact in enzymatic activity and oxidative reactions that help avoid a products deterioration. In addition, with ice crystal formation, less water will be available to support deteriorative reactions and microbial viability [2, 3].

In general, frozen foods are synonymous with high quality products and only small changes of quality attributes occur when correct freezing and storage procedures are followed. The characteristics of final frozen products are influenced by processing factors such as the freezing method, the freezing rate, the final temperature and frozen storage conditions. Quality attributes such as texture, color, flavor and nutritional content are mainly related to the way ice crystals are formed. Usually, when a plant or animal tissue is cooled, the ice crystals are initially formed at the product's surface and their growth strongly depends on the freezing rate. Some products require fast freezing rates (short freezing times) to assure the formation of many but small ice crystals within the product structure, avoiding cells shrinkage and reducing to minimal the degree of freeze damage. In this case, small texture changes and small loss of nutrients will be verified through drip on thawing. Additionally, a rapid freezing followed by a slow thawing inactivates more microorganisms. Other products, due to their geometric configurations and sizes, do not allow a fast freezing. If the product is cooled slowly (high freezing time), large ice crystals will be formed, causing maximum disruption of the tissues' structure. Besides the freezing rates, storage temperatures also play an important role in the frozen food quality. Fluctuations in the storage temperature may be harmful to the product's quality [2, 4–6].

4.2 Treatments: Pre-freezing

One should bear in mind that a freezing process only preserves the original attributes of a food and it will never improve quality. Therefore, it is crucial that products have high quality standards before the freezing stage. Food freshness, the relevance of variety for freezing, the soil composition, the dietary elements of animals, and the harvesting or slaughtering procedures have a huge impact on the final food quality. Although freezing reduces microorganisms loads, it is not enough to assure the safety of post-thaw products [7]. Thus, preparatory or pre-freezing treatments are usually required to inactivate undesirable microorganisms or to slow down deterioration reactions. These treatments for fruits and vegetables, and for fish and meat products are presented below.

4.2.1 Fruits and Vegetables

The removal of defective produce and inspecting, grading, cleaning, sorting, and in some cases, peeling, shelling, trimming, chopping and slicing are the most common preparatory treatments applied to fruits and vegetables [8–10]. Those procedures remove foreign products, minimize product variability and decrease microbial contamination. However, they may eliminate the protective barrier provided by cellular compartments and allow oxygen access, leading to leach of nutrients, browning, desiccation and interaction of enzymes that can cause loss of nutrients and texture as well as color and flavor changes [11, 12]. The deteriorative enzymes and microorganisms should be inactivated before freezing, thus allowing tissues stabilization and avoiding posterior quality degradation.

Blanching is a thermal treatment in which the products are heated by a brief immersion in hot water or by hot steam. Its major effect is related to enzymatic inactivation but there are other important benefits. It destroys vegetative cells of microorganisms at the food surface, removes any remaining insecticide residues, improves the color of green vegetables, and eliminates off-flavors produced by gases and other volatile substances that may have been formed during the period between harvesting and processing [13, 14]. However, blanching also causes cell membranes disruption, destroys cell turgor and removes intercellular air, filling these spaces with water. As a consequence, water crystallization can occur through the entire matrix of food, affecting texture, color, flavor, and nutritional quality of foods. Sometimes, due to the cellular turgor reduction, blanching and freezing may not be acceptable, mainly for products that are not cooked before consumption [7]. To reduce the negative effects of blanching, less severe heat treatments may be applied. Low temperatures and long-time treatments avoid excessive softness, improving the tissues firmness of frozen fruits and vegetables.

In fruits with sensitive tissues or/and that grow near or just above the soil, such as strawberries, an effective water washing must be carried out. Usually, fruits with low pH are protected from the microbial growth and blanching is not necessary [15].

Washing/sinking the products *in solutions of several compounds* may be required for maximum quality retention. Antioxidant solutions, such as ascorbic or citric acid or sulphur dioxide can be used to minimize the risk of browning; sugar solutions may also influence chlorophyll stability during storage; salt solutions remove intracellular air of tissues; and hydrogen peroxide and chlorine-based solutions contribute to microbial inactivation [5].

Other processes based on partial air drying, osmotic dehydration and immersion chilling and freezing in concentrated aqueous solutions are examples of alternatives to the commonly used treatments applied before freezing of fruits and vegetables.

Partial dehydration of foods is usually attained by air drying. The water removal is limited to 50–60% of the original content and the final products present water activity higher than 0.96. One of the major advantages of this technique is related to lower energy consumption of the freezing process, since the amount of water to be frozen is reduced. The costs with transport, storage and packaging also decrease. Products with high quality and stability (color and flavor) are obtained; the thawing process is also improved, i.e., less drip loss occurs [5, 16].

Osmotic dehydration consists in placing the food (whole or in pieces) in solutions of high sugar or salt concentration. The water inside the food moves to the concentrated solution and, simultaneously, the solute from the concentrated solution is transferred into the food. Osmotic concentration of fruits and vegetables prior to freezing improves their quality in terms of color, texture and flavor and the combination of this treatment with partial air drying requires less energy consumption than air drying alone [7, 17].

Immersion chilling and freezing in concentrated aqueous solutions (ICFCAS) is quite similar to osmotic dehydration. The main difference is related to the temperatures of the processes: ICFCAS occurs at temperatures lower (-20 to 0°C) than the ones of osmotic dehydration (30 to 80°C). The solute impregnation also improves color, flavor and nutritional content of foods, reducing the damage related with freezing and storage [16].

4.2.2 Fish Products

There are several factors that influence the quality of frozen fish. At the time of capture, the fish should be calm; if necessary, they should be anaesthetized to reduce strain and simplify handling and killing. Bleeding should take place immediately after killing, otherwise visible blood vessels will appear in the fish muscle. A careful and gentle handling will avoid physical damage and prevents enzymatic and bacterial activities. After being caught, the fish should be frozen as rapidly as possible, preferably before onset of rigor mortis. All intermediate storages will result in significant loss of fish quality. If rapid freezing is impossible, the fish should be chilled to temperatures below 0°C. Rapid chilling will slow down the enzymatic and microbial activities which occur post-mortem. However, this intermediate chill step (before freezing) will reduce the shelf life of the frozen product [18–21].

Fish muscle is very susceptible to freeze denaturation. Cryoprotectants can be added to protect the fish myofibrillar proteins. Sugars, amino acids, polyols, methyl amines, carbohydrates, some proteins and inorganic salts, such as potassium phosphates and ammonium sulfate, are examples of cryoprotectant compounds [7, 18]. Antifreeze proteins are specific cryoprotectants identified in a variety of fish species and cold tolerant insects and plants that may be used to improve the quality (flavor and texture) of frozen products. Antifreeze proteins lower the freezing temperature, inhibit ice crystal growth, including recrystallization, and affect crystal morphology. This method is a unique technique that directly improves the fish freezing process [5, 7].

Irradiation treatments, combined with freezing, have also been proposed as a means of retarding spoilage. However, high doses of irradiation can be adverse to product quality, due to changes in the chemical composition and alterations in the flavor of fish and seafood [7].

4.2.3 Meat Products

Animal feeding and the way that animals are handled and transported before slaughter affect meat quality and frozen storage life. Diets rich in highly unsaturated fatty acids or highly unsaturated vegetable oils reduce the frozen meat quality. Animal stress and exhaustion should be avoided since meat become unattractive for consumers: pale soft and exudative meat (in pigs) or dry, firm and dark meat (in beef and lamb), with alterations in flavor occur. Usually, meat is not frozen until *rigor mortis* is complete and an intermediate step of chilling should be applied.

Several techniques can be applied to allow meats to be frozen sooner after slaughter, producing a more stable frozen product. A rapid chilling reduces drip loss; however, if applied before rigor is attained, it adversely affects meat texture. The length of chilled storage prior to freezing affects the rate of deterioration during frozen storage. Shorter intervals between slaughter and freezing should be used. After slaughter, if carcasses are submitted to high voltage electric stimulation, the rigor will be faster thus allowing a rapid chilling without much of the toughening effect [22–25].

Cooking of meat can result in longer shelf life of the products. This can be explained by enzymatic and microbial inactivation, similar to blanching of vegetables, prior to freezing. However, cooking processes such as frying, which increase the fat content of the meat product, can lead to increased off-flavors during storage. Salt increases the rate of processes that lead to rancidity, which also reduces the quality of frozen stored foods.

Since many of the reactions leading to rancidity are oxidative, the addition of antioxidants can improve storage. Many herbs and spicy seasonings contain substances which help control rancidity in meats.

As in fish, cryoprotectant compounds can be used to promote the shelf life of frozen meat. It has been shown that the incorporation of antifreeze proteins is effective in controlling ice crystal size, reducing drip loss and retaining textural quality of frozen meats [5, 22–24].

For poultry meat, there is no evidence that chilling methods have influence on storage life. In terms of preservation, there are many antimicrobial compounds (salt, sodium nitrite), acidulants (sodium acetate, sodium dicetate and lactate) and antioxidants (butylated hydroxyanisole and butylated hydroxytoluene) that may be incorporated into poultry products to increase shelf life and prevent spoilage [26]. The use of antifreeze proteins in poultry muscles is more problematic, due to difficulties in finding an expedient route of perfusing the antifreeze proteins without causing disruption/damage of muscles structure [5].

4.3 Freezing Process

The freezing process involves four main stages (Figure 4.1): (i) pre-freezing stage –sensible heat is removed from the product, being the temperature reduced to the freezing point; (ii) super-cooling–temperature falls

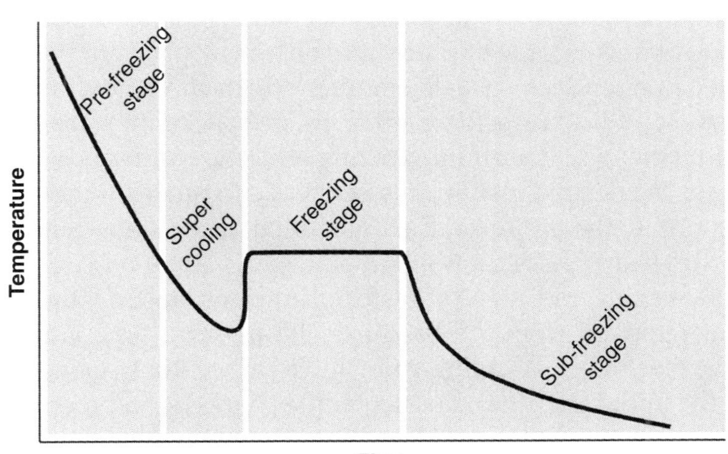

Figure 4.1 Typical cooling curve of a freezing process.

below the freezing point, which is not always observed; (iii) freezing – latent heat is removed and water is transformed into ice (i.e., crystallization) in all product; (iv) sub-freezing – the food temperature is lowered to the storage temperature.

The water must be cooled to temperatures substantially below the freezing point before ice begins to form. The nucleation should occur before ice crystals begin to grow. The nucleation process consists of the formation of a minimum crystal with a critical radius, i.e., the very fine particles formed, which are in equilibrium with the surrounding water and will be the site for further crystal expansion and growth. From a physical point of view, foods may be considered as dilute aqueous solutions with a freezing point below 0°C.

Two types of ice nucleation can occur: (i) homogeneous nucleation – occurs only in homogeneous particle-free liquids and happens due to random orientation and combination of water molecules, and (ii) heterogeneous nucleation – occurs in solid foods where the cells surfaces act as nucleation sites (the nucleus formations occurs around suspended particles or on the cell wall). The number of nucleation sites and the growth of ice crystal are strongly dependent on the heat transfer rate. High heat removal rates produce small and numerous ice crystals. Different foods, submitted to similar freezing rates and even with similar dimensions, have ice crystals with different sizes. This can be explained by different water availability of the foods. For the same foods, if different pre-freezing treatments are applied, the ice crystal sizes may also differ [1, 27, 28].

There are many factors that will determine the success of the freezing operation. Freezing methods and type of equipment used, composition and shape of product to be frozen, packaging materials, freezing rates and ice crystallization, products moisture content, specific heat, and heat transfer coefficients and packaging, are examples of factors that will determine freezing efficiency and product quality. To attain the desired results, it is necessary to relate all these factors. For example, the entire product has to be at the same temperature (superficies and mass center). However, this situation is dependent on the freezing rate, heat transfer coefficient, and on the amount of heat removed from the product. The freezing time is related to the freezing rate, packaging prior to freezing, the freezing method used, the initial and final product temperatures, food product shape, specific heat, thickness and food components. If the product initial temperature is just above the freezing point, a more controlled crystallization will occur when compared with products initially at room temperature and, consequently, a better product quality will be attained. The amount and rate of heat removal is dependent on the food chemical composition: more sugars, salt and/or alcohol involves longer freezing times and/or lower freezing temperatures. The wide variety of food products and their characteristics are important keys in the design and conception of freezing systems. No single freezing system can satisfy all freezing needs [7, 29]. However, several mathematical models have been developed to correlate the most important parameters of freezing processes [30, 31].

4.4 Freezing Methods and Equipment

A whole range of methods and equipment for freezing foods industrially is available. The most common ones are: blast freezers (batch and continuous), belt (spiral) freezers, cooled surface freezers, immersion freezers (batch and continuous), and cryogenic freezers.

4.4.1 Freezing by Contact with Cold Air

Freezing by contact with cold air is the most widely used method of freezing food products. Freezing foods by natural convection is not used industrially due to the low freezing rates (that results in high freezing times) occurring under such conditions. If heat is removed from product by forced convection (fans are used to increase the cold air speed), the efficiency of the process increases. The air temperature is more uniform and the air velocity can be controlled to promote heat transfer at the products surface, however the freezing time is always dependent on product characteristics/shapes. In thin products, with large exposure surfaces, the freezing time can be directly reduced by increasing cold air velocity. In thick products, with lower exposure surfaces, the freezing time will be limited essentially by the rate of heat conduction through product thickness [32]. The air temperature of a typical mechanical refrigeration freezer is usually between –32°C and –40°C (Miller and Butcher 2000; Rahman and Velez-Ruiz 2007).

4.4.1.1 Batch Air Blast Freezers

Air blast freezing is one of the oldest and most commonly used methods in the food industry. It is used to freeze a great variety of irregular shaped foods/products, such as fish, meat, fruits and vegetables, prepared meals, as well as packaged products.

Its major drawback is related to the cold air distribution. Also, as the freezing time is reduced with the increase of the air velocity, it is necessary to balance the costs associated to the decrease of freezing time and the increase of power related to the operation of fans.

Batch air blast freezers are related to the simplest technology that uses forced air convection. It consists of an insulated cabinet containing fans that force air flow through refrigerant evaporator coils and through the products to be frozen (Figure 4.2). Foods frozen in batch air blast freezers are usually stacked in racks or hung (carcasses). It is important to ensure that the cold air passes over the surface of each individual food piece [32].

In the situation of packaged foods, an additional physical barrier exists and long freezing times are required. The inability to circulate air over the product's surface and the temperature gradients between product and air will increase the freezing time [2]. Batch air blast freezers can also be considered as refrigerated rooms for storing food products under freezing conditions.

4.4.1.2 *Continuous Air Blast Freezers*

In continuous equipment, trays with food are stacked on trolleys or the food is moved through a freezing tunnel by conveyor belts. These freezing systems use a diversity of conveying arrangements.

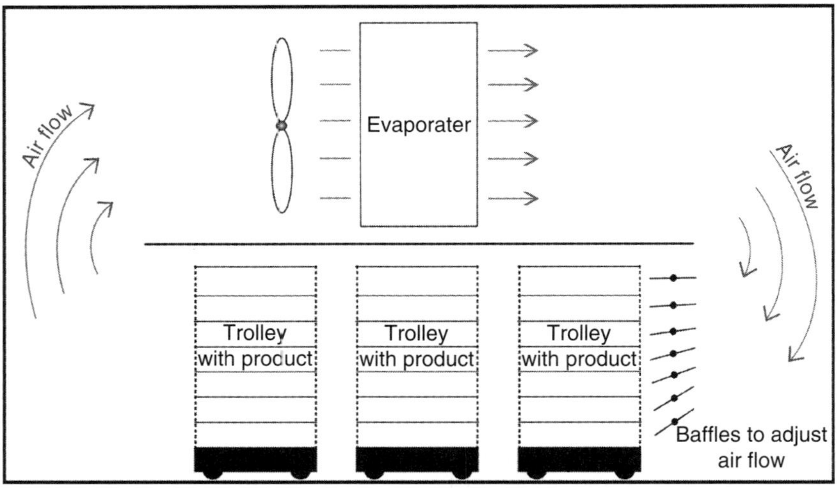

Figure 4.2 Schematic illustration of a batch air blast freezer.

The equipment available varies from a simple one pass belt systems, to more elaborate multipass, spiral belt or variable retention time systems [32]. The principle of a belt freezer is the same as that of a blast freezer, i.e., the product is frozen by cold air.

Spiral belt freezers (Figure 4.3) are widely used in the food industry to freeze chicken, fish, meat, bagels, prepared and processed foods on open trays or packages. The main convenience of this type of freezer is related to the reduced floor space required for installation of the equipment.

In tunnel freezers, the food products are placed in trays or racks that move continuously on conveyors (Figure 4.4). A vast variety of

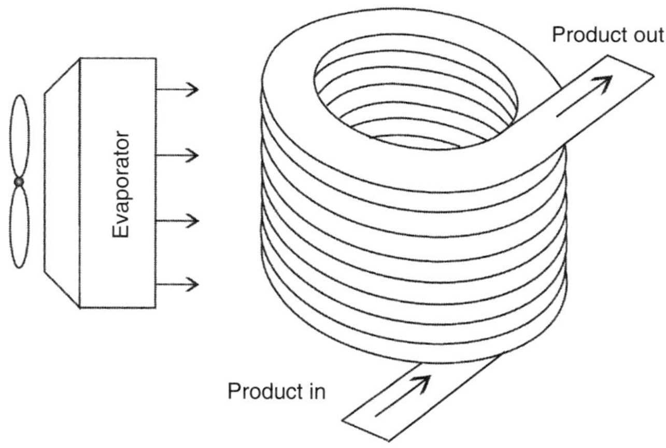

Figure 4.3 Schematic illustration of a spiral belt freezer.

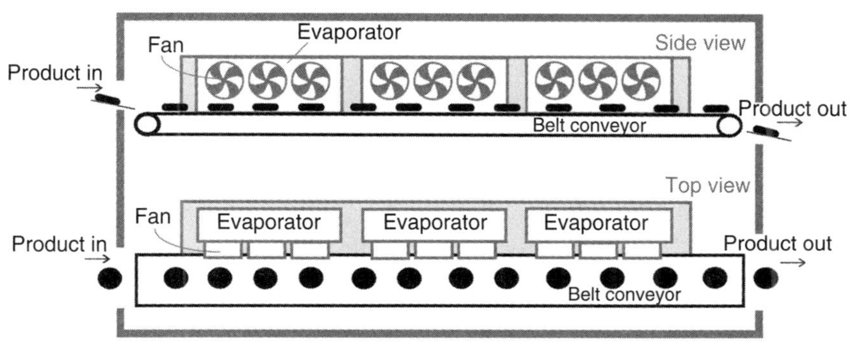

Figure 4.4 Schematic illustration of a tunnel freezer.

foods, with different sizes and geometries, packed or non-packed, can be frozen in this equipment. However, freezing operating conditions should be designed according to the product [33].

In recent years, the use of impingent technology in freezing processes has received special attention. Those freezers are usually continuous and are equipped with a jet system that impinges cold air directly onto the food surface. Generally, the air jets are applied perpendicularly to the product surface, which breaks the insulation air layer boundary, thereby increasing heat transfer coefficients and allowing a fast freezing [32, 34]. However, the reduction in freezing times is only relevant in thin food products [32].

The air impingement technique is also a versatile method that can be efficiently applied to freeze a vast variety of foods and food products, however, without small surface particles or toppings.

4.4.1.3 Fluidized Bed Freezers

The system consists of a perforated bed through which cold air, at high velocities, is blown vertically upward by the action of powerful fans (Figure 4.5). Fluidized bed freezers are appropriated for small food items (smaller than 15 mm), with uniform shape and size, such as peas, diced carrots and potatoes, corns kernels, and berry fruits [35]. The shape and size of the food pieces determine the air velocity for fluidization. In these freezers, food surfaces are in extended contact with cold air so food particles are frozen simultaneously and uniformly. When compared with air blast freezers, this process results in faster freezing and less dehydration of the products [1]. A high degree of fluidization will improve the heat

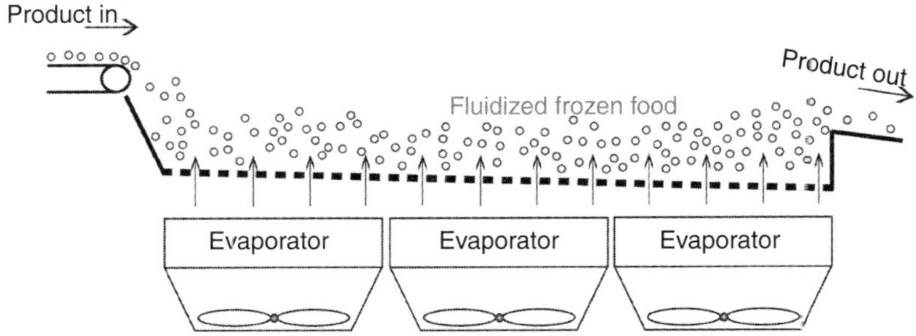

Figure 4.5 Schematic illustration of a fluidized bed freezer.

transfer. Some equipment produces an ice glaze on food surfaces, which is particularly useful for freezing products that have a tendency to clump together [1, 29].

4.4.2 Freezing by Contact with Cold Liquid

The immersion freezer consists of a tank with a cooled freezing media, such as glycol, glycerol, sodium chloride, calcium chloride, and mixtures of salt and sugar. The product is immersed in the solution while being conveyed through the freezer (Figure 4.6). This results in a rapid way of freezing, since liquids have higher heat conducting properties than air. The liquid can also be sprayed over the food, which makes heat transfer more efficient. The freezing solutions should be safe, without taste, odor and color.

In order to avoid product contact with the liquid refrigerant, flexible membranes can be used. This is important since solute of the solutions may be transferred to products.

4.4.3 Freezing by Contact with Cold Surfaces

In these freezing systems, the products are positioned between two metallic cold plates filled with evaporating refrigerant. Pressure is usually applied in plates to ensure a good contact between food products and cold surfaces. Plate freezers are composed of a stack of hollow plates that can be horizontal (Figure 4.7) or vertical, and they can operate in batch, semi-continuous or continuous conditions. Vertical plate freezers are generally used for bare product while horizontal freezers are mainly used for packaged or bare products. This type of equipment is only suitable for regular-shaped

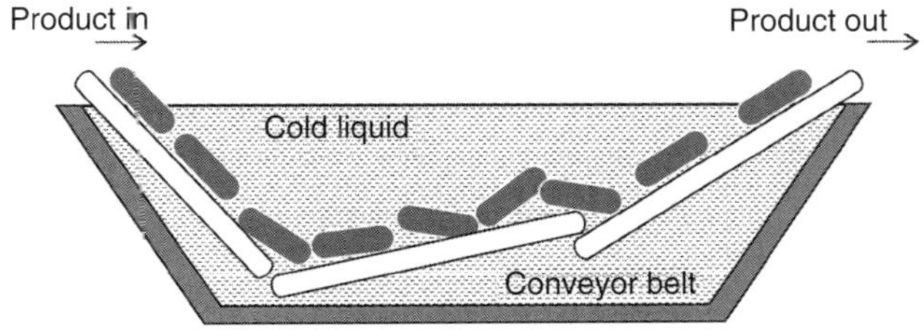

Figure 4.6 Schematic illustration of a batch liquid immersion freezer.

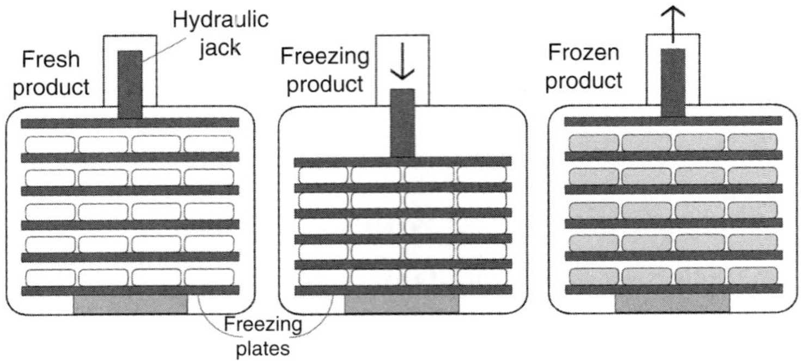

Figure 4.7 Schematic illustration of a horizontal plate freezer.

products or blocks, flat and relative thin foods such as filleted fish and fish fingers, or beef burgers [1].

Freezing by contact with cold air or liquid requires the step of cooling the freezing media. Freezing in contact with cold surfaces avoids this step and, if a good contact between plates and food products is achieved, it allows high heat transfer rates [32, 36].

4.4.4 Cryogenic Freezing

In cryogenic freezing the food is in direct contact with the refrigerant, through three different ways: (i) the cryogenic liquid is directly sprayed on the food in a tunnel freezer, (ii) the cryogenic liquid is vaporized and blown over the food in a spiral freezer or batch freezer, or (iii) the food product is immersed in cryogenic liquid in an immersion freezer. However, the most common method used is the direct spaying of cryogenic solutions over the product, while it is conveyed through an insulated tunnel [32].

In cryogenic freezing, food is exposed to an atmosphere below -60°C due to the phase change of the cryogenic liquids themselves [7]. The refrigerants used in the food industry are solid or liquid forms of carbon dioxide (boiling point of –78.5°C) and liquid nitrogen (boiling point of –196°C), which are odorless, colorless and chemically stable. The refrigerant evaporates or sublimes, removing heat from the product and causing a rapid freezing.

This process is very efficient due to the low freezing temperatures and high heat transfer rates. As a consequence, the ice crystals formed are small, which has a reduced impact in cell damage; flavor

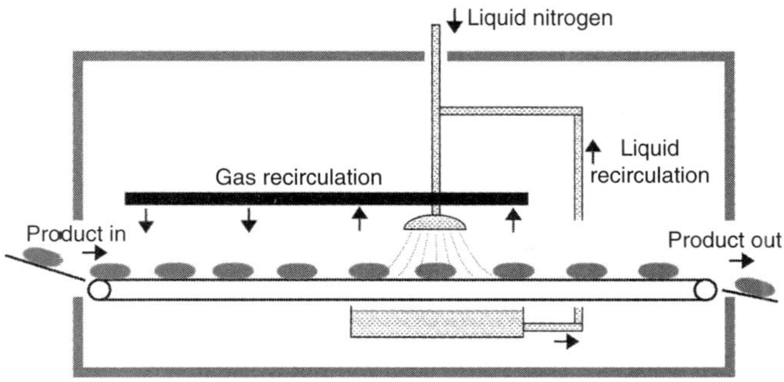

Figure 4.8 Schematic illustration of a cryogenic freezer.

and moisture losses are minimal; the maintenance equipment costs are low [29, 37].

Limitations of cryogenic freezing are mainly related to the high cost of the cryogenic liquid/solid refrigerants and with quality losses related to product cracking. This method is mainly used for high value products that must be rapidly frozen [29, 37].

4.4.5 Combination of Freezing Methods

Freezing methods may be combined in order to obtain high quality products with reduced freezing times and energy consumption [29].

Cryogenic freezing combined with air contact freezing through impingent technology, increases freezing rates whilst reducing process costs (Figure 4.9). A cold hard crust is formed on products by cryogenic freezing, after which the product is conveyed through a conventional mechanical freezer [7, 29, 36]. The heat transfer is typically three to five times higher than that obtained with conventional tunnels of axial flow fans [5, 22].

The combination of spraying and immersion cryogenic processes with impingement technology will allow lower temperatures and freezing times, uniformity of frozen products and higher production rates [29].

4.4.6 Innovations in Freezing Processes

Innovative freezing processes have been developed mainly with the goal of obtaining increased freezing rates, higher product quality

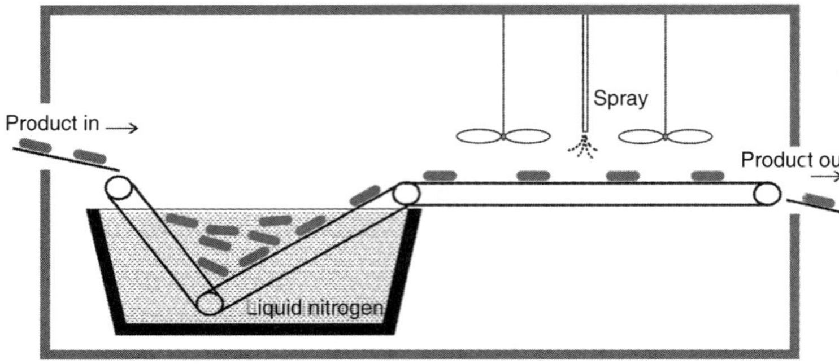

Figure 4.9 Schematic illustration of combined freezing processes.

and process cost reductions [38]. Examples of some new techniques are: (i) high pressure freezing, which leads to instantaneous and homogeneous formation of ice throughout the whole food product and thus improved quality; (ii) impingement air freezing, which promotes very rapid freezing processes without the high costs associated with cryogenic methods; (iii) the addition of antifreeze proteins, which lower the freezing temperature and slow down the recrystallization during frozen storage; (iv) the addition of bacterial ice nucleators, which increases the nucleation temperature, may reduce freezing time and improves the product quality and the dehydrofreezing. This reduces tissue damages by decreasing the water content of the products [13, 28]. Zheng *et al.* [39] points out that power ultrasound combined with freezing processes generates various effects upon the medium where it transmits that can be beneficial. For example, cavitation may lead to the production of gas bubbles that promote ice nucleation, and the occurrence of microstreaming accelerates heat and mass transfer processes. Thus, ultrasound technology can shorten the freezing process, and lead to better quality frozen products.

Several researchers have tested these and other novel methods, obtaining promising results. Li *et al.* [40] and Sun *et al.* [41] applied power ultrasounds during immersion freezing of potatoes and verified that, when ultrasound was applied to the phase change period, the freezing rate increased significantly. Jalté *et al.* [42] studied the effects of pulsed electric fields pretreatment on the freezing, freeze-drying and rehydration behavior of potatoes, and concluded that the quality and rehydration of the samples improved. LeBail *et al.* [43] reviewed the application of high pressure in freezing and thawing of foods. Alizadeh *et al.* [44] froze salmon fillets by pressure shift freezing and verified that ice crystals were smaller and more regular than the ones obtained with conventional freezing methods. Bunger *et al.* [45] verified that the combination of osmotic dehydration and freezing provided good results related to quality and acceptance of apples. Fagan *et al.* [46] combined modified atmosphere packaging with freeze chilling to extend the shelf life of raw whiting, mackerel and salmon fillets. The authors mentioned logistic benefits during frozen storage, product distribution and retailing.

4.4.7 Food Products and Freezing Methods

Small or thin food products, where heat conduction through the food itself does not have influence on the freezing velocity, are usually frozen in blast, tunnel and spiral freezers. If they are susceptible to high dehydration losses, a cryogenic tunnel or a blast freezer are recommended, previously optimized for quick freezing [37].

High value, wet, sticky, or delicate products (such as strawberries or shrimps) should be frozen in cryogenic or fluidised-bed freezers, where high gas velocities form a solid ice "crust" that results in a non-clumped product that can be handled without severe damage. These rapid freezing processes maximize the quality of many food products, but the costs are higher than the ones of blast or tunnel freezers. The internal part of the foods may be frozen at different rates using different types of freezers. Vertical or horizontal plate freezers can be used to freeze wet products in bulk, producing uniform blocks that are easy to handle [32, 37].

Prepackaged foods are frequently frozen in continuous blast and tunnel freezers. Alternatively, a stationary blast freezer or a horizontal plate freezer (operating in batch conditions) can also be used. Some cryogenic tunnels are also adapted to this type of food. For big prepackaged foods, where speed of freezing is limited by internal heat transfer (such as turkeys or chickens), a brine immersion freezer is the most adequate choice [37].

As mentioned before, slaughtered animals are not frozen until rigor is complete. Thus, air-blast freezing is a practical option to process carcasses, because freezing is not too rapid to allow muscle to be transformed into meat, and some surface evaporation occurs but not in excess [32].

In Table 4.1, food products were divided into categories and some of the most commonly applied freezing methods are presented.

Table 4.1 Freezing methods commonly applied to meat, fish, fruits and vegetables products [32].

Food product		**Freezing method**					
		Air blast	**Fluidized bed**	**Impingement**	**Liquid immersion**	**Plate**	**Cryogenic**
Meat	carcasses	x					
	cartons	x				x	
	large individually wrapped cuts	x			x		
	small or diced pieces				x		x
	cured or processed products	x			x		x
	hamburger patties	x		x		x	x
Poultry	whole or pieces	x			x	package food	x
	processed or breaded products	x		x		package food	x

Food product		**Freezing method**					
		Air blast	**Fluidized bed**	**Impingement**	**Liquid immersion**	**Plate**	**Cryogenic**
Fish	whole or eviscerated	x			x	x	x
	fillets or small diced pieces	x		x		x	x
	minced blocks					x	
	processed or breaded products	x		x		package food	x
Shellfish		x				package food	x
Prawns and shrimp		x		x			x
Fruits	small size (whole)	x	x			package food	x
	large size (sliced)	x				package food	
	purée or pulp	x				x	
Vegetables	small size	x	x			package food	x
	medium size	x				package food	
	leafy	x				package food	

4.5 Effect of Freezing and Frozen Storage on Food Properties

The ice crystallization that occurs during freezing processes, and along frozen storage, causes the major important physic and chemical modifications which decrease food quality.

4.5.1 Physical Changes

The main physical changes of foods verified during freezing processes are related to the risk of freeze cracking, moisture migration, recrystallization of ice crystals and drip loss during thawing.

4.5.1.1 Freeze Cracking

The small ice crystals formed with high freezing rates obtained with cryogenic freezers, allow preservation of food structure. However, products may crack under those conditions. This may happen when the internal stress of unfrozen food is higher than the frozen material strength at food surface. To avoid cracking, a previous cooling step should be applied prior to freezing. The reduction of the temperature gradients between the product and the freezing medium or a pre-cooling step decrease significantly the risk of freeze cracking [47, 48].

4.5.1.2 Moisture Migration

During freezing processes, when cell contents are super cooled, moisture movements may occur by an osmotic mechanism. The occurrence of temperature fluctuations results in vapor pressure differences, which are responsible for moisture migration. If frozen products are stored without an adequate moisture barrier, the ice on the food surface sublimes, since ice water pressure is higher than the environment vapor pressure. An opaque dehydrated surface is formed (microscopic cavities previously occupied by ice crystals) with an unsightly white color. This leads to freezer burn [1, 7, 47].

If temperature increases, water moves from the product; ice sublimes and water diffuses through the packaging film. If temperature decreases, the ice on the wrap tends to diffuse back to the food surface, however, the water reabsorption to the original location is very improbable. To reduce moisture migration, temperature fluctuations and internal temperature gradients should be minimized and internal barriers within the product and within the packaging should be included [47].

4.5.1.3 *Recrystallization*

Modifications in the size, shape or orientation of the ice crystals are known as "recrystallization" and usually lead to quality losses in some products. Recrystallization reduces the advantages of fast freezing leading to physico-chemical changes of food products. This process may happen in three different ways: (i) changes in surface shape or internal structure (isomass recrystallization); (ii) linkage of two adjacent ice crystals to form a large crystal (accretive recrystallization), and (iii) increase of the average size of the crystal (migratory recrystallization). Migratory recrystallization is the most important and it is mainly related to temperature fluctuations during storage. If temperature increases, the product's surface warms slightly, the ice crystals melt, moisture moves to regions of lower vapor pressure and some areas will be dehydrated. When temperature decreases, water vapor does not form new nuclei points and links to the existing ice crystals. This originates a reduction of the number of small crystals and an increase of large crystals, disrupting the cellular structure. The recrystallization during storage and transportation may lead to freeze-dried packaged product or to toughening of animal tissue [1].

4.5.1.4 *Drip Loss*

During ice formation, water is removed from the original location. However, during thawing, water may not be reabsorbed in the same regions, and usually drip loss is observed. Size and location of ice crystals, rate of thawing, the extent of water reabsorption, the status of the tissue before freezing, and the water-holding capacity of the tissue have a great influence on drip losses. The time required for thawing should be longer than the one used for freezing (for comparable temperature driving forces). In frozen meats, a slow thawing process at low temperatures will permit a better water diffusion in the thawed tissue and its relocation in the fibers. In vegetable tissues, the water is not reabsorbed [47].

4.5.2 Chemical Changes

During freezing, changes in temperature and concentration (due to ice formation) play an important role in enzymatic and nonenzymatic reactions rates. Ice crystals may release the enclosed contents of food tissues, such as enzymes and chemical substances, affecting the product quality during freezing and frozen storage. The main chemical changes verified during freezing and frozen storage are related with lipid oxidation, protein denaturation, enzymatic browning, and degradation of pigments and vitamins.

4.5.2.1 *Impacts on Texture, Color and Flavor*

Lipid oxidation and protein denaturation are the major important causes of quality loss in frozen meat and fish. Flavor, appearance, nutritional content and protein functionality are usually degraded by lipid oxidation. The solutes concentration during freezing processes catalyzes the initiation of oxidative reactions, which disrupt and dehydrate cell membranes, exposing membrane phospholipids to the oxidation process. Food products stored in contact with air, mainly fish and poultry that have significant amounts of polyunsaturated fatty acids, also are susceptible to oxidation. The decomposition of hydroperoxides of fatty acids in aldehydes and ketones results in the formation of volatile compounds that gives rise to the aroma and taste characterized as "rancid" [7, 47, 49]. Lipid oxidation also has an impact in terms of pigment degradation and color quality deterioration of the products. Freezing and thawing accelerate pigment oxidation. For example, the metmyoglobin formation in red meats (brown color) and the carotenoid bleaching in fish and poultry favor parallel fat oxidation. Hydrolytic rancidity, textural softening, and color loss are also direct consequences of hydrolytic enzyme activities, which can be inactivated by heat [47].

In relation to fruits and vegetables, the ice crystals formation leads to undesirable losses in texture, such as loss of turgor during thawing. The semi-rigid nature of the cells and the less orderly packaging of the cells are mainly responsible for the textural damage observed in frozen/thawed fruits and vegetables [1, 47]. Low storage temperatures and slow thawing should be guaranteed to minimize losses of membrane semi-permeability and cellular disruption. Also to avoid tissues softening, pretreatments can be applied (see Section 4.2). The most important chemical changes verified in frozen products are associated with the reactions that produce off-odors and off-flavors, pigment degradation, enzymatic browning and autoxidation of ascorbic acid. Water that does not freeze, even at very low temperatures, is responsible for deteriorative and enzymatic reactions, particularly during frozen storage [7]. In non-blanched products, enzymatic oxidation of phenolic compounds by polyphenoloxidase, leads to discoloration (browning) of food products. However, ascorbic acid can be introduced as an inhibitor of enzymatic reactions. The salts precipitation in concentrated solutions conduces to changes of anthocyanins color. During frozen storage of green blanched products, chlorophylls and carotenes are also degraded, the rate of pigment degradation being dependent on the extent of tissues damaged prior to freezing. The action of lipases and lipoxygenases leads to flavor alterations due to the accumulation of volatile compounds (carbonyl compounds and ethanol) in vegetable tissues [1, 47].

4.5.2.2 Impact on Nutritional Quality

Commonly, freezing is considered less destructive than any other preservation process and frozen products have a nutritional quality comparable to fresh products. Several unsaturated fatty acids (nutritionally essential or beneficial) are one of the major substrates for lipid oxidation, but the losses are not limiting in most of the frozen foods. Protein denaturation is mainly due to ice crystals formation and recrystallization, dehydration, solutes concentration and oxidation. Thus, several losses in protein functionality are reported in frozen fish, meat, poultry and egg products, and some texture deterioration in frozen muscle tissues may be attributed to protein damage. However, protein denaturation in frozen products is considered minimal when compared to the total available protein [47]. In terms of nutritional value, vitamins (essentially B and C) are the compounds that suffer a major negative impact with freezing and frozen storage conditions. Ascorbic acid losses are attributed to oxidative mechanisms during frozen storage. Blanching also affects negatively this quality indicator and the rates of deterioration are extremely slow when compared to ambient or chilled storage [47, 48].

4.5.3 Microbiological Aspects

During the pre-freezing stage, microorganisms can grow but very slowly (have a long generation time) when the temperature is approaching the minimum growth temperature. If the temperature is kept below the minimum temperature for growth, some microorganisms may die. However, above 0°C the loss of microorganisms' viability is limited and in practice, is negligible. When bacteria, in the exponential growth phase, are cooled quickly it is expected that microorganisms inactivation is more pronounced, but an abrupt temperature drop may lead bacteria to form cold shock proteins that protect them against other stresses such as heating, low pH or low water activity [50].

The freezing stage causes the apparent death of 10%–60% of the viable microorganisms and these values increase during frozen storage [51]. Factors such as low temperature, extracellular ice formation, intracellular ice formation, concentration of solutes and internal pressure may be involved in the microbial inactivation. The sensitivity of microorganisms to the freezing process differs considerably. Thus, the main concern is related to the microorganisms that survive during the freezing step, and with the ones that can grow when the product is thawed. Usually, the less resistant microorganisms are the Gram-negative bacteria followed by the Gram-positive bacteria. Nonsporulating rods and spherical bacteria are the most resistant ones, and spores (such as Clostridium and Bacillus) remain unaffected by freezing. Bacteria in the stationary phase are more resistant than those in the exponential phase [7, 52]. The freezing process causes damage mainly in the microorganisms membrane, which loses some barrier properties at temperatures below 15°C, leading to leakage of internal cell material. The dissociation of lipid-proteins may injure the cells during the freezing process. Cell membranes may also suffer mechanical damage due to ice crystals formation [50].

After storage at different temperatures, it is common to observe higher microbial inactivation for warmer storage (e.g., –8°C) temperatures than for colder storage temperatures (e.g., –18°C or lower). Freezing and storage at very low temperatures (–150°C or even colder) seems to result in increased survival. The long-time exposure to concentrated solutions (both internal and external) may lead to microbial death in both conditions. However, the recrystallization of ice observed if temperature fluctuations occur, increases the solutes concentration and consequently provokes damage to microorganisms. Temperature fluctuations at lower storage temperatures generate smaller ice crystals than at higher storage temperatures [50].

4.6 Final Remarks

Freezing is one of the oldest and most common processes used in food preservation and one of the best methods available in the food industry. There are several methods and types of equipment that can be used and adapted according to the different types of foods. Freezing usually retains the initial quality of the products. However, during freezing and frozen storage, some physical, chemical and nutritional changes may occur. To avoid this impact on fresh products, mainly in fruits and vegetables, some pretreatments may be required to inactivate enzymes and microorganisms.

References

1. P.J. Fellows. Freezing. In *Food processing technology: Principles and practice*, P.J. Fellows, ed. Woodhead Publishing Limited and CRC Press LLC: Cambridge, England, 418–451, 2000.
2. R.P. Singh, and D.R. Heldman. Food freezing. In *Introduction to food engineering*, R.P. Singh and D.R. Heldman, eds. Academic Press, Elsevier: California, USA, 501–541, 2009.
3. D.R. Heldman, and R.P. Singh. Thermodynamics of food freezing. In *Food process engineering*, D.R. Heldman and R.P. Singh, eds. AVI Publishing Company, INC.: Westport, Connecticut, 158–215, 1981.
4. C.J. Kennedy. Formation of ice in frozen foods and its control by physical stimuli. In *The properties of water in foods ISOPOW 6*, D.S. Reid ed. Blackie Academic & Professional: London, England, 1998.
5. C. Kennedy. Developments in freezing. In *Food preservation techniques*, P. Zeuthen and L. Bogh-Sorensen, eds. Woodhead Publishing Limited and CRC Press LLC: Cambridge, England, 228–240, 2003.
6. G.S. Tucker. Food biodeterioration and methods of preservation. In *Food and beverage packaging technology*, R. Coles and M.J. Kirwan, eds. Wiley-Blackwell: West Sussex, UK, 2011.
7. M.S. Rahman, and J. Velez-Ruiz. Food preservation by freezing. In *Handbook of food preservation*, M.S. Rahman, ed. CRC Press, Taylor & Francis Group: Boca Raton, USA, 635–665, 2007.
8. A. Cioubanu, and L. Niculescu. *Cooling technology in the food industry*, A. Cioubanu, et al., eds. Kent, England: Abacus Press, 1976.
9. F.P. Boyle, B. Feinberg, J.D. Ponting, and E.R. Wolford. Freezing fruits. In *Fundamentals of food freezing*, N.W. Desrosier and D.K. Tressler, eds. AVI Publishing Company, INC.: Westport, Connecticut, 135–214, 1977.
10. W.C. Deitrich, B. Feinberg, R.L. Olson, T.L. Roth, and F.H. Winter. Freezing vegetables. In *Fundamentals of food freezing*, N.W. Desrosier and D.K. Tressler, eds. AVI Publishing Company, INC.: Westport, Connecticut, 81–134, 1977.
11. P. Cano, M.A. Marin, and C. Fuster. Freezing of banana slices. Influence of maturity level and thermal treatment prior to freezing. *Journal of Food Science* 55(4): 1070–1073, 1990.
12. D.S. Reid. Optimizing the quality of frozen foods. *Food Technology* 44(7): 78–82, 1990.
13. C.L.M. Silva, E.M. Gonçalves, and T.R.S. Brandão. Freezing of fruits and vegetables. In *Frozen food science and technology*, J.A. Evans, ed. Blackwell Publishing Ltd: Oxford, UK, 165–183, 2008.

14. W.C. Parreno, and M.D.A. Torres. Quality and safety of frozen vegetables. In *Handbook of frozen food processing and packaging*, D.-W. Sun, ed. CRC Press, Taylor and Francis Group: Boca Raton, USA, 377–415, 2006.
15. D. Torreggiani, and A. Maestrelli. Quality and safety of frozen fruits. In *Handbook of frozen food processing and packaging*, D.-W. Sun, ed. CRC Press, Taylor & Francis Group: Boca Raton, USA, 417–440, 2006.
16. D. Torreggiani, T. Lucas, and A.-L. Raoult-Wack. The pre-treatments of fruits and vegetables. In *Managing frozen foods*, C.J. Kennedy, ed. Woodhead Publishing Limited and CRC Press LLC: Cambridge, England, 2000.
17. A. Collignan, A.L. Raoult-Wack, and A. Themelin. Energy study of food processing by osmotic dehydration and air-drying. *Agricultural Engineering Journal* 1(3): 125–35, 1992.
18. N. Hedges, and J. Nielsen. The selection and pre-treatments of fish. In *Managing frozen foods*, C.J. Kennedy, ed. Woodhead Publishing Limited and CRC Press LLC: Cambridge, England, 2000.
19. O.M. Magnussen, A.K.T. Hemmingsen, V. Hardarsson, T.S. Nordtvedt, and T.M. Eikevik. Freezing of fish. In *Frozen food science and technology*, J.A. Evans, ed. Blackwell Publishing Ltd: Oxford, UK, 151–164, 2008.
20. J. Jaczynski, A. Hunt, and J.W. Park. Safety and quality of frozen fish, shellfish and related products. In *Handbook of frozen food processing and packaging*, D.-W. Sun, ed. CRC Press, Taylor and Francis Group: Boca Raton, USA, 341–376, 2006.
21. A. Banks, J.A. Dassow, E.A. Feiger, A.F. Novak, J.A. Peters, J.W. Slavin, and J.J. Waterman. Freezing fish. In *Fundamentals of food freezing*, N.W. Desrosier and D.K. Tressler, eds. AVI Publishing Company, INC.: Westport, Connecticut, 273–317, 1977.
22. S. James. Freezing of meat. In *Frozen food science and technology*, J.A. Evans, ed. Blackwell Publishing Ltd: Oxford, UK, 124–150, 2008.
23. S.J. James. The pre-treatments of meat and poultry. In *Managing frozen foods*, C.J. Kennedy, ed. Woodhead Publishing Limited and CRC Press LLC: Cambridge, England, 2000.
24. S. Moorhead. Quality and safety of frozen meat products. In *Handbook of frozen food processing and packaging*, D.-W. Sun, ed. CRC Press, Taylor and Francis Group: Boca Raton, USA, 311–324, 2006.
25. L.J. Bratzler, A.M. Gaddis, and W.L. Sulzbacher. Freezing meats. In *Fundamentals of food freezing*, N.W. Desrosier and D.K. Tressler, eds. AVI Publishing Company, INC.: Westport, Connecticut, 215–239, 1977.
26. N. Kotrola. Quality and safety of frozen poultry and poultry products. In *Handbook of frozen food processing and packaging*, D.-W. Sun, eds. CRC Press, Taylor and Francis Group: Boca Raton, USA, 325–340, 2006.
27. P. Nesvadba. Thermal properties and ice crystal development in frozen foods. In *Frozen food science and technology*, J.A. Evans, ed. Blackwell Publishing Ltd: Oxford, UK, 1–25, 2008.
28. D.W. Sun, and L. Zheng. Innovations in freezing process. In *Handbook of frozen food processing and packaging*, D.-W. Sun, ed. CRC Press, Taylor & Francis Group: Boca Raton, USA, 175–195, 2006.
29. C.O.B. Wallens, and J. Venetucci. Emerging freezing technologies. In *Food processing: Recent developments*, A.G. Gaonkar, ed. Elsevier Science & Technology: Amsterdam, The Netherlands, 227–240, 1995.

30. S.E. Zorrilla, and A.C. Rubiolo. Mathematical modeling for immersion chilling and freezing of foods. Part I: Model development. *Journal of Food Engineering* 66(3): 329–338, 2005.
31. S.E. Zorrilla, and A.C. Rubiolo. Mathematical modeling for immersion chilling and freezing of foods. Part II: Model solution. *Journal of Food Engineering*, 66(3): 339–351, 2005.
32. M.F. North, and S.J. Lovatt. Freezing methods and equipment. In *Handbook of frozen food processing and packaging*, D.-W. Sun, ed. CRC Press, Taylor and Francis Group: Boca Raton, USA, 199–210, 2006.
33. P.O. Persson, and G. Londahl. Freezing technology. In *Frozen food technology*, C.P. Mallett, ed. Blackie Academic & Professional, Chapman & Hall: Glasgow, UK, 20–58, 1993.
34. C. James, and S.J. James. Freezing/Thawing. In *Handbook of meat processing*, F. Toldrá, ed. Blackwell Publishing: Iowa, USA, 105–124, 2010.
35. J. Chen, and A. Rosenthal. Food processing. In *Food science and technology*, G. Campbell-Platt, ed. Wiley-Blackwell: West Sussex, UK, 240–242, 2009.
36. J.M. Pardo, and K. Niranjan. Freezing. In *Food processing handbook*, J.G. Brennan, ed. Wiley-VCH: Weinheim, Germany, 125–145, 2006.
37. J.P. Miller, and C. Butcher. Freezer technology. In *Managing frozen foods*, C.J. Kennedy, ed. Woodhead Publishing Limited and CRC Press LLC: Cambridge, England, 2000.
38. R.M. George. Freezing systems. In *Quality in frozen food*, M.C. Erickson and Y.C. Hung, eds. Chapman & Hall: New York, USA, 3–9, 1997.
39. L. Zheng, and D.-W. Sun. Innovative applications of power ultrasound during food freezing processes – a review. *Trends in Food Science & Technology* 17(1): 16–23, 2006.
40. B. Li, and D.-W. Sun. Effect of power ultrasound on freezing rate during immersion freezing of potatoes. *Journal of Food Engineering* 55(3): 277–282, 2002.
41. D.-W. Sun, and B. Li. Microstructural change of potato tissues frozen by ultrasound-assisted immersion freezing. *Journal of Food Engineering* 57(4): 337–345, 2003.
42. M. Jalté, J.-L. Lanoisellé, N.I. Lebovka, and E. Vorobiev. Freezing of potato tissue pre-treated by pulsed electric fields. *LWT - Food Science and Technology* 42(2): 576–580, 2009.
43. A. LeBail, D. Chevalier, D.M. Mussa, and M. Ghoul. High pressure freezing and thawing of foods: A review. *International Journal of Refrigeration* 25(5): 504–513, 2002.
44. E. Alizadeh, N. Chapleau, M. de Lamballerie, and A. Le-Bail. Effect of different freezing processes on the microstructure of Atlantic salmon (Salmo salar) fillets. *Innovative Food Science & Emerging Technologies* 8(4): 493–499, 2007.
45. A. Bunger, P.C. Moyano, R.E. Vega, P. Guerrero, and F. Osorio. Osmotic dehydration and freezing as combined processes on apple preservation. *Food ScienceTechnology International* 10(3): 163–170, 2004.
46. J.D. Fagan, T.R. Gormley, and M.M. Uí Mhuircheartaigh. Effect of modified atmosphere packaging with freeze-chilling on some quality parameters of raw whiting, mackerel and salmon portions. *Innovative Food Science & Emerging Technologies* 5(2): 205–214, 2004.
47. N.E. Zaritzky. Factors affecting the stability of frozen foods. In *Managing frozen foods*, C.J. Kennedy, ed. Woodhead Publishing Limited and CRC Press LLC: Cambridge, England, 2000.

48. D. Martínez-Romero, S. Castillo, and D. Valero. Quality control in frozen vegetables. In *Handbook of vegetable preservation and processing*, Y.H. Hui, et al., eds. Marcel Dekker, Inc: New York, USA, 2004.
49. M. Berry, J. Fletcher, P. McClure, and J. Wilkinson. Effects of freezing on nutritional and microbiological properties of food. In *Frozen food science and technology*, J.A. Evans, ed. Blackwell Publishing Ltd: Oxford, UK, 26–50, 2008.
50. L. Bogh-Sorensen. Maintaining safety in the cold chain. In *Managing frozen foods*, C.J. Kennedy, ed. Woodhead Publishing Limited and CRC Press LLC: Cambridge, England, 2000.
51. Y.G. Moharram, and S.D. Rofael. Shelf life of frozen vegetables. In *Shelf life studies of foods and beverages: Chemical, biological, physical, and nutritional aspects*, G. Charalambous, ed. Elsevier Science Publishers B.V.: Amsterdam, 1993.
52. C.O. Gill. Microbiology of frozen foods. In *Handbook of frozen food processing and packaging*, D.-W. Sun, ed. CRC Press, Taylor & Francis Group: Boca Raton, USA, 85–100, 2006.

5

Chemical and Functional Properties of Food Components

Campos-Montiel R.G.[1], Pimentel-González D.J.[1] and Figueira A.C.[2]

[1]*Institute of Agricultural Sciences, Autonomous University of Hidalgo State, Hidalgo, México*
[2]*CIEO, Research Center for Spatial and Organisational Dynamics, ISE, Department of Food Engineering, University of the Algarve, Faro, Portugal*

Abstract
The relationship between food and human health has been empirically known for centuries. Correlations between both have, however, only been systematically investigated since the second half of the last century, giving rise to a new area of knowledge within the food and nutrition sciences named functional foods. This chapter brings together notions about the functional and chemical properties of different components of food. This is followed by a review of the nutritional value and sensory properties of food. The effects of post-harvest storage and processing techniques on the food's bioactive compounds are also reported. From all of this some conclusions are finally drawn.

Keywords: Functional food, food chemistry, nutraceuticals, probiotics, prebiotics, bioactive compounds, health claims, post-harvest storage, sensory properties of food, nutrition

5.1 Introduction

In the last decades, the consumers' perspective of food has shifted from that of a nutrient and energy-supplier, towards that of a health-promoter, influencing systemic physiological

Visakh P. M., Sabu Thomas, Laura B. Iturriaga, and Pablo Daniel Ribotta (eds.) Advances in Food Science and Technology, (151–184) © 2013 Scrivener Publishing LLC

functions and processes. This has resulted in the rise of the concept of functional foods as a new nutrition paradigm. Health-conscious consumers are increasingly taking control of their own health, and thus constantly exerting pressure on the scientific community, governments, and on the food industry. Indeed, scientists are constantly pressed for the identification and determination of "healthier" compounds, which also has been made possible by a remarkable increase in analytical and manufacturing possibilities. Most of these findings are then translated by the food industry into new, "healthier" commercial products, which has prompted governments to both promote and implement legislation to safeguard food safety and the health of the consumer.

5.2 Functional and Chemical Properties of Food Components

5.2.1 Functional Foods: Historical Perspective and Definitions

The study of the medicinal effects of foods has been traced-back to Chinese Medicine to at least 1000 BC, with the use of these foods in the Orient having been a cultural practice for centuries [1]. On the other hand, in Europe, Hippocrates (460–377 BC), the Greek father of modern medicine, reportedly said, "Let food be thy medicine and medicine be thy food [2]." But it was only more recently, in 1984, that in-depth research on the health benefits of specific foods was started in Japan. Lately, in 1991, this resulted in the establishment, by the Japanese Ministry of Health, Labour and Welfare (MHLW), of the first system for the evaluation of functional food and health claims (Foods for Specified Health Use – FOSHU). A further requirement for FOSHU products is that they have to show an ordinary food form, and not that of food supplements (namely extracts, tablets or capsules) [3–5].

The concept of functional foods has spread around the world, having become increasingly popular [6–8]. However, at present, an internationally accepted definition for functional foods is nonexistent. Within the European Union (EU), the Functional Food Science in Europe (FUFOSE) project, coordinated by the International Life Sciences Institute (ILSI) stated that, "a food can be regarded as functional if it has been satisfactorily demonstrated to affect beneficially one or more target functions in the body beyond adequate nutritional effects in a way that is relevant to either an improved state of health and well-being and/or a reduction of risk of disease." In addition, "a functional food must remain food and it must demonstrate its effects in amounts that can normally be expected to be consumed in the diet: it is not a pill or a capsule, but part of the normal food pattern." [9–11].

In China, the guideline of registration for functional foods states that, "Health (functional) food means that a food has special health functions or is able to supply vitamins or minerals. It is suitable for consumption by special groups of people and has the function of regulating human body functions but is not used for therapeutic purposes. And it will not cause any harm whether acute or subacute or chronic [12]." Contrary to that specified by EU regulation, in China, functional foods are available in eleven formats, which include capsules, tablets, powders and granules, liquids, and foods (the last representing less than 1% of all functional foods) [6].

In the USA, the Food and Drug Administration (FDA) has adopted the definition of the Institute for Food Technologists (IFT), "food and food components that provide a health benefit beyond basic nutrition…" [13]. Health Canada defines it as, "similar in appearance to, or may be, a conventional food, is consumed as part of a usual diet, and is demonstrated to have physiological benefits and/or reduce the risk of chronic disease beyond basic nutritional functions [14]."

5.2.2 Legislation on Functional Food Claims

Consumers' interest and acceptance of functional foods has been increasing globally. This has resulted in a growing demand for better and more reliable information, namely on claims made in relation to various product health benefits [15, 16]. This has led to the formulation of legislation worldwide, some of which is shown in Table 5.1.

Table 5.1 Legislation on functional food claims in different countries.

	Functional food claims	**Permissible claim relationship between a food product and a reduction of a disease state**
Canada	Risk-reduction claims (a description of the link between a food or food constituent and the reduction of risk of a particular disease, which includes restoring, correcting or modifying bodily functions is required). Only the exact wording indicated in the regulations is permissible for these risk-reduction claims.	• a healthy diet low in sodium and high in potassium and reduced risk of high blood pressure; • a healthy diet with adequate calcium and vitamin D and reduced risk of osteoporosis; • a healthy diet low in saturated and trans fat and reduced risk of heart disease; • a healthy diet rich in vegetables and fruit and reduced risk of some types of cancers; and • non-fermentable carbohydrates in gums and hard candies and the non-promotion of dental caries.
	Nutritional or functional claims (a specification of the type or quantity of a particular nutrient within the product, and the making of claims about the nutrient's well-established role in the maintenance or support of specific bodily functions is required. Functional claims must not state that a product has an effect on a specific disease or its signs and symptoms. These claims may only state the food's effects on the normal functioning of the human body).	Claims that a product provides "100 percent of an individual's daily vitamin C intake" and that "Calcium aids in the formation and maintenance of bones and teeth," are examples of acceptable nutritional content claims. This is in contrast to a claim such as "Milk helps build strong bones and teeth," which would not be permissible because the claim is directed to the food product itself, rather than the nutrient within the food. Nutritional-type claims have fewer requirements than disease-risk-reduction claims. Any food with a nutrient or functional claim must generally contain five percent or more of the recommended daily intake of the nutrient. For foods without recommended daily intakes, claims such as "high in" or "good source of," generally may not be made because the consumer cannot place the statement into a proper context.

	Functional food claims	Permissible claim relationship between a food product and a reduction of a disease state
	General health claims (no specific rules)	Examples of general health claims would be "healthy" and "include probiotic yogurt in your diet as part of healthy eating."
Codex Alimentarius	**Health claim** means any representation that states, suggests, or implies that a relationship exists between a food or a constituent of that food and health. Health claims include the following:	
	1. **Nutrient Function Claims** are nutrition claims that describe the physiological role of the nutrient in growth, development and normal functions of the body.	Example: "Nutrient A (naming a physiological role of nutrient A in the body in the maintenance of health and promotion of normal growth and development). Food X is a source of/ high in nutrient A."
	2. **Other Function Claims** are claims that concern specific beneficial effects of the consumption of foods or their constituents, in the context of the total diet on normal functions or biological activities of the body. Such claims relate to a positive contribution to health or to the improvement of a function or to modifying or preserving health.	Examples: "Substance A (naming the effect of substance A on improving or modifying a physiological function or biological activity associated with health). Food Y contains x grams of substance A."

(Continued)

Table 5.1 (cont.)

	Functional food claims	Permissible claim relationship between a food product and a reduction of a disease state
	3. **Reduction of disease risk claims** are claims relating the consumption of a food or food constituent, in the context of the total diet, to the reduced risk of developing a disease or health-related condition. Risk reduction means significantly altering a major risk factor(s) for a disease or health-related condition. Diseases have multiple risk factors and altering one of these risk factors may or may not have a beneficial effect. The presentation of risk reduction claims must ensure, for example, by use of appropriate language and reference to other risk factors, that consumers do not interpret them as prevention claims.	Examples: "A healthful diet low in nutrient or substance A may reduce the risk of disease D. Food X is low in nutrient or substance A". "A healthful diet rich in nutrient or substance A may reduce the risk of disease D. Food X is high in nutrient or substance A".

	Functional food claims	Permissible claim relationship between a food product and a reduction of a disease state
Japan	**Health claims** are presentations that state, suggest, or imply that a relationship exists between a food or the constituents of a food and health. Health claims include nutrient–function claims, enhanced function claims, and reduction of disease risk claims. This definition is the same as that included in the Proposed Draft Guidelines for Use of Health and Nutrition Claims of the Codex Alimentarius in 1999.	
	Generic health claims are claims based on well-established, generally accepted knowledge derived from evidence in the scientific literature and/or on recommendations from national or international public health bodies.	
	Product-specific claims are claims that concern certain physiological effects other than a generic health claim, which requires demonstrations based on scientific evidence for individual products.	

(Continued)

Table 5.1 (cont.)

	Functional food claims	**Permissible claim relationship between a food product and a reduction of a disease state**
	Enhanced function claims are claims that concern specific beneficial effects regarding the consumption of foods and their constituents in the context of the total diet regarding physical or psychological functions or biological activities but that do not include nutrient function claims.	
	Structure/function claims are any statements regarding the effects of dietary supplementation on the structure or function of the body, that is defined by the Dietary Supplement, Health and Education Act in the USA in 1994. These claims are generally similar to the enhanced function (or other) claims.	
FDA	Five types of health-related statements or claims are allowed on food and dietary supplement labels: 1. **Nutrient content claims** indicate the presence of a specific nutrient at a certain level.	

	Functional food claims	Permissible claim relationship between a food product and a reduction of a disease state
	2. Structure and function claims describe the effect of dietary components on the normal structure or function of the body.	
	3. Dietary guidance claims describe the health benefits of broad categories of foods or diets and do not refer to a disease or a health related condition.	
	4. Qualified health claims convey a developing relationship between components in the diet and reduced risk of disease, as reviewed by the FDA and supported by the weight of credible scientific evidence available.	
	5. Health claims confirm a relationship between components in the diet and reduced risk of disease or health condition, as approved by FDA and supported by significant scientific agreement.	

(Continued)

Table 5.1 (cont.)

	Functional food claims	Permissible claim relationship between a food product and a reduction of a disease state
European Union	Health claims should comply with the specified in Articles 13 and 14 of the Regulation (EC) No 124/2006 **Article 13 - Health claims other than those referring to the reduction of disease risk and to children's development and health**, include: the role of a nutrient/substance in growth, development and the functions of the body; psychological and behavioral functions; slimming and weight control or reduction of hunger, increase of satiety or the reduction of available energy from the diet.	
	Article 14 - Reduction of disease risk claims and claims referring to children's development and health, may be made where they have been authorized in accordance with the procedure laid down in Articles 15, 16, 17 and 19 of Regulation (EC) No 124/2006.	

5.2.3 Classification of Functional Foods

A worldwide accepted classification for the functional foods that have been developed and are available couldn't be found to date. Kaur and Das [15], Kotilainen *et al.* [17], Klimas *et al.* [18], and Siró *et al.* [19] amongst others have, however, suggested a common classification based on the functional foods' origin or modification that can be seen in Table 5.2 and Figure 5.1 [20].

Table 5.2 Classification of functional foods.

Type of functional food	Examples
Food products in which the original recipe has been modified to include ingredients which have a beneficial effect on diseases and health.	Calcium fortified bread; ω-3 fortified breads; Phytosterol fortified margarine; Fruit juices fortified with vitamin C.
Foods from which a harmful ingredient has been removed, reduced, or replaced to counteract anti-nutritional compounds produced by processing.	Fibers as fat releasers in meat or ice cream products; Chewing gum to which xylitol has been added, instead of sugar.
Food in which the ingredients are improved by increasing specific components, by changing the animals' feeds, different growing conditions or post-harvest technologies for fruits or vegetables, or innovative processing methodologies.	Eggs, meats or fish high in ω-3 fatty acids; Beef high in conjugated linoleic acid; Functional grapes with improved antioxidant activities; Fermentation with specific bacteria to yield bioactive peptides.
Novel foods with an enhanced health benefits, produced by genetic modifications or the consumption of varieties not previously used.	Rice with high iron or B-vitamin content; Vegetable oils with an enhanced fatty acid composition; foods free from food allergens; Canola oil with an high carotenoid content; wheat with enhanced lutein concentrations; Berries with improved antioxidant activities.

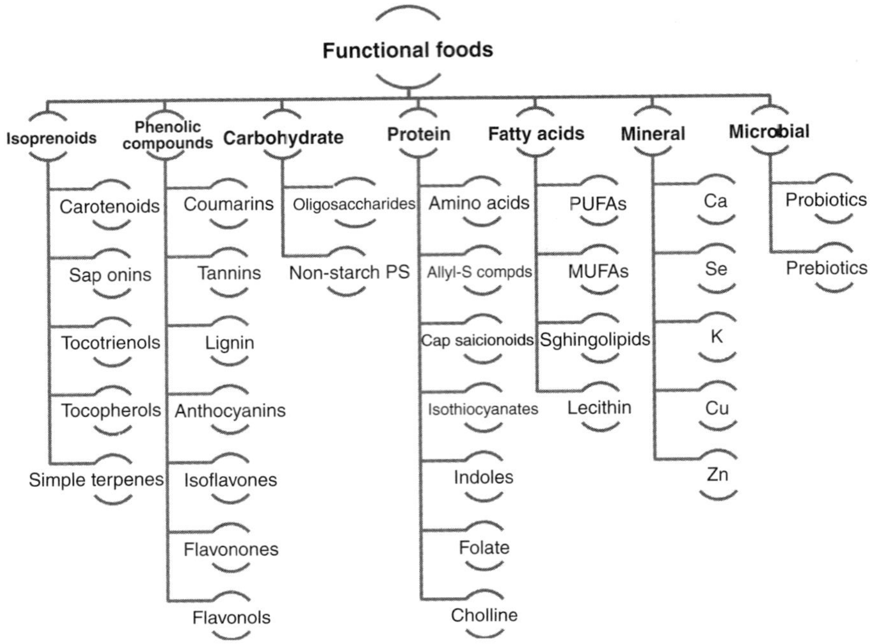

Figure 5.1 Organization for Functional Foods [20].

5.2.4 Functional Properties of Food Components

In recent years, there has been a global trend toward the use of natural phytochemicals present in natural resources as antioxidants and functional ingredients (Table 5.3) [2].

5.2.4.1 Phenolic Compounds

Polyphenols are classified into phenolic acids, flavonoids, and less common stilbenes and lignans. Many studies have focused on the antioxidant activities of flavonoids. Although several flavonoids are highly efficacious free radical scavengers *in vitro,* there is little information on the importance of dietary flavonoids as antioxidants *in vivo,* or evidence for such activity *in vivo.* Moreover, there have been few studies on phenolic acids compared to the number of studies on flavonoids, despite the high contents of phenolic acids in fruits, cereals, and some vegetables [21].

Flavonoids, perhaps the most important single group of phenolics in foods, comprise a group of over 4000 aromatic plant compounds, which include anthocyanins, proanthocyanidins, flavonols

Table 5.3 Chemical constituent and their potential human health [2].

Chemical constituents	Food	Potential benefits
Isoprenoids	Carrots, various fruits, oat, vegetables, corn, avocado, egg yolk , spinach, tomatoes, watermelon, pink grapefruit, guava, papaya, grains, palm oil, chickpeas and soybeans	Lowers cholesterol; Effective against colon cancer; Protects the eyes against the development of Age-related Macular Degeneration, Cataracts; Anticancer (colon); Powerful antioxidant, protects against formation of cancers (Prostate, Bladder, Cervical, Leukemia, reduces cholesterol levels; Anticancer (breast cancer); Promotes cardiovascular health; Lowers cholesterol, effective against colon cancer.
Polyphenolic Compounds	Citrus fruits, onions, apples, tea, broccoli, fruits, vegetables, soyabean, blueberries, blackberries, black raspberries, berries, legumes, dark grapes, raisins, berries, peanuts, turmeric root	Antioxidants; Reduces risk of cancer; Counteracts inflammation in the body; Lower blood sugar levels in people with diabetes; Phenolic acids reduce oxidation of LDL cholesterol; Reduces formation of cancer; Lowers total serum cholesterol increasing HDL; Strongly anti-inflammatory and strongly anti-oxidant; Effective anti-clotting agent.
Carbohydrates	Legumes, oats, barley, some fruits whole grain foods wheat and corn bran, nuts	Contribute to maintenance of a healthy digestive tract; Anticancer (colon).
Fatty acids	Salmon, flax seed, tree nuts	Potent controllers of the inflammatory processes; Maintenance of brain function; Reduce cholesterol disposition; Reduce risk of coronary heart disease.
Minerals	Food	Important constituents of balanced diet.
Microbial	Yogurt, other dairy and nondairy applications	May improve gastrointestinal health and systematic immunity.

and catechins. Phenolic acids, on the other hand, include hydroxy-cinnamic acids (e.g., caffeic or ferrulic acid conjugates, sinapic acid) and hydroxybenzoic acids (e.g., benzoic, gentisic or *p*-anisic acids) [22]. Phenolic acids constitute about one-third of the dietary phenols and they are present in plants in the free and bound forms. Bound-phenolics may be linked to various plant components through ester, ether, or acetal bonds [23]. Clifford [21] estimated that the daily consumption of phenolic acids ranged from 25 mg to 1 g. An increasing interest in determining the antioxidant activities exhibited by phenolic acids and their derivatives should also be noted [24–25]. The content of phenolic substances in food is of valuable interest for a number of reasons: There is a correlation between taste (astringency, bitterness) in fruits and content of phenolic compounds. Phenolics seem to play an important role in the natural defense mechanisms in fruit (e.g., antifungal effects), and increasing interest in the health benefits of fruits and fruit products is associated with the content of different groups of phenolic compounds with antioxidative effects.

5.2.4.2 *Carbohydrates*

The soluble polysaccharides have been correlated with hypercholesterolemia and hypoglycemic effect, whereas water insoluble polysaccharides are mainly associated with decreases in digestive tract transit time.

5.2.4.3 *Fatty Acids*

Fatty acids are organic compounds formed by a hydrocarbonated chain and a carboxylic group that is normally bounded with glycerol forming acylglycerides (mono-, di- or triglycerides). Depending on the nature of the hydrocarbonated chain, fatty acids can be saturated or unsaturated, which in turn can be monounsaturated or polyunsaturated fatty acids (PUFA) [26]. Many of the fatty acids can be synthesized by humans, but there is a group of PUFA, the essential fatty acids, that the human body cannot produce: omega-3 (n−3) and omega-6 (n−6) fatty acids. The parent omega-6 fatty acid is linoleic acid (C18:2n−6, LA) and the parent omega-3 fatty acid is α-linolenic acid (C18:3n−3, ALA). Omega-6 fatty acids such as arachidonic acid (C20:4n−6; AA) can be synthesized by humans from LA, and omega-3 fatty acids, such as eicosapentaenoic acid (C20:5n−3; EPA), docosapentaenoic acid (C22:5n−3, DPA) and docosahexaenoic acid (C22:6n–3, DHA), from ALA; however, the conversion of ALA in EPA, DPA and DHA is low and these omega-3 fatty acids are considered essential fatty acids too [20].

Fatty acids are important for human and animal health and they are of interest because they are precursors in the eicosanoids' biosynthesis. They are viewed as important bioregulators of many cellular processes, and have potential mechanisms of action in some diseases (Table 5.4).

Table 5.4 Diseases affected by ω -3 fatty acid intake and potential mechanisms of action [27].

Disease	Potential mechanisms of action of ω-3 fatty acids
Coronary heart disease and stroke	Prevent arrhythmias (ventricular tachycardia and fibrillation); Are prostaglandin and leukotriene precursors; Have anti-inflammatory properties; Inhibit synthesis of cytokines and mitogens; Stimulate endothelium-derived nitric oxide; Are antithrombotic; Have hypolipidemic properties with effects on triglycerides and VLDLs; Inhibit atherosclerosis.
Essential fatty acid deficiency during development	Are an important constituent of the membrane phospholipids in the brain and retina.
Autoimmune disorders including lupus and nephopathy	Are involved in suppression of cell-mediated immune responses; Inhibit the function monocytes; Inhibit the production or action of cytokines and eicosanoids; Stabilize renal function.
Inflammatory bowel disease	Have anti-inflammatory properties; Inhibit interleukin-1; Inhibit tumor necrosis factor production; Are free radical scavengers; Decrease platelet responsiveness.
Breast, colon and prostate cancers	Inhibit tumor growth.
Rheumatoid arthritis	Alter eicosanoid metabolism; Ameliorate inflammation.

5.2.4.4 *Microbial (Prebiotics and Probiotics)*

5.2.4.4.1 Prebiotics

The concept of a prebiotic arose from two observations:

- Bacteria like any other living organism have (sometimes specific) nutrient requirements.
- Some nutrients, particularly complex carbohydrates, pass undigested into the colon where they are utilized by resident bacteria [20].

Gibson and Roberfroid [25] defined a prebiotic as a non-digestible food ingredient that beneficially affects the host by selectively stimulating the growth and/or activity of a limited number of bacteria in the colon.

5.2.4.4.2 Probiotics

In accordance with Farnworth [28], Roberfroid [5] and Ranadheera *et al.* [29], probiotic is a live microbial food ingredient that is beneficial to health. The concept of probiotics is not new; Hippocrates and other scientists in the early ages reported that fermented milks could cure some disorders of the digestive system [28, 29].

As of now, probiotics are almost exclusively consumed as fermented dairy products such as yogurt or freeze-dried cultures, fermented vegetable beverages, cereals, meats, cheese and chocolate products [5, 28].

The selection of microorganisms included in food/drinks depends on different criteria, such as:

- Microorganism of human origin;
- Resistance to acid conditions of stomach, bile and digestive enzymes normally found in the human gastrointestinal tract;
- Ability to colonize human intestine;
- Safety for human consumption;
- Scientifically proven efficacy [28].

Since these microorganisms are not expected to survive and grow in the host's intestinal tract, they are not categorized as probiotics by most scientists and are considered as yogurt cultures [30]. Regardless of the diversity of these microorganisms, the main probiotic preparations currently available on the market belong to a group of bacteria designated as lactic acid bacteria (e.g., Lactobacilli, Streptococci and Bifidobacteria), which are important normal constituents of the human gastrointestinal microflora and produce lactic acid as a major metabolic product [31, 32]. These probiotics used in foods have previously been primarily added as part of the fermentation process, however increasingly they are added as supplements. Furthermore, there is also an increasing trend in using probiotics as nutraceuticals which are available in various forms, such as in capsules. This changing trend in probiotic delivery may lead to a reduced functional efficacy, due to exclusion of the potential synergistic effect of the food (Table 5.5).

Table 5.5 Beneficial effects of prebiotics on probiotic bacteria in foods [29].

Food	Prebiotics	Probiotics	Effect
Yogurt	Hi-maize/resistant starch Inulin Fructooligo-saccharides	*L. acidophilus* *L. casei* *L. acidophilus* *L.casei* *L. rhamnosus* *L. reuteri* *Bifidobaceterium* *L. acidophilus* *L.casei* *L. rhamnosus* *Bifidobaceterium* *B. animalis* *B. longum*	↑Growth and viability ↑Growth and viability ↑Viability and fatty acid production
Fermented milk	Polydextose Oligofructose	*L. acidophilus* *L. rhamnosus* *B. animalis subsp. lactis* *L. acidophilus* *L. rhamnosus* *B. animalis subsp. lactis*	↑Growth, viability and fatty acid production ↑Growth, viability and fatty acid production
Ice cream	Inulin	*L. acidophilus* *B. lactis*	↑Viability
Cheese and cheese-based products	Oligofructose Inulin Carboxy methyl cellulose	*L. acidophilus* *B. animalis subsp. lactis* *L. acidophilus* *B. animalis subsp. lactis* *P. freudenreichii subsp. shermanii*	↑Growth, viability, sensory and fatty acid production ↑Growth, viability, sensory and fatty acid production ↑Growth

5.2.4.4.3 Beneficial Health Effects and Therapeutic Value of Probiotics

Probiotics may provide a number of potential health benefits [29, 33]:

- mainly through maintaining a good balance and composition of intestinal flora, helping to increase the body's ability to resist the invasion of pathogens and maintain the host's wellbeing;
- maintenance of normal intestinal gut microflora, protection against gastrointestinal pathogens;
- enhancement of the immune system, reduction of lactose intolerance;
- reduction of serum cholesterol level and blood pressure [33];
- anti-carcinogenic activity;
- improved utilization of nutrients and improved nutritional value of food are some of these identified benefits;
- prevention of urogenital diseases (candidal vaginitis);
- prevention of the alleviation of constipation;
- protection against traveller's diarrhea;
- prevention of infantile diarrhea;
- reduction of antibody-induced diarrhea, the control of inflammatory bowel diseases and of irritable bowel syndrome;
- reduction of hypercholesterolemia, the protection against colon and bladder cancer, the prevention of osteoporosis and the prevention of food allergy and of atopic diseases.

5.3 Nutritional Value and Sensory Properties of Food

The goals of food processing are to focus on ensuring chemical and microbiological safety in foods, nutritional value and acceptability to the consumer, and attention to sensory properties of food. However, food processing may present effects on these properties of food.

Beyond the aforementioned characteristics food-processing techniques may influence food quality in regard to physical, biological, sensory and chemical properties.

Factors included in physical properties that may be affected by food processing are the following: shape, color, size, surface condition, texture, freshness, total solids, etc., and these can change the appearance of the product. In biological terms, we can talk about total bacteria, total coliform bacteria, total mold, free from pathogenic microorganisms, etc. Regarding the sensory aspects, flavor, aroma, taste, texture, etc., are involved; finally, in the chemical properties are included the nutritional value, moisture content, functional value, pH, chemical contaminants and food additives, among others.

Food additives are important factors due to their great promotion and development of by the food industry, and are regarded as the soul or pillar of modern food industries. This basically brings many advantages to the food industry. They can: 1) reduce food spoilage and therefore keep the food fresh, reduce food loss and reduce the risk of food poisoning, 2) improve sensory properties of food, 3) maintain and improve the nutritional value of food, 4) increase food varieties and convenience, 5) be advantageous to food, the production mechanization and automation, 6) meet other special needs, and 7) improve the economic and social benefits. Examples of the last items are foods with added probiotics, prebiotics, fiber, vitamins, etc. Nevertheless there are examples of food without additives or substitutes such as fat free, sugar free, etc.

5.3.1 Nutritional Value of Food

Food composition is determined by proximate analysis of carbohydrate, lipid, and protein contents, as well as minerals and vitamins. Actually researchers have focused on further evaluating their amino acid content and quality, fatty acid profiles, simple and complex carbohydrates, soluble and insoluble fibers, and other contents like functional additives such as antioxidants, known as nutraceutical ingredients. In the food industry there are foods processed with or without nutraceutical value, it depends on the nature and intensity of food processing techniques which can either improve or worsen the nutritional quality of food. The most common food processing technique is heat treatment at low or moderate temperature, and this generally leads to improved digestibility and inactivation of anti-nutritional factors. By contrast, the most severe conditions of high temperature or extreme pH may impose severe nutritional losses and induce the formation of toxic derivates in food. In other cases, the ingredient with low nutraceutical value delivers as a result food of low quality. In recent years, further research has studied this concern and results have shown that they are focused on the improvement or substitution of the nutraceutical value.

The generation of transgenic animals and plants, the utilization of encapsulated nutrients, or the simple addition of bioactive compounds into the final product, are different strategies that are available to improve the nutritional value of food products [34].

Actually, consumers reject the addition of some antioxidants that are very effective in controlling lipid oxidation, whereas they accept natural products with antioxidant activity, since they are often perceived as safer and more nutritious than food containing additives or food coming from animals fed ingredients from a non-natural origin. While natural products are desired by many consumers, these products can be difficult to define since some man-made food additives and feed ingredients can be completely identical to those present in nature, slightly different, or modified for a better use [35].

Consumers demand safer and more nutritious food products exempt of non-natural origin preservatives or other food additives. For example, products with lower fat contents, with higher ratio of unsaturated fatty acids, especially n-3 fatty acids, are desired because these lipids can help prevent the development of cardiovascular and inflammatory pathologies [35]. Nowadays there is a lot of research involved in the improvement of the nutritional value of foods. One of the species used more in development in order to improve the nutritional value of foods is the soybean. Soybean is a good substitute since it is a good source of protein (about 40%), is an edible oil of high quality that is cholesterol free (about 21%), and is a carbohydrate (34%) [36]. It is one of the most promising foods in the world available to improve the diet of millions of people.

Cereals are the most important source of food and have a significant impact in the human diet throughout the world. Since the 90s, in India and Africa, cereal products have comprised 80% or more of the average diet, 50% in Central and Western Europe, and between 20–25% in the US [37]. Cereals like maize, rice, millet and sorghum can supply sufficient qualities of carbohydrate, fat, protein and many minerals, but diets consisting primarily of cereals are high in carbohydrate and deficient in vitamins and protein.

Research has been carried out on the fortification of carbohydrate-rich foods with protein-rich food, especially soybeans, in order to improve their nutritional value. These improved carbohydrate foods with soybean have helped to combat malnutrition in children and maintain and repair the body tissues of adults. Soybean is also an excellent economical source of nutrients and the cheapest source of protein for rural households in a nutritional and economic comparative analysis with other major sources of protein like eggs, beef, milk and cowpea. Thus, it is a cost-efficient source of quality protein. Most anti-nutritional factors of soybean are eliminated by heat treatment [38]. It is also a good source of many required vitamins and minerals. Among cereals and other legumes, it has the highest protein content, about 40%, whereas other legumes have 20–30% and cereals have a protein content of 8–15% [39].

Soy protein has been used and accepted as a food ingredient to enhance the value of finished foods. Soybeans and soyfoods have been identified with their protein content from a nutritional perspective, and as such there is much interest among clinicians and researchers in their potential role in preventing and treating chronic diseases [40].

The development of high-protein foods of plant origin is essential in developing countries due to the shortage and high cost of animal protein [41]. Consumption of such products plays a major role in combating malnutrition, which is a serious problem in these countries. Various plant protein sources may be combined to obtain products with improved protein quality [42].

As a matter of fact, the above mentioned cereals are important sources of plant protein throughout the world. Maize constitutes an important percentage of the cereals consumed in many countries. The grain is often processed into a fermented product known as "ogi," which can also be prepared from millet and sorghum, and is consumed in many parts of West Africa. During ogi manufacture, nutrients including protein and minerals are lost from the grain thereby affecting nutritional quality adversely [41]. Akinrele and Bassir [43] found that this cereal product was incapable of supporting the growth of rats. A number of studies have been carried out to improve the nutritive value of ogi. A reduction in protein loss was achieved by using an improved wet-milling technique [44], while no nutrient losses occurred during production from high-lysine corn using an improved method [45]. The nutritive value of ogi was also improved by fortification with amino acids [46] and plant proteins [43]. Similarly, the protein content of maize meal was increased by combination with soy flour [47], blends of roasted soybean and peanut meals [41] and blends of cashewnut, African locust bean and sesame oil meals [48].

In summary, the goal of food technology is to maintain and/or improve the quality of food nutrient content and bioavailability and organoleptic characteristics in order to support human nutrition in keeping with the acceptability of consumers.

5.3.2 Sensory Properties of Food

In food production consumer satisfaction is increasingly taken into account. Thus, the concept of quality has evolved from being "an adaptation to internal (intrinsic) specifications," to "the ability of an organization to meet the needs, both explicit and implicit, that the client has" [49].

The methods used to assess quality are: 1) objective scales based on measuring instruments, and 2) subjective scales based on human assessment (sensory analysis) [50]. Whenever the safety and hygiene of a food is guaranteed, the satisfaction of its organoleptic properties becomes the most important criterion; it determines its choice and, even more importantly, the consumer's loyalty to a product or brand. Quality, viewed as the consumer's acceptability of a product, is composed by different aspects covered by the senses: sight (color and defects), smell (aroma and taste), touch (manual and buccal), sound (touch and during mastication), and taste (flavor). All quality attributes, both external and internal, are contemplated and evaluated by the consumer at the time to decide on the purchase of a raw product.

Sensory attributes are of great importance for engendering preference. This fact is obvious to all consumers, food producers and retailers, and to researchers in meat science and technology. The relationships between sensory attributes and preference are also investigated by research teams from all over the world [51]. The number of reports that include sensory perception in one form or another is thus large, and a review of all of these is impossible in such a short chapter.

Preference is very often considered to be a spot measure for liking and not a good predictor for repeated consumption, since this is affected by the individuals' values and attitudes, as well as cultural factors and other cognitive structures [51]. Still, the product attributes, both describing usage and the sensory perception of the product, are considered to be decisive in the determination of one product preference over another. Although the cost of a trained sensory panel is high, it can be utilized for the description of a large spectrum of attributes, including appearance, color, flavor, odor and texture. Instruments are also increasing in price, and are often limited to a small spectrum of parameters. However, the potential of rapid non-destructive techniques, such as NIR spectroscopy, will perhaps give new impetus for instrument development [52]. In addition, with the inclusion of multivariate statistics in the interpretation of data, the complexity of human perception might be simulated well enough for usage in a variety of instrumental applications [53].

The sensory characteristics of foods, especially appearance, texture, and flavor influence the food purchasing decisions of consumers. Therefore, a major concern is to increase the nutritional composition of products without negatively compromising the sensory qualities [35].

Among processed meat industries, substitution of some ingredients with other non-meat ingredients has been practiced. This replacement is done due to several reasons such as for quality, health or economic purposes. As an example, the replacement of ingredients from animal origin with those of plants has been applied in food industries [54]. Starches, such as maize, tapioca, rice, potato, and wheat, have been used in processed meat products as meat filler and water binder [55]. The other ingredients that may contribute to the carbohydrates' nutrient in burgers are non-starch hydrocolloids. Carrageenan, konjac, alginate, and xanthan gum are such good sources of non-starch hydrocolloids which are able to work with proteins to help in retaining moisture content and thus modify the texture of meat products [56]. Another good source of carbohydrates that can be incorporated in burgers is dietary fiber. The usage of dietary fiber in processed meat formulations is especially practiced where the economical, nutritive, and technological issues are concerned. Some of the dietary fibers that have commonly been used are cellulose, oat fiber, wheat fiber, potato fiber, carrot fiber, sugar beet fiber, soy and pea fiber [57].

Babji *et al.* [58] have reported on the quality assessment of brands of chicken burgers available in Malaysia without evaluation in texture profile and sensory analysis. In addition, Ramadhan *et al.* [59] studied the quality of commercial chicken burgers currently available in Malaysia by evaluating their quality attributes such as texture and color, and consumer acceptance through sensory evaluation. Results showed that all of the commercial chicken burgers produced locally in Malaysia are significantly different on several quality attributes such as chemical composition and textural and color properties due to variations in formulation. Some brands contained lower fat and a lesser concentration of cholesterol. The majority of the chicken burger brands complied with Malaysia's food regulations in several aspects such as meat percentage, fat and protein content. Sensory evaluation showed that the chicken burger with yellowish color, moderate hardness and chewiness are preferred by the panelists.

5.4 Postharvest Storage and Processing

5.4.1 Bioactive Compounds Postharvest

The increased intake of fruits and vegetables has been associated with a reduced incidence of degenerative diseases due to their antioxidant activities [60]. In this sense, the fruit and vegetables have bioactive compounds or phytochemicals such as vitamins (A, C and E), anthocyanins, and other phenolic compounds and carotenoids which contribute to the antioxidant capacity [61].

Some of the postharvest technology used avoids changes in bioactive compounds in different fruits and vegetables in cold storage, modified atmosphere packaging, organic solutions and irradiation.

A food's bioactive compound is any compound that provides a health benefit beyond basic nutritional benefits. These compounds are secondary plant metabolites [62].

The best known and studied activity of the bioactive compounds is its antioxidant capacities; in addition, these compounds have an anti-inflammatory activity and may act as regulators of both the genes involved and the inflammatory, neurodegenerative and carcinogenic processes, among others.

It is well known that the bioavailability of the bioactive compounds is different when consumed pure, or within its original matrix; thus, it must be taken into account that in the same food several bioactive compounds may interact and have a synergistic effect [62].

The body has various ways to mitigate or neutralize free radicals and thus protect itself from their harmful actions. In a first line of antioxidant defense, we can find antioxidant enzymes such as superoxide dismutase, catalase, glutathione peroxidase, and so on, which are able to neutralize reactive oxygen species [63]. In this regard, it is crucial to note the importance of proper nutrition, as the enzymes require certain trace elements such as zinc, copper, and manganese which act as prosthetic groups. In the second line are included the antioxidants that eliminate free radicals. These substances are antioxidant vitamins, such as ascorbic acid (vitamin C), tocopherols (vitamin E), -carotene and other bioactive compounds mainly present in plant foods, such as the phenolic compounds [64].

Most of the antioxidants isolated from higher plants are polyphenols, which show antioxidant properties, as well as antibacterial, anticarcinogenic, anti-inflammatory and antiviral properties [65].

The total hydrophilic antioxidant activity (H-TAA) was different during cold storage for some commercial plums, with a high correlation (R^2=0.949) between H-TAA and total phenolics, and a lower relationship with anthocyanins (R^2=0.84). The lipophilic total antioxidant activity (L-TAA) behavior was different during postharvest storage for different plum cultivars. The correlation between L-TAA and total carotenoids was high (R^2=0.88) [66].

The use of modified atmosphere packaging (MAP) in plum cultivars retarded the increases of H-TAA production. The L-TAA had a significant delay in the plums stored under MAP conditions [67].

The H-TAA levels in pomegranates treated with acetyl salicylic acid were significantly higher than in controls during storage. No effect was observed in L-TAA during storage of pomegranates when acetyl salicylic acid was used [68].

The antioxidant capacity of fresh-cut mango cubes treated with ascorbic acid, citric acid and calcium chloride solution was significantly higher than in controls over the whole storage period [69].

5.4.1.1 *Phenols*

Phenolic compounds constitute a large group of secondary metabolites widely distributed in the plant kingdom. For the past 10 years, these compounds have received enormous attention from researchers and food manufacturers. More than 8000 polyphenols have been identified, and evidence for a role in the prevention of degenerative diseases including cancer and cardiovascular diseases is emerging [70].

Low temperature has been found to increase total phenolic content in pomegranate arils [71], dark-puple and yellow plums [66], and apples [72], probably due to stimulation of the activity of some enzymes involved in phenolic biosynthesis by cold storage [73]. But in red strawberry, when compared to white varieties, the total phenolic content decreased [74].

When plum cultivars were stored under modified atmosphere packaging, the results revealed that the increases in total phenols were delayed [67]. This might be due to the effect of low O_2 and high CO_2 in retarding postharvest ripening, as can be inferred by a reduced ethylene production, fruit softening, color change and acidity loss [67] and possible delay in phenylalanine ammonia lyase, chalcone synthase or anthocyanidin synthase, the key enzymes in the biosynthesis pathway of phenolic compounds [75].

The content of total phenolic compounds in pomegranates diminished throughout storage in control fruit, while no significant changes were observed with the use of acetyl salicylic acid under storage [68].

The total phenolic content on fresh-cut mango cubes treated with an ascorbic acid, citric acid and calcium chloride solution was significantly higher than that observed in control cubes during storage [69].

5.4.1.2 Anthocyanins

Anthocyanins are the general products of flavonoids' metabolism, with their difference from flavonoids residing in the absence of the carbonyl group(s). They are responsible for the flower, fruit and leaf color of all angiosperms [76], and are found in greater amounts in grapes and berries [62].

During cold storage their amounts were similar in different plum cultivars. The increase in peel anthocyanin was parallel to the reduction in hue values showing that these pigments contribute to the color changes associated with the postharvest ripening process [66]. Similar results have been found in other commodities such as blueberry [77], raspberry and strawberry [78], fresh prunes [79] and cherry [80]. Manganaris *et al.* [81] reported increases in anthocyanin content in the pulp of "Harrow Sun" plums.

The concentration of anthocyanins was retarded in plums kept under modified atmosphere packaging conditions, when compared with the control fruit [67].

The treatment with acetyl salicylic acid of pomegranates incremented the total anthocyanins in storage for 84 days with respect to the control fruit [68].

5.4.1.3 Carotenoids

Carotenoids are lipophilic molecules synthesized by plants and act as color pigments in fruit.

During low temperature storage the levels of carotenoids of only yellow plums increased, which was correlated to the decrease in hue color parameter. This carotenoid decrease couldn't be found in other plum varieties [66]. The increase in carotenoid content has also been observed in stored kiwifruit [82], watermelon [83] and sapote [84].

The use of modified atmosphere packaging in plums induced a delay in the change of total carotenoids during storage [67].

Statistical differences ($P<0.05$) could not be observed between the levels of carotenoids in mangos treated with either an ascorbic acid, citric acid or calcium chloride solution and control samples [69].

The irradiation treatment of early season grapefruit resulted in significantly ($P<0.05$) higher levels of β-carotenoid content of grapefruit before or after storage conditions, when compared to their initial (0 day) level. On the contrary, in late season fruit, no effect could be found for the β-carotenoid content of irradiated grapefruit, before or after 35 days of storage [85]. Sebastião *et al.* [86] reported that gamma irradiation also didn't affect the levels of β-carotenoid in parsley.

5.5 Conclusion

Although an enormous amount of work has already been done, the study of functional foods is still at an early stage. Due to its intrinsic nature, and the global world in which we're living, it is felt that the stakeholders would benefit from a harmonization of the existing legislation on functional foods' definition, and health claims on these products.

A presently ongoing discussion on this deals with the foreseen European Union's position on article 13 general function health claims, which is expected to pass 222 claims, whilst 2000 others will most certainly be rejected. This will place multinational industries in a dilema: how to explain to consumers that a FDA-accepted claim (EUA) has been rejected by the European Food Safety Authority (EFSA).

Acknowledgements

A.C. Figueira has been partially financed by the Foundation for Science and Technology (FCT).

References

1. FAO. Food Quality and Standards Service (AGNS) Food and Agriculture Organization of the United Nations (FAO) November, 2007.
2. S. Dharti, S. Gandhi, and M. Shah. Nutraceuticals-Portmanteau of Science and Nature. *International Journal of Pharmaceutical Sciences Review and Research* 5 (3), 33–38, 2010.
3. T. Shimizu. Health claims on functional foods: The Japanese regulations and an international comparison. *Nutrition Research Reviews* 16, 241–252, 2003.
4. T. Shimizu. Health claims and scientific substantiation of functional foods – Japanese regulatory system and the international comparison, 2011.
5. M.B. Roberfroid. 2000. Prebiotics and probiotics: Are they functional foods? *The American Journal of Clinical Nutrition* 71(6 Suppl), 1682S-7S; discussion 1688S-90S, 1994.
6. Y. Yang. Scientific substantiation of functional food health claims in China. *The Journal of Nutrition* 138, 1199S–1205S, 2008.
7. A. Ikeda, A. Moraes, and G. Mesquita. Reflections on trends and opportunities of functional foods. *Revista P & D Engenharia de Produção* 8(2), 40–56, 2010.
8. N. Sutar, P.P. Sutar, and D. Mohapatra. New horizons in functional food sector: An Indian perspective. *J. Dairying, Foods & H.S.* 29 (3/4), 166–172, 2010.
9. A.T. Diplock, P.J. Agget, M. Ashwell, F. Bornet, E.B. Fern, and M.B. Roberfroid. Scientific concepts of functional foods in Europe: Consensus document. *British Journal of Nutrition* 81, 1–27, 1999.
10. M. Blades. Functional foods or nutraceuticals. *Nutrition and Food Science* 30(2), 73–75, 2000.
11. ILSI Europe. Concepts of functional foods. ILSI Europe Concise Monograph, 2002.
12. SFDA: Special approval procedures for drugs. China Laws and Regulations of Foods, Drugs, and Cosmetics. Order No. 21; Promulgation date: 2005-11-18; Effective date: 2005-11-18.
13. IFT. Expert Report. Functional foods: opportunities and challenges, 2005. http://members.ift.org/IFT/Research/IFTExpertReports/
14. Health Canada website: http://www.hc-sc.gc.ca/fn-an/label-etiquet/claims-reclam/nutra-funct_foods-nutra-fonct_aliment-eng.php (accessed in 31.08.2011).
15. S. Kaur, and M. Das. Functional foods: An overview. *Food Science and Biotechnology* 20 (4), 861–875, 2011.
16. L. Katan. Health Claims & Functional Foods website. Food Ethics Council. Report of the business forum meeting on 17th March 2009. www.foodethicscouncil.org.

17. L. Kotilainen, R. Rajalahti, C. Ragasa, and E. Pehu. Health enhancing foods: Opportunities for strengthening the sector in developing countries. Agriculture and Rural Development Discussion Paper 30, 2006. The International Bank for Reconstruction and Development/The World Bank.
18. M. Klimas, C. Brethour, and D. Bucknell. Introduction and background. In *International market trends analysis for the functional foods and natural health products industry in the United States, Australia, the United Kingdom, and Japan*. March 17, p. 3, 2008. Nutri-Net Canada, Ontario, Canada.
19. I. Siró, E. Kápolna, B. Kápolna, and A. Lugasi. Functional food. Product development, marketing, and consumer acceptance – a review. *Appetite* 51, 456–467, 2008.
20. R. Wildman. Chapter 25: Probiotics and prebiotics. In *Handbook of nutraceuticals and functional foods*, 407–422, 2001.
21. M.N. Clifford. Chlorogenic acids and other cinnamates – nature, occurrence, and dietary burden. *J. Sci. Food Agric.* 79, 362–372, 1999.
22. H. Li, K. Cheng, and C. Wong. Evaluation of antioxidant capacity and total phenolic content of different fractions of selected microalgae. *Food Chemistry* 102(3), 771–776, 2007.
23. J. Chalas, C. Claise, M. Edeas, C. Messaoudi, L. Vergnes, A. Abella, and A. Lindenbaum. Effect of ethyl esterification of phenolic acids on low-density lipoprotein oxidation. *Biomed Pharmacother.* 55, 54–60, 2001.
24. M. Lodovici, F. Guglielmi, M. Meoni, and P. Dolara. Effect of natural phenolic acids on DNA oxidation in vitro. *Food and Chemical Toxicology* 39, 1205–1210, 2001.
25. C.A. Rice-Evans, N.J. Miller, and G. Papanga. Structure-antioxidant activity relationships of flavonoids and phenolic acids. *Free Radicical Biology and Medicine* 20, 933–956, 1996.
26. N. Rubio-Rodríguez, S. Beltrán, and I. Jaime. Production of omega-3 polyunsaturated fatty acid concentrates: A review. *Innovative Food Science & Emerging Technologies* 11(1), 1–12, 2010.
27. A.M. Abdel-Salam. Functional foods: Hopefulness to good health. *American Journal of Food Technology* 5, 86–89, 2010.
28. E.R. Farnworth. The beneficial health effects of fermented foods – potential probiotics around the world. *Journal of Nutraceuticals, Functional & Medical Foods* 4, 93–117, 2005.
29. R.D.C.S. Ranadheera, S.K. Baines, and M.C. Adams. Importance of food in probiotic efficacy. *Food Research International* 43(1),1–7, 2010.
30. A.C. Senok, A.Y. Ismaeel, and G.A. Botta. Probiotics: Facts and myths. *Clinical Microbiology and Infection* 11, 958–966, 2005.
31. R. Penner, R.N. Fedorak, and K.L. Madsen. Probiotics and nutraceuticals: Non-medicinal treatments of gastrointestinal diseases. *Curr. Opin. Pharmacol.* 5, 596–603, 2005.
32. G. Reddy, M. Altaf, B.J. Naveena, M. Venkateshwar, and E.V. Kumar. Amylolytic bacterial lactic acid fermentation – A review. *Biotechnology Advances* 26(1), 22–34, 2007.
33. J.L. Rasic. Microflora of the intestine probiotics. In B. Caballero, L. Trugo, & P. Fings, eds. *Encyclopedia of food sciences and nutrition*, pp. 3911–3916, 2003. Oxford: Academic Press.

34. M.H. Moghadasian. Advances in dietary enrichment with n-3 fatty acids. *Critical Reviews in Food Science and Nutrition* 48, 402–410, 2008.
35. R. Bou, R. Codony, A. Tres, E.A. Decker, and F. Guardiola. Dietary strategies to improve nutritional value, oxidative stability, and sensory properties of poultry products. *Critical Reviews in Food Science and Nutrition* 49, 800–822, 2009.
36. S.R. Singh, K.O. Rachie, and K.E. Dashiell. *Soybeans for the tropics: Research, production and utilization*. John Wiley and Sons Ltd, Chichester, UK, p. 230, 1987.
37. I.C. Onwueme, and T.D. Sinha. Field crop production in tropical Africa. Michael Health Ltd. Reigate Survey RH2 9EL, Technical Centre for Agricultural and Rural Cooperation, CTA. p. 190–192, 1991.
38. O.A. Sowonola, T.Y. Tunde-Akintunde, and F. Adedeji. Nutritional and sensory qualities of soymilk kunnu blends. *African Journal of Food and Nutritional Sciences* 5(2), 1–12, 2005.
39. D.K. Salunkhe, S.K. Sathe, and N.R. Reddy. Legume lipids. In *Chemistry and biochemistry of legumes*, S.K. Arora, ed. Edward Arnold Pub. Ltd, London: 5–20, 1983.
40. M. Messina, V. Messina, and K.D.R. Setchell. *The simple soybean and your health*. Avery Pub. Group. New York. pp. 260, 1994.
41. E.R. Aminigo, and J.O. Akingbala. Nutritive composition and sensory properties of ogi fortified with okra seed meal. *Journal of Applied Sciences and Environmental Management* 8 (2), 23–28, 2004.
42. A.P. Rodríguez-Bürger, A. Mason, and S.S. Nielsen. Use of fermented black beans combined with rice to develop a nutritious weaning food. *Journal of Agricultural and Food Chemistry* 46, 4806–4813, 1998.
43. I.A. Akinrele, and C.C.A. Edwards. An assessment of the nutritive value of a maize-soya mixture "soy-ogi" as a weaning food in Nigeria. *British Journal of Nutrition* 26(2), 177–185, 1971.
44. E.O.I. Banigo, and H.G. Muller. Manufacture of ogi (a Nigerian fermented porridge): Comparative evaluation of corn, sorghum and millet. *Canadian Institute of Food Science and Technology Journal* 5, 217–221, 1972.
45. E.O.I. Banigo, J.M. deMan, and C.L. Duitschaever. Utilization of high-lysine corn for the manufacture of ogi using a new, improved processing system. *Cereal Chemistry* 51, 559–572, 1974.
46. A.O. Adeniji, N.N. and Potter. Properties of ogi powders made from normal fortified and opaque-2 corn. *Journal of Food Science* 43(5), 1571–1574, 1978.
47. W.A. Plahar, and H.K. Leung. Comparison of Ghanaian fermented maize meal and the effect of soya fortification on sensory properties. *Journal of the Science of Food Agriculture* 34, 407–411, 1983.
48. T.E. Ekpenyong, B.L. Fetuga, and V.A. Oyenuga. Fortification of maize flour based diets with blends of cashewnut meal, African locust bean meal and sesame oil meal. *Journal of Food and Science and Agriculture* 28 (8), 710–716, 1977.
49. J. Ferratto. Importancia de la gestión de la calidad en frutas y hortalizas, situación y perspectivas. Presentación Feria Internacional de la Alimentación. FIAR. Rosario, 2003.
50. A.A. Kader. Postharvest technology of horticultural crops. University of California. Agriculture and Natural Resources, pp. 296, 1992.
51. S.F. Siegel, and E. Risvik. Cognitive set and food acceptance. *Journal of Food Science* 52, 825–826, 1987.

52. T. Nœs, and B. Kowalski. Predicting sensory profiles from external instrumental measurements. *Food Quality and Preference* 1 (4-5), 135–147, 1989.
53. E. Risvik. Sensory properties and preferences. *Meat Science* 36:67–77, 1994.
54. W.R. Egbert, and C.T. Payne. Plant proteins. In *Ingredients in meat products: Properties, functionality and applications*, R. Tarte, ed. Springer Science Business Media, LLC. New York: pp. 111–129, 2009.
55. G. Joly, and B. Anderstein. Starches. In *Ingredients in meat products: Properties, functionality and applications*, R. Tarte, ed. Springer Science Business Media, LLC. New York: pp. 25–55, 2009.
56. J.W. Lamkey. Nonstarch hydrocolloids. In *Ingredients in meat products: Properties, functionality and applications*, R. Tarte, ed. Springer Science Business Media, LLC. New York: pp. 57-82, 2009.
57. J.M. Bodner, and J. Sieg. Fiber. In *Ingredients in meat products: Properties, functionality and applications*, R. Tarte, ed., Springer Science New York: pp. 83–109, 2009.
58. A.S. Babji, M.N. Nuri, J. Suherman, and M.Y. Seri Chempaka. Quality assessment of local and franchise beef and chicken burgers. *Pertanika Journal of Tropical Agricultural Science* 23(2), 103–112, 2000.
59. K. Ramadhan, N. Huda, and R. Ahmad. Physicochemical characteristics and sensory properties of selected Malaysian commercial chicken burgers. *International Food Research Journal* 18(4), 1349–1357, 2011.
60. M. Schreiner, and S. Huyskens-Keil. Phytochemicals in fruit and vegetables: Health promotion and postharvest elicitors. *Crit. Rev. Plant Sci.* 25, 267–278, 2006.
61. M. Stacewicz-Sapuntzakis, P.E. Bowen, E.A. Hussain, B.I. Damyanti-Wood, and N.R. Famsworth. Chemical composition and potential health effects of prunes: A functional food? *Crit. Rev. Food Sci. Nutr.* 41, 251–286, 2001.
62. H. Gil. Tratado de nutrición. Composición y calidad nutritiva de los alimentos. 2da. Edición. *Editorial Panamericana, México*, 2010.
63. A.E. Veiga, D.J.A. Aguilar, V.B. Calvo, and M.L. Llanes. Radicales libres, formación y daño celular. El sistema antioxidante como protector frente a los radicales libres. *Análisis Clínicos. México*, 89, 201–216, 1997.
64. P. Zafrilla, J. Morillas, A. Martínez-Cachá, J. Mulero, J.M. Cayuela, and J.M. López Nicolás. Radicales libres y antioxidantes. *Alimentación, Equipos y Tecnología* 167, 109–11, 2002.
65. L.M. Muchuweti, A.N. Mupure, T. Murenje, and M.A.N. Benhura. Screening of antioxidant and radical activity of Vigna ungiculata, Bidens pilosa and Cleome gynandra. *American Journal of Food Technology* 2, 161–168, 2007.
66. H.M. Diaz-Mula, P.J. Zapata, F. Guillen, D. Martínez-Romero, S. Castillo, M. Serrano, and D. Valero. Changes in hydrophilic and lipophylic activity and related bioactive compounds during postharvest storage of yellow and purple plum cultivars. *Postharvest Biol. Technol.* 51, 354–363, 2009.
67. H.M. Diaz-Mula, D. Martínez-Romero, S. Castillo, M. Serrano, and D. Valero. Modified atmosphere packaging of yellow and purple plum cultivars 1. Effect on organoleptic quality. *Postharvest Biol. Technol.* 2011. In Press, doi:10.1016/j.postharvbio.2011.02.010.
68. M. Sayyari, S. Castillo, D. Valero, and M.M. Días. Acetyl salicylic alleviates chilling injury and maintains nutritive and bioactive compounds and

antioxidant activity during postharvest storage of pomegranates. *Postharvest Biol. Technol.* 60, 136–142, 2011.

69. R.M. Robles-Sánchez, M.A. Rojas-Graü, I. Odriozola-Serrano, G.A. Gónzalez-Aguilar, and O. Martín-Belloso. Effect of minimal processing on bioactive compounds and antioxidant activity of fresh-cut "Kent" mango (Mangifera indica L.). *Postharvest Biology and Technology* 51, 384–390, 2009.
70. P. Kroom, and G. Williamson. Polyphenols: Dietary components with established benefits to health? *J. Sci. Food Agric.* 85, 253–273, 2005.
71. S.H. Mirdehghan, M. Rahemi, M. Serrano, F. Guillen, D. Martinez-Romero, and D. Valero. The application of polyamines by pressure or immersion as a tool to maintain functional properties in stored pomegranates. *J. Agric. Food Chem.* 55, 755–760, 2007.
72. M. Leja, A. Mareczek, and J. Bem. Antioxidant properties of two apple cultivars during long-term storage. *Food Chem.* 80, 303–307, 2003.
73. Y. Hamauzu. Role and evolution of fruit phenolic compounds during ripening and storage. *Stewart Postharvest Rev.* 2, 5, 2006.
74. Y. Shin, J.A. Ryu, R.H. Lin, J.F. Nock, and C.B. Watkins. Harvest maturity storage temperature and relative humidity affect fruit quality antioxidant contents and activity and inhibition of cell proliferation of strawberry fruits. *Postharvest Biology and Technology* 49, 201–209, 2008.
75. Y. Desjardins. Physiological and ecological functions and biosynthesis of health-promotion compounds in fruit and vegetables. In F.A. Tomás-Barberan and M.I. Gil, eds. *Improving the health-promoting properties of fruit and vegetables products*, CRC Press-Taylor & Francis, Boca Raton, FL, USA, pp. 201–247, 2008.
76. G.E. Castillo, and S.I. Martínez. *Manual de fitoterapia*. Elsevier Masson, pp. 29–38, 2007.
77. Y. Zheng, C.Y. Wang, S.Y. Wang, and W. Zheng. Effect of high-oxygen atmospheres on blueberry phenolics, anthocyanins and antioxidant capacity. *J. Agric. Food Chem.* 51, 7161–7169, 2003.
78. W. Kalt, C.F. Forney, A. Martin, and R.I. Prior. Antioxidant capacity vitamin C, phenolics and anthocyanins after storage of small fruits. *J. Agric. Food Chem.* 47, 4638–4644, 1999.
79. Y. Hamauzu, and C. Cune. Changes in fruit quality phenolic compounds and antioxidant capacity of fresh prunes during storage. *Acta Hort.* 682, 557–563, 2005.
80. B. Gonçalves, A.K. Landbo, D. Knudsen. A.P. Silva, J. Moutinho-Pereira, E. Rosa, and A.S. Meyer. Effect of ripeness and posthaevest storage on the phenolic profiles of cherries (Prunus aviom L.). *J. Agric. Food Chem.* 55, 523–530, 2004.
81. G.A. Manganaris, A.R. Vicente, C.H. Crisosto, and J.M. Labavitch. Effect of dips in a 1-methylcyclopropeno generating solution of "Harrow Sun" plums stored under different temperature regimes. *J. Agric. Food Chem.* 55, 7015–7020, 2007.
82. S. Tavarini, E. Degl'Innocenti, D. Remorini, R. Massai, and L. Guidi. Antioxidant capacity, ascorbic acid, total phenols and carotenoids changes during harvest and after storage of Hayward kiwifruit. *Food Chem.* 107, 282–288, 2008.
83. P. Perkins-Veazie, and J.K. Collins. Carotenoid changes of intact watermelons after storage. *J. Agric. Food Chem.* 54, 5868–5874, 2006.

84. L. Alia-Tejacal, R. Villanueva Arce, C. Pelayo-Zaldivar, M.T. Colinas-León, V. López Martínez, and S. Bautista-Baños. Postharvest physiology and technology of sapote mamey fruit (Pouteria sapota (Jacq) H.E. Moore ** Stearn). *Postharvest Biol. Technol.* 45, 285–297, 2007.
85. B.S. Patil, J. Vanamala, and G. Hallman. Irradiation and storage influence on bioactive components and quality of early and late season "Rio Red" grapefruit (Citrus paradise Macf.). *Postharvest Biology and Technology* 34, 53–64, 2004.
86. K.I. Sebastiao, L.B. Almeida-Muradian, M.F. Romanelli, P.M. Koseki, and A.L.C.H. Villavicencio. Effect of gamma-irrdiation on the levels of total and cis/trans isomers of beta-carotene in dehydrated parsley. *Radiat. Phys. Chem.* 63, 333–335, 2002.

6

Food: Production, Properties and Quality

Yantyati Widyastuti[1], Tatik Khusniati[2] and Endang Sutriswati Rahayu[3]

[1]Reseach Center for Biotechnology, Indonesian Institute of Sciences, Cibinong, Indonesia
[2]Microbiology Division, Research Center for Biology, Indonesian Institute of Sciences, Cibinong, Indonesia
[3]Faculty of Agricultural Technology, Gadjah Mada University, Yogyakarta, Indonesia

Abstract
Food is any solid or liquid material consumed by a living organism for maintaining life and keeping healthy. Food production is mainly from land and follows the Good Agriculture Practices. The source of foods generally derive from plants and animals and basically contain a lot of nutrition which is good for human health. Plant source foods are rich in carbohydrate and a good source of dietary proteins, vitamins, minerals and fiber. Animal source foods are an excellent source of high quality and easily digested protein and are considered the highest quality available, as they contain a full complement of essential amino acids. The properties of foods were basically related to water activity and affected by the treatments of the foods. Processing and preservation will certainly affect food properties. Food quality, particularly safe and healthy foods, are a priority for meeting the requirements and expectations of the customer.

Keywords: Food product, production, properties, quality, nutrients

6.1 Introduction

Food is defined as any solid or liquid material consumed by a living organism to supply energy, build and replace tissue or participate in such reactions [1]. According to another definition by the FAO/WHO

Visakh P. M., Sabu Thomas, Laura B. Iturriaga, and Pablo Daniel Ribotta (eds.) Advances in Food Science and Technology, (185–200) © 2013 Scrivener Publishing LLC

Codex Alimentarius Commission, "food is a substrate whether processed, semi-processed or raw, that is intended for human consumption and includes drink, chewing gum and any substance that has been used in the manufacture, preparation or treatment of food." Foods are needed everyday because food consumption is a basic activity necessary for human survival. Basically, people have the right to expect the food they eat to be safe with enough good nutrient content so that it is suitable for consumption. It is clearly shown that some nutrients are a requirement of a food. Food should contain substances which have a positive effect on humans, especially for maintaining life and keeping healthy after being consumed, and therefore consumption of food will certainly guarantee human survival.

Raw foods are mainly from plants and animals, and they will often be ready for consumption after cooking. However, there has also been a tradition of eating raw fish in some parts of the world for a million years. It is accepted that fish can be consumed raw much better than meat because it contains far less connective tissue. Recently, food preparation from raw materials is made easier with the availability of processed food. Processed foods have been altered from their natural state for safety and preservation reasons. The methods used for processing foods include canning, freezing, refrigeration and dehydration. All these methods sound user-friendly and safe. However, there are many processed foods that are not good for our health and should be avoided, i.e., those that are made with trans-fats, saturated fats, and large amounts of sodium and sugar. Examples of good processed foods are pasteurized milk and frozen vegetables. Pasteurized milk is certainly free from pathogenic bacteria and frozen vegetables preserve their vitamins and minerals for a long period of time.

This chapter addresses the issues relating to food production, properties and quality needed to meet consumer demand. Properties and quality have been recognized as an important essential component of food product related to healthy food, because food spoilage is wasteful, costly and can adversely affect trade and consumer confidence.

6.2 Food Production

Most production of food comes from land, although there is great potential for the sea to provide various seafoods. From land, food production traditionally is closely related to agriculture and generally refers to cultivation of plants or crops and rearing of animals. Their productivity is strongly affected by the genotype of plants or crops and animals. Food production may follow the directions of Good Agricultural Practices, as defined by the Food and Agriculture Organization (FAO) of the United Nations. The term Good Agricultural Practices can refer to any collection of specific methods for on-farm production and post-production processes, which when applied to agriculture, produces results that are in harmony with the values of the proponents of those practices. Good Agricultural Practices may be applied to a wide range of farming systems at different scales and sites. They are applied through sustainable agricultural methods, such as integrated pest management, integrated fertilizer management and conservation agriculture. Furthermore, they also rely on principles that:

1. economically and efficiently produce sufficient, safe and nutritious food;
2. sustain and enhance natural resources;
3. maintain viable farming enterprises and contribute to sustainable livelihoods;
4. meet cultural and social demands of society.

6.3 Factors Affecting Production and Improvement of Food

Food production and its availability depends on several factors including soil, climate, population, income per capita and technology.

6.3.1 Soil and Climate

Food production is faced with a very difficult situation related to climate change all around the world. The impact of climate change is very severe and one of the impacts is the increase in temperature. Drought affects all stages of crop growth and development, since absorption of nutrients from the soil is influenced by temperature condition and moisture. Soil and climatic conditions including the physical, chemical and biological properties of soil, rates at which nutrients are supplied and applied fertilizer affect the growth of crops and their product. The deficiency of nutrients needed by crops limits their growth and production. In many countries in Europe there is a tendency towards cereal grains yield stagnation and increased yield variability that may have been influenced by the negative impact of climatic changes. Consequently, farmers are currently adapting to climate change, in particular in terms of changing the timing of cultivation and selecting other crop species and cultivars. Certain regions suffer from increase incidents of heat waves and droughts without possibilities for shifting crop cultivation [2]. The physiological responses of crops suggest that they will grow faster, with slight changes in development, such as flowering and fruiting, depending on the species. Changes in food quality in a warmer and high CO_2 situation are to be expected, for example, decreased protein and mineral nutrient concentration as well as altered lipid composition [3].

Increase in temperature will cause severe damage to the physiology, metabolism and the health of animals. A hot environment impairs production including growth, meat, milk and egg yield and quality, as well as reproduction performance, metabolic and health status and immune response. Rising environmental temperatures pose a greater risk to animal product, in particular meat spoilage and carcass contamination with *E. coli* and *Salmonella* in poultry. *Bos indicus* cattle sire lines could lead to produce tougher, less juicy beef with less marbling [4].

6.3.2 Population and Income Per Capita

Food sufficiency or efforts in overcoming deficiencies in food quantity and quality are major nutritional challenges globally. Tremendous increase of human population followed by increases in per capita have changed food demand in some parts of the world, putting strong pressure on food production [5]. Per capita quantity of crop consumption remains relatively constant and tends to decline across all income levels, while there is a different situation for livestock products consumption. Per capita consumption of beef, dairy, pork, poultry, eggs and fish continues to increase among high income levels (Table 6.1).

6.3.3 Technology

Organic farming is a method in agriculture based on ecology and naturally occurring biological processes. In this technology the

Table 6.1 Estimated per capita food consumption by food item and per capita income level.

Real income	**$ 1500**	**$ 5000**	**$ 15,000**	**$ 25,000**
(tons of cereal equivalents per capita per year)				
All food	0.56	0.99	1.67	1.94
Crops	0.23	0.25	0.25	0.25
Cereals	0.13	0.13	0.11	0.09
Rice	0.04	0.03	0.02	0.01
Wheat	0.04	0.07	0.07	0.07
Others	0.05	0.03	0.02	0.01
Root crops	0.03	0.02	0.01	0.01
Vegetable oils	0.02	0.03	0.04	0.04
Sweeteners	0.02	0.04	0.05	0.05
Other	0.03	0.03	0.04	0.06
Livestock	0.30	0.69	1.32	1.59
Beef	0.12	0.25	0.43	0.48
Dairy	0.05	0.14	0.31	0.41
Pork	0.02	0.08	0.20	0.26
Poultry meat	0.01	0.06	0.10	0.10
Eggs	0.01	0.02	0.04	0.05
Other	0.09	0.14	0.24	0.29
Fish	0.03	0.05	0.08	0.10

Per capita real GDP (PPP) in 2002 US dollars. Source: Rask & Rask (2011) based on regression results, FAO and World Bank data from 159 countries (1975–2002).

perception among consumer is that organically produced crops possess higher nutritional quality. Herencia *et al.* [6] found that organic crops showed higher phosphorus and dry matter content and lower nitrogen and nitrate content than conventional crops. They also found crops with opposite trends in nutrient content depending on the cultivation cycle, which seems to indicate that conditions in which crops develop have more of an influence than the type of fertilization. The limitation to fertilization that is applied in organic farming can lead to an available nitrogen shortage for plants and possibly less nitrogen content.

The aim to improve the production of food can be directed towards producing food in a more efficient way with an emphasis on quantity and quality improvement. The technology of plant genetic engineering plays an important role in generating new plants with better productivity. Genetic engineering can be defined as the manipulation of plant development structure or composition by insertion of specific DNA sequence [7]. These sequences may be derived from the same species or even the same variety of plant. This may be done with the aim of altering the levels of expression of specific endogenous genes to make them more or less active, or to alter when and where in the plant they are switched on or off. Alternatively, the aim may be to change the biological properties of the proteins they encode. However, in many cases genes are derived from other species, which may be plants, animals or microbes, with the objective of introducing novel biological properties or activities. Numerous transgenic plants have been generated, including many crop species. Transgenic plants will have an impact on conventional breeding programs because they can significantly decrease the time to develop a new variety.

Functional foods are foods eaten for specified health purposes because of their rich content of one or more nutrients or non-nutrient substances which may confer health benefits [1]. Cereals such as barley and oats are good sources for functional ingredients of soluble fiber such as (1-3,1-4)-ß-D-glucan, referred to as ß-glucan. These ingredients affect the glycaemic, insulin, and cholesterol response to foods. The inclusion of ß-glucan in both cereal and dairy-based foods illustrate their potential as ingredients to manipulate the structure and texture of those foods. Therefore, ß-glucan from barley, oat and other cereals represents an important functional ingredient for the cereal-based food industry [8].

Recent technology in animal reproduction, including multiple ovulation and embryo transfer (MOET) as well as semen predetermined sex, have significantly increased the rate of reproduction of in farm animals. Sexed semen will contribute to increased profitability of dairy and beef production. It could be used to produce offspring of the desired sex from a particular mating to take advantage of differences in the value of males and females for specific marketing purposes [9]. Use of sexed semen in conjugation with *in vitro* embryo production is a potentially efficient way of obtaining offspring of a predetermined sex. There are a number of issues that appear to influence the success rate of using sexed semen to produce bovine embryos *in vitro*, including a reduction in fertilization rates, lower cleavage rates, blastocyst rates and pregnancy rate. Large scale transfer of *in vitro* produced Holstein embryos to beef recipients is a feasible production scheme [10]. The use of sexed frozen-thawed sperm was economically viable for the commercial MOET program in Holstein heifer [11]. The effort in selecting animals that have been primarily oriented towards productive traits, from now on must be oriented toward robustness and above all adaptability to heat stress [12].

An alternative to eating more whole grains could be to consume functional cereal products. Functional cereal products are grains, such as wheat, maize, rice and oats, that have been modified to provide health benefits over and above basic nutrition or grain that are similar in appearance to conventional foods; they are intended to be consumed as part of a normal diet, but have been modified to aid physiological functions beyond the provision of simple nutritional requirements. Golden rice is genetically modified rice that produces carotenoids in the endosperm of the grain. Carotenoids are a group of plant pigments important in the human diet as the only precursors of vitamin A.

6.3.4 Plant Source Foods

Basically, plants and crops can provide all human dietary macro- and micronutrients needed to live a healthy life as a vegetarian. Cereals, fruits and vegetables provide the nutrients in a complementary basis. Cereal grains are rich in carbohydrates and a good source of dietary proteins, vitamins, minerals and fiber. However, the nutritional quality and sensorial properties of cereals are sometimes low or poor if they are compared to that of animal products. The reasons behind this are the lower protein content, the deficiency of certain essential amino acids, lysine in particular, the low availability of starch and the presence of anti-nutrients such as phytic acid, tannins, and polyphenols. Major cereal grains, wheat and rice, represent the preferable source of dietary nutrients for humans that were widely consumed as staple foods in some parts of the world.

Tabel 6.2 World cereal market (FAO, 2011).

Year	Cereal	Wheat	Rice
	---million tonnes---		
2001	1907.9	589.3	400.6
2002	1836.6	574.0	380.8
2003	1894.4	561.5	393.4
2004	2074.2	632.6	406.9
2005	2052.2	625.5	424.2
2006	2019.8	600.9	428.6
2007	2133.4	610.7	440.1
2008	2288.6	683.7	458.5
2009	2263.4	685.1	455.9
2010	2239.6	685.2	467.0
2011	2307.0	680.6	478.8

The production based on the report of FAO [13] increased every year, as shown in Table 6.2, as a result of intensified crop management [14].

Fruits and vegetables are rich in minerals and vitamins which serve an array of important functions in the body. Vitamin A maintains eye health and boosts the body's immunity to infectious diseases. B-vitamins are necessary for converting food into energy. Folate, one of the most common B-vitamins, can also significantly reduce the risk of neural tube birth defects in newborns and contribute to the prevention of heart disease. Vitamins C and E are important micronutrients in fruits and vegetables that serve as powerful antioxidants that can protect cells from cancer-causing agents. Vitamin C, in particular, can increase the body's absorption of calcium and iron from other foods. Calcium is an essential mineral for strong bones and teeth, while low iron levels can lead to anemia, one of the most severe nutrition-related disorders. Many fruits and vegetables are also very high in dietary fiber which can help move potentially harmful substances through the intestinal tract and lower blood cholesterol levels. Much of the potency of fruits and vegetables is believed to also come from substances known as phytochemicals. Phytochemical antioxidants from fruits, vegetables and legumes can significantly inhibit the development of cardiovascular disease. Combinations of phytochemical antioxidants from different plant categories such as fruits, vegetables and legumes may possess complementary cardiovascular disease fighting activities [15].

6.3.5 Animal Source Foods

Animals (livestock) make an important contribution to human welfare, because they provide foods of high nutritive value, including milk, meat and eggs. They represent an excellent source of high quality and readily digested protein [16] which is suitable for human consumption (Table 6.3) [17]. Protein of animal products is considered the highest quality available, as it contains a full complement of essential amino acids and most resembles the amino acids of the human body in its amino acid composition. The micronutrients in meat have a high level of absorption and utilization by the body. Beef is a nutrient-rich food, providing good quality protein, vitamins B-6 and B-12, niacin, iron, and zinc. However, animal fats have gained the reputation of being less healthy. Beef cattle produce conjugated linoleic acid (CLA) which is known for its anticarcinogenic effects and deposit these compounds in the meat so that beef consumers can receive bioformed CLA. To increase the CLA yield in beef it is essential to provide cattle an appropriate substrate for formation of CLA [18].

Table 6.3 Nutritional benefits and risks of animal source foods (Neumann *et al.*, 2002).

Benefits	Risks
High energy density and low dietary bulk Dietary diversity Quality protein Micronutrients in bioavailability form Better maternal nutrition (in pregnancy and lactation)	Bacterial food contamination Zoonotic infections (animal parasites infecting people) Milk substitutes before 6 months of age increases risk of disease and may displace breast-feeding

Analysis of global production and consumption of animal source food showed that supply of animal source food depends largely on demand. The FAO data show that livestock production is growing rapidly, which is interpreted to be the result of the increasing demand for animal products [19]. The amount of meat production and consumption in eastern Asian countries, particularly in the northeast and some in the southeast, has grown rapidly due to the globalization of the food industry and rapid economic growth of the countries [20]. Poor people everywhere are eating more animal products as their incomes rise above poverty level and as they become urbanized [21]. Although there is a great rise in global livestock production, the pattern of consumption is very uneven. The countries that consume the least amount of meat are in Africa and South Asia. The main determinant of per capita meat consumption appears to be wealth. There has been a rise in the production of livestock products and this is expected to continue in the future, particularly in developing countries, with the greatest increase being in the production of poultry and pigs as well as eggs and milk [19].

Polkinghorne and Thompson [22] have reviewed the principles of world meat standard and grading which is strongly related to the demand for and requirements of meat. Meat classification is defined as a set of descriptive terms describing the features of the carcass that are useful to those involved in the trading of carcasses; while grading is defined as the placing of different values on carcasses for pricing purposes, depending on the market and requirements of traders. Early systems only needed to describe intact carcasses as the breakdown of the carcass into cuts and was done by the buyer of the carcass. Then, key parameters to describe the characteristics of the carcass changed to be more detailed to meet the requirements of consumers. There are several major grading schemes being developed as shown in Table 6.4. Differences in the priority of beef classification from selected countries may have resulted from changing consumer demand for meat. Several factors influencing the changes in consumer demand for meat include health concerns, changes in demographic characteristics, the need for convenience, and changes in distribution and price [23].

Production of animal products is strongly affected by the diet consumed by the animals. The use of agro-industrial by-products or novel pasture species has been adopted to reduce feed cost.

Table 6.4 Principal component of selected beef classification and grading schemes in selected countries around the world.

Country	Canada	Europe	Japan	South Korea	The Rep. of South Africa	USA	Australia	
Scheme	Canada	EUROP	JMCA	Korea	South Africa	USDA	AUS-MEAT	Meat Standards Australia
Grading unit	Carcass	Carcass	Carcass	Carcass	Carcass	Carcass	Carcass	Cut
Classification	Yes	Yes	-	-	Yes	-	Yes	-
Quality grade	Yes (4)+(5)	-	Yes (5)	Yes (5)	-	Yes (8)	-	Yes (3)
Yield grade	Yes (3)	-	Yes (3)	Yes (3)	-	Yes (5)	-	-
Pre slaughter	-	-	-	-	-	-	Grainfed	*Bos indicus*% HGP implants
Slaughterfloor	Carcass weight Sex Conformation Marbling score Meat color	Carcass weight Sex Fat cover Conformation	Carcass weight Sex Marbling score Meat color Meat brightness Fat color	Carcass weight Sex Marbling score Meat color Fat color	Carcass weight Dentition Rib fat Sex	Carcass weight Sex Marbling Ossification score Meat color	Carcass weight Dentition P8 fat Sex Butt shape Marbling score	Carcass weight Sex Electrical stimulation Hang Marbling score Ossification score
Chiller	Texture Fat color Fat thickness	-	Fat luster Fat texture Fat firmness Rib thickness Fat thickness	Firmness Texture Lean maturity Fat thickness	-	Meat texture Rib fat Kidney and perirenal fat	Meat color Fat color	Meat color Hump height Ultimate pH
Post chiller	-	-	-	-	-	-	-	Ageing time Cooking method

Source: Polkinghorne and Thompson (2010) with slight modification. HGP: hormone growth promotant.

Tannin-containing feeds result in sheep and goat meat of a lighter color and tend to increase milk yield and protein content, probably because they protect dietary proteins from ruminal degradation. Conjugated linoleic acid (CLA) in kid meat can be increased by feeding animals chopped cactus cladodes. Olive cake silage in lamb and ewe diets may increase linoleic and oleic content in meat and milk fat, respectively [24]. Dietary forage, such as grass or legume hay, appears to facilitate the establishment of microorganisms in the digestive tract that enhance the formation and deposition of CLA in the tissues. The provision of modest amounts of grain is more conducive to CLA synthesis rather than high levels of grain [18]. In hens, inclusion of humate and probiotics to their diet late in the laying period increased egg production, reduced mortality, and improved feed conversion efficiency [25], and supplementation of dietary microbial phytase 500 U/kg to normal corn-soybean diet improved egg production [26].

6.4 Food Properties

A food property is a particular measure of food behavior as a matter; or its behavior with respect to energy; or its interaction with human senses; or its efficacy in promoting human health and well-being [27]. An understanding of food properties is essential for scientists and engineers who have to solve problems, especially in food production related to consumption. Food preservation and processing affects the properties of foods in a positive or negative manner. The influence of water on the physical properties of food is dependent on the state of water in food which is expressed as water activity [28]. The water activity (a_w) of a food is the ratio between the vapor pressure of the food itself when in a completely undisturbed balance with the surrounding air media, and the vapor pressure of distilled water under identical conditions. The water activity increases with temperature.

Processed fruits and vegetables are often low moisture, sugar-rich foods, characterized by color, flavor and structural properties. There are relationships between a_w and some important chemical, physical and structural changes that occur during the processing and preservation of fruits and vegetables and their derivatives [29]. In food powders, a_w affected heat resistance of microorganisms.

The factors and mechanism involved in microorganisms' death or resistance to temperature in low-water-activity environments were detected by checking the efficiency of a rapid heating-cooling treatment to destroy microorganisms dried after mixing with wheat flour or skim milk [30].

6.5 Food Quality

Food quality can be described as the requirement necessary to satisfy the needs and expectations of the customer [31]. The scope of discussion on quality is very wide and complex. In agricultural and food products, typical quality parameters are sensory properties, shelf life, safety, health, nutritional value, crop yield per area and disease resistance. Shelf life is such an important requirement it should be of interest to everyone involved in the food chain, and safe food is a basic human right. There must be shared responsibility for the availability of safe food for consumers including the government, food industry and consumers themselves. The government is responsible for regulations and enforcement, advice to the industry and consumer education. The food industry has to implement good practices for food production related to quality assurance, appropriate technology and training of managers and food handlers. On the other side, consumers with their expectations and demands for safe food may be aware of the properties and quality of safe food.

More attention is being paid to the role of food in human health and in food safety and security [15, 32, 33], and that secondary metabolite content is a factor which must be considered during the assessment of agriculture systems. Antioxidants and probiotics have recently attracted the attention of the consumer and industry because of their potential health benefits. The natural dietary antioxidants in fruits, vegetables and legumes promote vascular health. The different food categories possess different bioactive compounds with various antioxidant capacities. When those foods are consumed together they may produce synergistic antioxidant interactions and more positive physiological effects on cardio health than if consumed alone. The potential of phytochemicals found in fruits and vegetables, mainly the polyphenol flavonoids including flavanols, flavanones, flavones, isoflavones and anthocyanin, will reduce the risk of cardiovascular diseases [15]. Probiotic microorganisms and the selection of suitable types of cereal grains were required to produce new cereal-based probiotic foods with suitable aroma, flavor and pH [34].

Food quality is presented as a system of product requirements, both the material and immaterial, related to the product itself, the production context, the product-packaging system, and the product-market system. There are two sets of approaches for food quality, which may come from the consumer and the producer. Consumers express their expectations and needs as requirements for food products. These requirements must be satisfied by the performance of the food products, which are functional and subjective. Performance must derive from characteristics of the product, which are structural and objective. The concept of performance and characteristics is illustrated in Figure 6.1 [31]. A set of product performance is greatly needed by consumers for their acceptance and satisfaction.

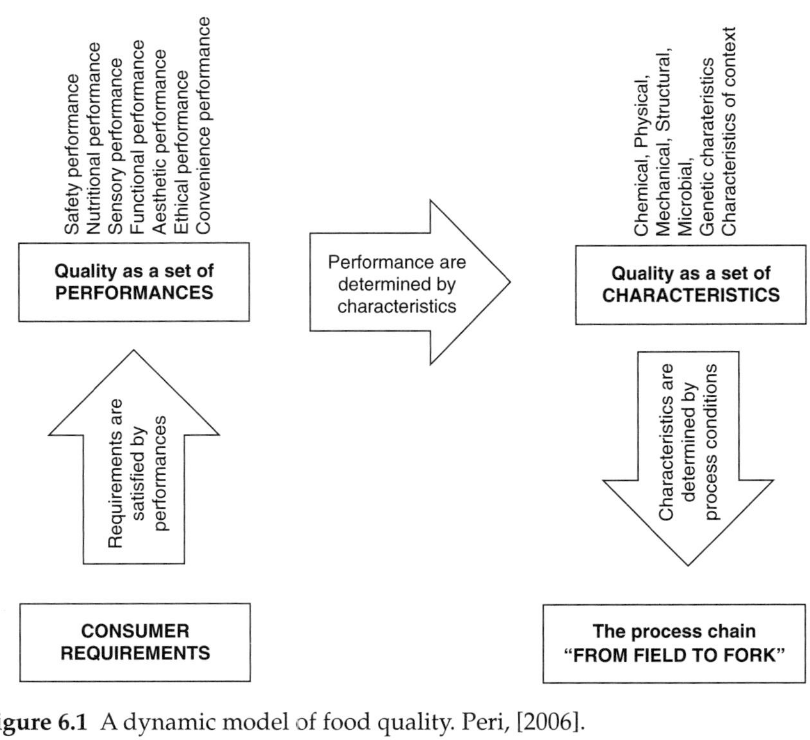

Figure 6.1 A dynamic model of food quality. Peri, [2006].

References

1. D.A. Bender. *Benders dictionary of nutrition and food technology*, 8th ed. Woodhead Publishing Ltd. Cambridge: England, 2006.
2. J.E. Olesen, M. Trnka, K.C. Kersebaum, A.O. Skjelväg, B. Seguin, P. Peltonen-Sainio, F. Rossi, J. Kozyra, F. Micale. Impacts and adaptation of European crop productivity systems to climate change. *European Journal of Agronomy* 34:96–112, 2011.
3. F.M. DaMatta, A. Grandis, B.C. Arenque, M.S. Buckeridge. Impact of climate changes on crop physiology and food quality. *Food Research International* 43:1814–1823, 2010.
4. N.G. Gregory. How climatic changes could affect meat quality. *Food Research International* 43:1866-1873, 2010.
5. K.J. Rask and N. Rask. Economic development and food production–consumption balance: A growing global challenge. *Food Policy* 36:186–196, 2011.
6. J.F. Herencia, P.A. Garcia-Galavi., J.A.R. Dorado and C. Maqueda. Comparison of nutritional quality of the crops grown in an organic and conventional fertilized soil. *Scientia Horticulturae* 129:882–888, 2011.
7. N.G. Halford, and P.R. Shewry. Genetically modified crops: Methodology, benefits, regulation and public concerns. *British Med. Bulletin* 56:62–73, 2000.
8. C.S. Brennan, and L.J. Cleary. The potential use of cereal (1-3,1-4)-ß-D-glucans as functional food ingredients. *Journal of Cereal Science* 42:1–13, 2005.
9. W.D. Hohenboken. Application of sexed semen in cattle production. *Theriogenology* 52:1421–1433, 1999.
10. M.B. Wheeler, J.J. Rutledge, A.F. Brown, T. VanEtten, S. Malusky, D.J. Beebe. Application of sexed semen technology to in vitro embryo production in cattle. *Theriogenology* 65:219–227, 2006.
11. H. Hayakawa, T. Hirai, A.Takimoto, A. Ideta, and Y. Aoyagi. Superovulation and embryo transfer in Holstein cattle using sexed sperm. *Theriogenolgy* 71:68–73, 2009.
12. A. Nardone, B. Ronchi, N. Lacetera, M.S. Ranieri, and U. Bernabucci. Effect of climate change on animal production and sustainability of livestock systems. *Livestock Science* 130:57–69, 2010.
13. FAO Cereal Supply and Demand Brief. 2011.WWW. fao.org.
14. K.G. Cassman. Ecological intensification of cereal production systems: Yield potential, soil quality and precision agriculture. Proceedings of the National Academy of Science, USA, Vol. 96, 5952–5959, 1999.
15. S.Wang, J.P. Melnyk, R. Tsao, and M.F. Marcone. How natural dietary antioxidants in fruits, vegetables and legume promote vascular health. *Food Research International* 44:14–22, 2011.
16. A. Bender. Meat and meat products in human nutrition in developing countries. FAO Food and Nutrition Paper #53. Food Policy and Nutrition Division of FAO, 2:1–88, 1992.
17. C. Neumann, D.M. Harris, and L.M. Rogers. Contribution of animal source foods in improving diet quality and function in children in the developing world. *Nutrition Research* 22:193–220, 2002.

18. P.S. Mir, P.A. McAllister, S. Scott, J. Aalhus, V. Baron, D. McCartney, E.Charmley, L. Goonewardene, J. Basarab, E. Okine, R.J. Weselake, and Z. Mir. Conjugated linoleic acid-enriched beef production. *American Journal of Clinical Nutrition* 79 (supl): 1207S-11S. 2004.
19. A.W. Speedy. Global production and consumption of animal source foods. *Journal of Nutrition* 133:4048S-4053S, 2003.
20. K.-C. Nam, C. Jo, and M. Lee. Meat products and consumption culture in the East. *Meat Science* 86:95–102, 2010.
21. C.L. Delgado. Rising consumption of meat and milk in developing countries has created a new food revolution. *J. Nutr.* 133:3907S-3910S, 2003.
22. R.J. Polkinghorne, and J.M. Thompson. Meat Standards and grading: A world review. *Meat Science* 86:227–235, 2010.
23. A.V.A. Resurrecion. Sensory aspects of consumer choices for meat and meat products. *Meat Science* 66:11–20, 2003.
24. V. Vasta, A. Nudda, A. Cannas, M. Lanza, and A. Priolo. Alternative feed resources and their effects on the quality of meat and milk from small ruminants. *Animal Feed Science and Technology* 147:23–246, 2008.
25. M.A. Yörűk, M. Gűl, A.Hayirli, and M. Macit. The effects of supplementation of humate and probiotic on egg production and quality parameters during the late laying period in hens. *Poultry Science* 83:84–88, 2004.
26. J.S. Um, and K. Paik. Effects of microbial phytase supplementation on egg production, eggshell quality, and mineral retention of laying hens fed different levels of phosphorus. *Poultry Science* 78:75–79, 1999.
27. M.S. Rahman, and O.J. McCarthy. Classification of food properties. *International Journal of Food Properties* 2(2):1–6, 1999.
28. P.P. Lewicki. Water as the determinant of food engineering properties: A review. *Journal of Food Engineering* 61:483–495, 2004.
29. E. Maltini, D. Torreggiani, E. Venir, and G. Bertolo. Water activity and the preservation of plant foods. *Food Chemistry* 82:79–86, 2003.
30. C. Laroche, F. Fine, and P. Gervais. Water activity affects heat resistance of microorganisms in food powders. *International Journal of Food Microbiology* 97:307–315, 2005.
31. C. Peri. The universe of food quality. *Food Quality and Preference* 17:3–8, 2006.
32. A. Hoisington, M.M. Manore, C. Raab. Nutritional quality of emergency foods. *J. American Dietetic Assoc.* 111:573–576, 2011.
33. P. Combris, R. Goglia, M. Henini, I.G. Soler, M. Spiteri. Improvement of the nutritional quality of foods as a public health tool. *Public Health*, doi: 19.1016/j.puhe, 2011.07.004.
34. G. Kedia, R. Wang, H. Patel, and S.S. Pandiella. Use of mixed cultures for the fermentation of cereal-based substrates with potential probiotic properties. *Process Biochemistry* 42:65–70, 2007.

7

Regulatory Aspects of Food Ingredients in the United States: Focus on the Safety of Enzyme Preparations Used in Food

Shayla West-Barnette and Jannavi R. Srinivasan

U.S. Food and Drug Administration, Center for Food Safety and Applied Nutrition, Office of Food Additive Safety, Maryland, USA

Abstract

Enzyme preparations have long been used throughout the world as ingredients in various foods such as cheeses, yogurts, breads, and alcoholic beverages. In the United States, the Food and Drug Administration (FDA) is responsible for ensuring the safety of the use of food ingredients that are either added to food, used in food processing, or otherwise become a component of food. In this regard, the FDA uses a science-based approach to evaluate the safety of the uses of enzyme preparations in food and food processing. This chapter discusses the FDA's regulatory framework for food ingredients from a historical perspective, and provides the agency's current thinking on safety evaluations of enzyme preparations added to food or used in food processing. This chapter also discusses how FDA's safety evaluations of enzyme preparations have kept pace with current technologies that are used by enzyme manufacturers.

Keywords: Enzyme, enzyme preparation, food ingredients, recombinant DNA technology, microorganism, regulatory, GRAS, GMP, exposure, safety studies

Visakh P. M., Sabu Thomas, Laura B. Iturriaga, and Pablo Daniel Ribotta (eds.) Advances in Food Science and Technology, (201–226) © 2013 Scrivener Publishing LLC

7.1 Introduction

Since ancient times, enzymes have been used in the preparation of various foods such as cheeses, yogurts, breads, and alcoholic beverages [1]. Although these uses have spanned thousands of years, scientific understanding of how enzymes function did not formally develop until the 19th century [1]. One of the earliest observations of enzyme activity occurred in 1814, when Kirchoff noted the decomposition of starch by germinated barley [2]. In 1833, the first clear observance of a specific enzyme-catalyzed reaction was made by Puyen and Persey, who found that a precipitate from malt extract contained a heat-stable substance that could convert starch to sugar [3]. This substance was named "diastase" based on its ability to separate soluble dextrins from insoluble starch granules [4]. Later, diastase was renamed malt alpha amylase [4]. Further observations in the late 19th century elucidated a variety of reactions catalyzed by enzymes, thereby enhancing knowledge in this area [5].

Given the array of reactions that involve enzymes, it is not surprising that much effort has been dedicated to characterizing their biochemical nature. To date, there are 3,540 enzymes, many of whose structures and activities have been identified [5]. Of these, many are used in food production and processing to achieve a variety of desired technical effects.

In the United States (U.S.), the Food and Drug Administration (FDA) is responsible for ensuring the safety of the use of food ingredients that are either added to food, used in food processing, or otherwise become a component of food. In this regard, the FDA uses a science-based approach to evaluate the safety of the uses of enzyme preparations in food and food processing. A discussion of what constitutes an enzyme preparation is discussed later in this chapter. This chapter discusses the FDA's regulatory framework for food ingredients from a historical perspective and lays out the agency's current thinking on safety evaluations of enzyme preparations added to food or used in food processing. This chapter also discusses how FDA's safety evaluations have kept pace with current technologies used by enzyme manufacturers.

7.2 Regulatory History of Food Ingredients: Guided by Safety

In 1906, the U.S. Congress passed the nation's first comprehensive consumer protection law in response to serious abuses in the consumer marketplace [6]. This law, named the Pure Food and Drug Act (the 1906 Act), defined "food" as "all articles used for food, drink, confectionery, or condiment by man or other animals, whether simple, mixed, or compound(ed)." The statutes in the 1906 act focused on postmarket surveillance with the intention of prohibiting the sale to the consumer of harmful or mislabeled food and drugs [7, 8]. Since the law was limited in scope, many hazardous foods and drugs continued to be marketed. A pivotal case occurred when several deaths were reported after the use of a medical preparation known as "Elixir of Sulfanilimide" in 1937. The resulting public outrage led to congressional action that allowed for tighter controls over food and drugs. In 1938, Congress passed the Federal Food, Drug, and Cosmetic Act (1938 Act). The 1938 Act included provisions for premarket safety evaluations for drugs and enhanced postmarket surveillance for food and drugs [9, 10]. Importantly, the 1938 Act represented a shift toward premarket controls for drugs; however, it did not provide the FDA with similar authority for foods [8]. Food ingredients could be placed in the food supply without the FDA's knowledge or safety review. According to the 1938 Act, when the FDA questioned the safety of a food ingredient, the agency was responsible for proving that the food ingredient was unsafe.

During the early 1950s, a committee led by James Delaney held hearings to address the use of food ingredients [6]. In a report based on these hearings, the committee estimated that nearly 840 ingredients were used in food. Of these, only about 420 were considered safe, and many had never been evaluated for safety. This report, along with incidents of chemical contamination of food that occurred in 1954 and 1958, prompted Congress to amend the 1938 Act with the 1958 Food Additives Amendment. The 1958 Amendment gave the FDA the authority to conduct premarket safety reviews and issue regulatory approvals for "food additives" [11]. The 1958 Amendment defined food additives as "all substances...the intended use of which results or may reasonably be expected to result, directly or indirectly, either in their becoming a component of food or otherwise affecting the characteristics of food." Under the 1958 Amendment, new food additives are considered to be unsafe for their intended uses until they are proven safe based on data and other scientific information [12]. Thus, the 1958 Amendment placed the burden of proving safety on the manufacturer, and the FDA was tasked with reviewing the safety information and making a safety decision.

Excluded from the food additive definition were "substances that are generally recognized, among experts qualified by scientific training and experience to evaluate their safety as having been adequately shown...to be safe under the conditions of intended use." Based on this exclusion, a new concept to food—the Generally Recognized as Safe (GRAS) paradigm—was created. Under this paradigm, any food ingredient that is GRAS based on a history of safe use in food prior to January 1, 1958 is exempt from the mandatory premarket safety review and regulatory approval required for food additives [13]. Also exempt as GRAS are food ingredients that have been scientifically shown to be safe for their intended uses based on publicly available data and information reflecting the consensus of scientific opinion.

In 1959, the FDA published a list of about 180 food ingredients whose uses were considered to be GRAS in Volume 21 of the Code of Federal Regulations (21 CFR), Part 182 (formerly §121.101(d)) [14]. The FDA did not intend for this list to be a comprehensive one including all GRAS food ingredient uses, as many commonly used food ingredients such as water and salt had long been recognized as safe by experts and consumers [6, 15]. Instead, the agency intended that the list include food ingredients whose uses were recognized as safe by experts, but were not easily recognized as safe by consumers.

In 1969, a private laboratory conducted animal studies on cyclamate (a sweetener), which had previously been included in the GRAS list [16]. The results of the studies suggested that cyclamate was a carcinogen. This led to a comprehensive review of the uses of cyclamate in food and prompted the removal of this food ingredient use from the GRAS list (the Delaney Clause, which was part of the 1958 Amendment, prohibited the use in food of any ingredient found to induce cancer in man, or, after tests, found to induce cancer in animals). The ensuing public concern over the safety of food ingredient uses considered to be GRAS led to a presidentially-mandated GRAS review [17]. The review led to what was termed the GRAS affirmation process. Under this process, the FDA responded to GRAS affirmation petitions by conducting comprehensive safety evaluations of GRAS ingredient uses in food. If the FDA concluded that there were sufficient data and information to support the GRAS status of a food ingredient's use, then the FDA affirmed the GRAS status of the ingredient's use through notice and comment rulemaking [6, 18]. GRAS-affirmed food ingredient uses were then listed in 21 CFR Parts 184 and 186.

The GRAS affirmation process proved to be resource-intensive for the agency. Therefore, in 1997 the agency published a proposal to have a voluntary GRAS notification program replace the GRAS affirmation process [15]. Under the proposed rule, a manufacturer may make its own GRAS determination for a food ingredient use and may then choose to contact the FDA about the determination by submitting a notice containing the data and information supporting the manufacturer's GRAS determination. When a manufacturer submits a GRAS notice to the FDA describing its conclusion that the use of a food ingredient is GRAS, the FDA evaluates the submitted data and information. The FDA also considers whether the safety data are generally available (i.e., published in the scientific literature) and reflect a consensus of scientific opinion. At the conclusion of the evaluation, the FDA responds to the GRAS notice with a letter. If the FDA finds that the data and information in the GRAS notice meet the standards for a GRAS determination, then the agency responds with a "no questions" letter. If the FDA finds that the notice does not meet the standards for a GRAS determination, then the agency responds with a "no basis" letter. These agency opinion letters differ from the regulations published as part of the older GRAS affirmation process and after FDA's safety evaluations and premarket approvals of food additive uses.

Importantly, the safety standard for food additive uses and GRAS food ingredient uses is the same, and, as a matter of principle, a food additive use is not safer than a GRAS food ingredient use [8]. The quality and quantity of data needed to support the safety of a food additive use and the quality and quantity of data needed to support the safety of a GRAS food ingredient use are equivalent. The key element distinguishing GRAS food ingredient uses from food additive uses is the common knowledge of the safety data and information. For GRAS food ingredient uses, the data and information relied on to establish safety must be generally available *and* there must be a basis to conclude that there is a consensus among qualified experts about the safety of the food ingredient for its intended use [15]. These concepts are graphically illustrated in Figure 7.1.

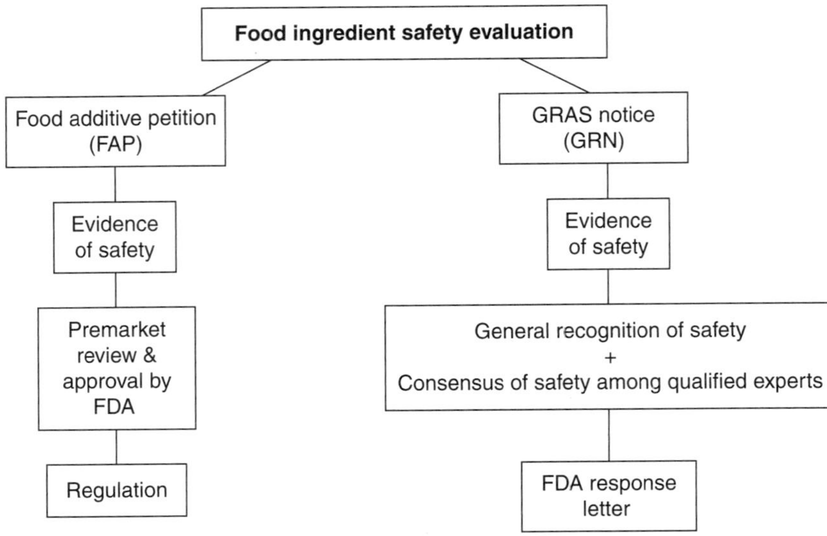

Figure 7.1 Comparison of safety evaluations for food additives and GRAS food ingredients.

7.3 Scientific Advancement as Part of the Regulatory History of Enzyme Preparations

Given the wide variety of reactions that enzymes catalyze, enzyme preparations are commonly used in food processing and in some instances in food itself. Enzyme preparations share their regulatory history in the U.S. with other food ingredients. The technology with which some enzymes are produced has also been a part of this regulatory history.

As early as 1969, the FDA had regulated some enzyme preparations as food additives under 21 CFR Part 173. These are listed in Table 7.1.

Later, numerous enzyme preparations were affirmed as GRAS in 21 CFR Part 184. These are listed in Table 7.2. The enzyme preparations listed in these regulatory categories have a wide range of technical effects and contain enzymes derived from a variety of sources including plants, animal tissues, and microorganisms (most were derived from microorganisms). In the past, microorganisms used in the production of enzyme preparations were either naturally occurring microbial strains or had been improved by selection of spontaneous mutants or by traditional mutagenesis.

Table 7.1 Enzyme preparations approved as secondary direct food additives permitted for human consumption.

Regulation	Name of Enzyme Preparation	Intended Use	Year
173.110	Amyloglucosidase derived from *Rhizopus niveus*	For degrading gelatinized starch into constituent sugars, in the production of distilled spirits and vinegar	1975
173.115	Alpha-acetolactate decarboxylase (α-ALDC) enzyme preparation derived from a recombinant *Bacillus subtilis*	As a processing aid in the production of alcoholic malt beverages and distilled liquors	2001
173.120	Carbohydrase and cellulase derived from *Aspergillus niger*	For removal of visceral mass (bellies) in clam processing; as an aid in the removal of the shell from the edible tissue in shrimp processing	1970
173.140	Esterase-lipase derived from *Mucor miehei*	As a flavor enhancer	1982
173.145	Alpha-Galactosidase derived from *Mortierella vinaceae* var. *raffinoseutilizer*	For use in the production of sugar (sucrose) from sugar beets	1974
173.150	Milk-clotting enzymes, microbial (derived from *Endothia parasitica, Bacillus cereus, Mucor pusillus, Mucor miehei Cooney et Emerson, Aspergillus oryzae*	In the production of those cheeses for which it is permitted by standards of identity	1969
173.170	Aminoglycoside 3´-phosphotransferase II	Catalyzes the phosphorylation of certain aminoglycoside antibiotics and is used as a selectable marker in the development of genetically modified cotton, oilseed rape, and tomatoes	1994

Table 7.2 Enzyme preparations affirmed as GRAS.

Regulation	Name of Enzyme Preparation	Intended Use	Year
184.1012	Alpha-amylase enzyme preparation from *Bacillus stearothermophilus*	Hydrolysis of edible starch to produce maltodextrins and nutritive carbohydrate sweeteners	1995
184. 1024	Bromelain (an enzyme preparation derived from the pineapples *Ananus comosus* and *A. bracteatus*)	To hydrolyze proteins or polypeptides	1995
184.1027	Mixed carbohydrase and protease enzyme product	To hydrolyze proteins or carbohydrates	1983
184.1034	Catalase (bovine liver)	To decompose hydrogen peroxide	1995
184.1148	Bacterially-derived carbohydrase enzyme preparation	To hydrolyze polysaccharides	1999
184.1150	Bacterially-derived protease enzyme preparation	To hydrolyze proteins or polypeptides	1999
184.1250	Cellulase enzyme preparation derived from *Trichoderma longibrachiatum*	For the breakdown of cellulose	1999
184.1316	Ficin (enzyme preparation derived from the latex of species of the genus *Ficus*)	To hydrolyze proteins or polypeptides	1995
184.1372	Insoluble glucose isomerase enzyme preparations	To convert glucose to fructose	1983
184.1387	Lactase enzyme preparation from *Candida pseudotropicalis*	To convert lactose to glucose and galactose	1996
184.1388	Lactase enzyme preparation from *Kluyveromyces lactis*	To convert lactose to glucose and galactose	1984
184. 1415	Animal lipase (enzyme preparation obtained from edible forestomach tissue of calves, kids, or lambs, or from animal pancreatic)	To hydrolyze fatty acid glycerides	1995

Regulation	Name of Enzyme Preparation	Intended Use	Year
184.1420	Lipase enzyme preparation derived from *Rhizopus niveus*	For the interesterification of fats and oils	1998
184.1443a	Malt (enzyme preparation derived from barley)	To hydrolyze starch or starch derived polysaccharides	1995
184.1583	Pancreatin (enzyme preparation obtained from porcine or bovine pancreatic tissue)	To hydrolyze proteins or polypeptides	1995
184.1585	Papain (proteolytic enzyme derived from *Carica papaya L.*)	As an enzyme, processing aid, and texturizer	1983
184.1595	Pepsin (enzyme preparation obtained from the glandular layer of hog stomach)	To hydrolyze proteins or polypeptides	1995
184.1685	Rennet (animal-derived) and chymosin preparation (fermentation-derived)	As an enzyme, a processing aid, a stabilizer, and thickener	1990
184.1914	Trypsin (enzyme preparation obtained from purified extracts of porcine or bovine pancreas)	To hydrolyze proteins or polypeptides	1995
184.1924	Urease enzyme preparation from *Lactobacillus fermentum*	To convert urea to ammonia and carbon dioxide	1992
184.1985	Aminopeptidase enzyme preparation derived from *Lactococcus lactis*	As an enzyme, as an optional ingredient for flavor development in the manufacture of cheddar cheese, and in the preparation of protein hydrolysates	1995

As the food processing industry became more sophisticated and moved toward responding to increased product demand, it was faced with several challenges. Among these was the impetus to optimize the chemical attributes of enzymes used in various applications in the food industry [19, 20, 21]. In addition, there was a need to develop enzymes that have uniform composition and consistent activity in higher amounts in order to respond to industry needs [1, 22]. The emergence of recombinant DNA techniques during the 1990s, including gene cloning, protein engineering, sequencing, and bioinformatics, helped the enzyme manufacturing industry address these challenges. Recombinant enzyme systems allow for insertion of DNA encoding desired enzymes into known strains that can be genetically manipulated. One advantage of using these systems is that some enzyme encoding genes can be manipulated to produce enzymes that are optimized for the conditions of industrial use. For example, alpha amylase is used in the production of sweeteners from starch, a process which involves high temperatures [19]. The native alpha amylase is unstable at these temperatures. To address this issue, a recombinant form of the enzyme with a modified amino acid sequence was developed. This recombinant enzyme has increased thermal stability and other improved properties. Another advantage of recombinant enzyme systems is the ability to produce higher enzyme yields. For example, chymosin, an enzyme commonly used in the dairy industry, was historically derived from calf tissues [23]. Genetically manipulated microorganisms were shown to produce recombinant chymosin at higher levels due to lower proteolysis. Reflective of the emergence of recombinant DNA techniques, in 1991 bovine chymosin derived from *Escherichia coli* strain K-12 became the first recombinant food enzyme to be GRAS-affirmed by FDA in 21 CFR Part 184, Paragraph 1685 [19, 24]. This recombinant chymosin served as an example of an emerging technology that in the years to follow would be increasingly used to manufacture enzymes intended for use in food and food processing.

The enzyme preparations with GRAS claims that have not been questioned under the FDA's GRAS Notification Program are listed in Table 7.3 [25]. Notably, all of the enzymes listed in this table are microbially-derived, and enzymes from recombinant microorganisms are the subjects of nearly half of these GRAS notices. FDA's evaluations of these notices demonstrate that the agency's scientific and regulatory evaluative framework is flexible, addressing both

Table 7.3 List of GRAS notices that received a "no questions" letter from the FDA as of August 2011.

GRAS Notice No.	Enzyme	Source	Intended Use
20	Pullulanase	*Bacillus subtilis*	In hydrolyzing starch and starch-related compounds in the production of corn sweeteners, baked goods, and alcoholic beverages
32	Pectin lyase	*Trichoderma reesei*	In the preparation of fruit and vegetable juices, purees, and concentrates
43	Lipase	*Aspergillus oryzae*	In dough, baked goods, and the fats and oil industry as a processing aid for the interesterification or hydrolysis of glycerides and as an enzyme in brewing beer
68	Lipase	*Penicillium camembertii*	In fats and oils to produce fatty acids or glycerides
79	Alpha-amylase	*Bacillus licheniformis*	For the liquefaction of starch in the production of syrups and for the thinning of starch in distilling mashes in the production of alcohol
81	Lipase	*Candida rugosa*	In fats and oils to produce fatty acids or glycerides; in the esterification of fatty acids to produce glycerides
85	Isoamylase	*Pseudomonas amyloderamosa*	As a debranching enzyme that hydrolyzes alpha-1,6-glucosidic linkages in glycogen, amylopectin, and their alpha-limit dextrins
88	Invertase and Lactase	*Saccharomyces cerevisiae* and *Kluyveromyces marxianus*	In foods in general

(Continued)

Table 7.3 (cont.)

GRAS Notice No.	Enzyme	Source	Intended Use
89	Carbohydrase, catalase, glucose oxidase, pectinase, and protease	*Aspergillus niger*	In foods in general
90	Carbohydrase, protease, and carbohydrase	*Aspergillus oryzae*, *Aspergillus oryzae*, and *Rhizopus oryzae*	In foods in general
103	Lipase	*Aspergillus oryzae*	In bakery products, egg yolks, whole eggs, and fats and oils
106	Glucose oxidase	*Aspergillus oryzae*	In baking applications and in the manufacture of foods such as cheese, beer, carbonated beverages, and fruit juice
111	Lipase	*Aspergillus niger*	In dairy-based flavoring preparations, cheeses, liquid and dried egg white, bread, flour, unstandardized bakery products, modified triglycerides, hydrolyzed lecithin, edible fats and oils, and modified egg yolk
113	Lipase	*Aspergillus oryzae*	In dairy-based flavoring preparations, cheeses, liquid and dried egg white, bread, flour, unstandardized bakery products, modified triglycerides, hydrolyzed lecithin, edible fats and oils, and modified egg yolk
114	Pectate lyase	*Bacillus subtilis*	In fruit and vegetable purees and concentrates
122	Laccase	*Aspergillus oryzae*	In breath freshening products (such as breath mints and chewing gum)

GRAS Notice No.	Enzyme	Source	Intended Use
126	Alpha-amylase	*Pseudomonas fluorescens* Biovar1	For the hydrolysis of edible starch to produce various starch hydrolysis products and to produce fermentable sugars for use in the production of distilled ethanol for alcoholic beverages
132	Lactase	*Aspergillus niger*	In the dairy industry to hydrolyze lactose found in milk, whey, cheese, yogurt, and other dairy products
142	Phospholipase	*Aspergillus oryzae*	In thc production of cheese
145	Phospholipase A2	*Streptomyces violaceoruber*	To hydrolyze soy and egg yolk lecithins
149	Beta-glucanase	*Trichoderma harzianum*	To improve the clarification and filtration of wines
158	Lipase	*Aspergillus niger*	In the production of triglyceride products
183	Phospholipase A2		To hydrolyze phospholipids in bread dough, fine bakery wares, and egg yolk-based products
195	Mixed beta-Glucanase and xylanase	*Humicola insolens*	In the brewing industry for clarifying beer
201	Asparaginase	*Aspergillus oryzae*	In reducing L-asparagine levels in wheat dough-based products such as cookies and crackers, fabricated potato chips, and cut or sliced potato products
204	Phospholipase C	*Pichia pastoris*	In degumming vegetable oils for food use
205	Pullulanase	*Bacillus subtilis*	In the brewing industry (to hydrolyze 1-6- alpha-D-glucosidic linkages in pullulan, amylopectin, and glycogen)

(Continued)

Table 7.3 (cont.)

GRAS Notice No.	Enzyme	Source	Intended Use
212	Phospholipase A2	*Streptomyces violaceruber*	To hydrolyze soy and egg yolk lecithins
214	Asparaginase	*Aspergillus niger*	To lower free L-asparagine levels in breads, cereal-based products, potato-based products, and reaction flavors
216	Lipase	*Rhizopus oryzae*	To produce tailored triglycerides for use in infant formula
230	Chymosin	*Trichoderma reesei*	For milk coagulation during cheese making
238	Lipase	*Hansenula polymorpha*	To modify lipids in dough for bakery and noodle applications, in egg yolks for bakery applications and mayonnaise production, and in the refining process of soy bean oil
265	Glycerophospholipid cholesterol acyltransferase (GCAT)	*Bacillus licheniformis*	To modify phospholipids to lyso-phospholipids and cholesterol ester in egg yolks to avoid product separation during mayonnaise production; processed meat products for emulsification, better consistency, and reduced cooking loss; cheese for increased yield; eggs to give a softer and more tender crumb in bakery products, and degumming of vegetable oils; as an enzyme in the production of ultra-high temperature processed milk, powdered milk, and yogurt
267	Protein glutaminase	*Chryseobacterium proteolyticum*	To deamidate vegetable proteins (cereal, soy, and pea), milk proteins, and yeast proteins; and, to deamidate proteins in baked goods, dairy foods such as yogurt, cheese, and ice-cream, egg-based foods such as mayonnaise, and cakes

GRAS Notice No.	Enzyme	Source	Intended Use
274	Branching glycosyltransferase	*Bacillus subtilis*	In the starch industry to obtain dextrins with improved physical properties, such as higher solubility, lower viscosity, and reduced retrogradation
277	Maltotetraohydrolase	*Bacillus licheniformis*	In bread and other baked goods to delay the staling process
292	Cellulase	*Myceliophthora thermophila*	In the production of wine, beer and fruit juices
296	Lipase	*Aspergillus niger*	In baked goods to enhance the gas holding capacity of the dough, leading to an increased stability of the dough upon proofing
315	Transglucosidase	*Trichoderma reesei*	In the production of isomalto-oligosaccharide syrups from starch and potable ethanol from molasses
333	Acid fungal protease	*Trichoderma reesei*	In grain processing (corn steeping), alcoholic beverage (potable alcohol) manufacture, and degumming of membranes during orange juice manufacturing
345	Carboxypeptidase	*Aspergillus niger*	In production of cheese to accelerate the ripening process, in production of enzyme-modified cheese as a debittering aid, and in fermented meat to accelerate the development of flavor during the ripening process
372	Glucoamylase	*Trichoderma reesei*	In grain processing, including the manufacture of corn sweeteners such as high fructose corn syrup, brewing, potable alcohol manufacture, and lactic acid production

conventionally-produced enzyme preparations and those produced using advanced technologies.

7.4 Safety Evaluation of Enzyme Preparations

In its review of submissions for enzyme preparations, the FDA considers the identity of the enzyme (including the enzyme source), the manufacturing process and composition, intended use and technical effect, estimates of dietary exposure, and relevant safety studies. In general, the same safety considerations apply to all enzyme preparations. However, additional information pertaining to genetic modification of the enzyme source is expected in submissions for recombinant enzyme preparations [26].

7.4.1 Identity of the Enzyme

A description of an enzyme's identity can include: the accepted name, systematic name, Enyzme Commission (EC) number according to the recommendations of the International Union of Biochemistry and Molecular Biology [5], other names by which the enzyme may be classified, and a CAS registry number, if available. The EC number is used to classify an enzyme based on the reaction(s) it catalyzes, and the CAS registry number is a unique numeric identifier that links a substance to specific chemical information [27]. The physical and chemical properties that define an enzyme include its activity, substrate specificity, and the key reaction(s) catalyzed by the enzyme. Other properties that may be used to identify an enzyme include specific activity, molecular weight, amino acid sequence, and stability and activity as a function of temperature and pH, if available. The primary structure of the enzyme can be modified via chemical or genetic methods. Such an alteration can affect enzyme performance under the intended conditions of use, as in the case of the modified alpha amylase discussed earlier.

Information on the source of an enzyme is another key component relating to the enzyme's identity. The enzyme preparations that the FDA has reviewed for safe use in food have been derived from a wide variety of sources. These include animal tissues (e.g., porcine and bovine livers), plants and plant products (e.g., pineapple, papaya, barley, and fig), and bacteria and fungi. Enzyme sources should comply with the principles outlined in the monograph "Enzyme Preparations" (section "Other Requirements") of the 6th (2008) or current edition of the Food Chemicals Codex (FCC) [28]. These principles are discussed in subsequent paragraphs.

When animal tissue is used as an enzyme source, the tissue should comply with the applicable U.S. meat inspection requirements and should be handled in accordance with good hygienic practices [29]. Under the Federal Meat Inspection Act of 1906, the United States Department of Agriculture has jurisdiction over meat and meat products. When plant material is used as an enzyme source, components of the material should not leave harmful residues in the finished food under normal conditions of use. Examples of enzymes derived from animal tissue and plant material are included in Table 7.2. Since the vast majority of enzyme preparations produced in the industry and reviewed by the FDA are from microbial sources, the remainder of this section will focus on the safety evaluations of microbially-derived enzyme preparations [22].

When an enzyme is derived from a microorganism, the production microorganism must be well characterized and demonstrated to be nonpathogenic and nontoxigenic [20, 22]. Characterization of the source microorganism generally include relevant information about the microorganism's taxonomy, morphology, and growth characteristics.

A discussion of the source microorganism's taxonomy usually includes information about the organism's origin and isolation, as well as information about its taxonomic classification. The field of microbial classification is continuously evolving. In the past, many microorganisms were classified according to their morphological characteristics. However, applications of gene-based analyses have resulted in the reclassifications of microorganisms at the species and genus levels. For example, *Bacillus stearothermophilus* was recently reclassified as *Geobacillus stearothermophilus* using 16S rRNA gene sequencing and bioinformatic analysis, among other methods [30].

Information about the production microorganism's morphology may include microscopic observations such as cell shape and colony appearance. The discussion of the microorganism's growth characteristics may include information about its growth requirements.

It is generally accepted that pathogenic microorganisms would not be used in the production of enzymes intended for use in food [20]. A nonpathogenic microorganism is "one that is very unlikely to produce disease under ordinary circumstances [22]." The nonpathogenic nature of a microorganism is often demonstrated using information about its natural occurrence in food or prior industrial use. For example, *Bacillus licheniformis* strains are common in soil, and as such can be found in cereals and other agricultural products. Consequently, spores of the microorganism are commonly found in processed or dried foods, as well as in herbs and spices [31]. Additionally, *B. licheniformis* has been used to produce several enzyme preparations that have been reviewed by the FDA (see Tables 7.1–3). In cases where production microorganisms are not commonly found in foods and do not have prior industrial uses, studies conducted using animal models may be used to demonstrate the nonpathogenic nature of the microorganism.

A nontoxigenic microorganism is "one which does not produce injurious substances at levels that are detectable or demonstrably harmful under ordinary conditions of use or exposure [22]." It is widely understood that some microbial strains (mainly fungal strains) normally considered to be nontoxigenic are capable of producing toxins when cultured under certain growth conditions. For example, *Aspergillus oryzae* strain A1560 can produce low levels of mycotoxins when cultured in certain media. However, the strain has been genetically modified to eliminate the pathways involved in mycotoxin production. Many other commercial strains have been modified in this manner. In some cases, the growth conditions for fungi that are capable of producing mycotoxins can be adjusted and monitored to minimize or eliminate mycotoxin synthesis. For example, published reports show that mycotoxin production by *A. niger* can be minimized by controlling the fermentation conditions [32]. When applicable, such adjustments to the growth conditions should be discussed to support the safety of the fungal enzyme source. Also, appropriate analytical tests should be conducted and specifications set to assure that enzyme preparations intended for use in food do not contain mycotoxins at unsafe levels.

Once a microorganism is shown to be nonpathogenic and nontoxigenic, it may either be used in enzyme production as is or may be used to develop other production microorganisms via recombinant DNA techniques or classical mutagenesis. If the microorganism is used in the development of other production microorganisms, a discussion of the modifications is necessary for FDA's safety evaluation.

In the case of genetically modified (also referred to as genetically engineered) microorganisms (GMMs), thorough characterization of the introduced DNA sequences, as well as the source(s) of the sequences is important. All introduced sequences should be identified, including genes encoding the enzyme and any selectable markers, and regulatory DNA sequences. The introduced sequences may be derived from laboratory-adapted organisms, organisms sampled from the environment, or may be generated from a pool of genes from various sources. The "donors" of the DNA sequences should be well-characterized as described above.

In some cases, the enzyme-encoding genes themselves may be modified by classical mutagenesis techniques such as ultraviolet radiation or chemical mutagenesis. This was the case for the previously-described recombinant alpha-amylase that had improved thermostability, which was critical for its use in the production of sweeteners.

Regardless of the techniques used to modify the production microorganism or the enzyme itself, all approaches and steps involved should be described in a submission to FDA.

7.4.2 Manufacturing Process and Composition

Enzyme preparations should be produced in accordance with the current good manufacturing practice (cGMP) [33]. When enzyme preparations are obtained from microorganisms, the details of the fermentation process should be described. This includes all steps and controls necessary to maintain the proper growth conditions, and assure the purity and genetic stability of the culture. Some enzymes are isolated from the cellular mass (e.g., chymosin), while most enzymes are secreted to the fermentation broth and subsequently purified and concentrated. All of the procedures used to isolate the enzyme from the cellular material or the fermentation broth should be described, including chemical and physical treatments and quality controls. All materials used in the fermentation and subsequent downstream processing (including antifoaming and flocculating agents, if used) should be identified as suitable for use in food processing.

It is important to distinguish the enzyme itself from the enzyme preparation which it is a component of. The active enzyme responsible for the intended technical effect is the functional component of an enzyme preparation. Enzyme preparations may contain a blend of two or more active enzymes. For the manufactured enzyme to successfully catalyze a given chemical reaction during food processing or in the final food, other components may be required. These typically include formulating agents intentionally added to the preparation such as diluents, preservatives, stabilizers, or other substances suitable for use in food. These ingredients are added to the enzyme to stabilize and adjust the enzyme activity and prevent microbial contamination. An enzyme preparation may also contain the residues of compounds used in the manufacturing process (e.g., fermentation medium) or cellular constituents derived from the production microorganism.

Since the enzyme is the active component of an enzyme preparation, it is important to know how much enzyme is present in a preparation. This information is critical for estimating dietary intake of the enzyme. The total organic solids (TOS) of an enzyme preparation refers to the sum of all organic compounds in the enzyme preparation derived from the enzyme source and manufacturing process including the enzyme. The percent TOS is calculated as follows:

$$(\%)\ \text{TOS} = 100 - \text{A} - \text{W} - \text{D}$$

where: A = % ash, W = % water, D = % diluents and other formulation ingredients.

All enzyme preparations used for food processing should conform to specifications for purity as outlined in the monograph, "Enzyme Preparations" of the 6th (2008) or current edition of the Food Chemicals Codex (FCC) [28]. Conformance to set specifications for enzyme preparations used in food processing should be shown by relying on analysis of several manufacturing lots. Standard analytical methods (such as those described in the FCC) used to meet the specifications should be referenced. If used, non-standard methods (such as those established internally by the manufacturer) should be validated and described. The enzyme activity in the final enzyme preparation should be measured and the unit of enzyme activity should be defined.

7.4.2.1 *Intended Use(s) and Technical Effect(s)*

The technical effect(s) of the enzyme as well as its intended use(s) and use level(s) in foods should be described. It is also important to discuss whether the active enzyme is likely to be present in the final food or will be inactivated or removed. The identity and safety of the products of the enzymatic reaction should also be discussed, if appropriate.

7.4.2.2 Estimates of Dietary Exposure

An estimate of dietary exposure to the enzyme preparation should be discussed as a component of an overall safety assessment. Enzyme preparations are used in food processing at very low levels and often are removed from the final food or inactivated. For example, enzymes used in processing starch into glucose or high fructose corn syrup are removed during purification of the syrup. Also, enzymes used in baked goods are inactivated by high temperatures during baking. Although most enzyme preparations are not expected to be carried over in their entirety to the final food, they may still be present at residual levels and should thus be assessed for safety. Even if the enzyme preparation is removed from food, the residual level of the enzyme in TOS, "as consumed" should be estimated if possible.

It is generally accepted that the estimated daily intake (EDI) of the enzyme preparation is calculated on the basis of TOS. It would be optimal to use the level of TOS in the final food. However, in most instances it is not possible to estimate the TOS content in food. For this reason, the EDIs for enzyme preparations are usually calculated on the basis of TOS use levels, i.e., the levels of TOS added to food or used in the production of food ingredients. This approach substantially overestimates exposure to enzyme preparations.

7.4.2.3 Toxicological Considerations

The need for toxicological assessment of an enzyme in an enzyme preparation should be established on a case-by-case basis. For example, enzymes derived from sources with a history of safe use in the production of other enzyme preparations or food ingredients may not require the same level of toxicological testing as enzyme preparations derived from uncharacterized sources in order to demonstrate safety. If toxicological testing of an enzyme is conducted, the test article is usually the enzyme concentrate from the manufacturing process before the addition of the formulation ingredients. The content of TOS of the tested concentrate is determined and used to derive the no observed adverse effect

Table 7.4 Toxicological tests typically provided in enzyme submissions to FDA.

Test Type	Toxicological Endpoints
Genotoxicity	
Bacterial Reverse Mutation Assay (Ames Test)	Mutagenicity
Chromosomal Aberration Test	Clastogenicity
Gene Mutation Test	Mutagenicity
Short-term	
14-day repeat dose feeding study	Range finding
28-day repeat dose feeding study	Range finding
90-day subchronic study	NOAEL determination
Irritation	
Acute dermal irritation	Local irritant potential
Acute ocular irritation	Local irritant potential

level (NOAEL) calculated as TOS per kilogram bodyweight per day. The safety margin is then calculated by dividing the NOAEL by the EDI calculated on the basis of TOS. The toxicological tests used to confirm safety of enzymes in most enzyme preparations are listed in Table 7.4.

7.4.2.4 Enzyme Preparations Containing Allergenic Ingredients

If an enzyme preparation contains proteins derived from a major food allergen, the enzyme preparation may fall under the provisions of the Food Allergen Labeling and Consumer Protection Act of 2004 (FALPCA), unless it is granted an exemption from allergen labeling as a result of a petition or a notification. According to FALCPA, a major food allergen is defined as one of the following foods and ingredients that contain protein from them: milk, egg, peanuts, tree nuts, soybeans, wheat, fish, and Crustacean shellfish. The food source names of the major food allergens are milk, egg, peanuts, the specific type of tree nut (e.g., almonds), soybeans, wheat, the specific species of fish (e.g., flounder) and the specific species of Crustacean shellfish (e.g., crab). More information on food allergen labeling requirements may be found in the FDA guidance documents for food labeling and nutrition [34].

The assessment of an enzyme that is derived from an allergenic food or has a potential to cause an allergic reaction when consumed should include information that is consistent with the current views of the scientific community. Considerations included in this assessment may include the enzyme source, a comparison of the amino acid sequence of the enzyme to the amino acid sequences of all known allergens, susceptibility of the enzyme to pepsin digestion, and other relevant information, if available.

7.5 Conclusion

Enzymes are ubiquitous in nature and have been used in foods and in food processing for millennia. In response to changes in consumer demand, new developments in molecular biology and manufacturing technologies have paved the way for faster, more efficient routes in food enzyme manufacturing and in the production of food using enzymes. These new developments have also allowed for adjustment of enzyme properties to manufacturing conditions and production of enzyme preparations that contain lower levels of undefined contaminants from the production process. The FDA has continuously adjusted its regulatory procedures to keep up with these evolving technologies. However, regardless of the technology used to manufacture food enzymes, safety has been and will always remain at the core of the FDA's evaluations.

Acknowledgements

The authors acknowledge guidance and support received from Dr. Zofia Olempska-Beer and the management in the Division of Biotechnology and GRAS Notice Review for their review of this manuscript.

References

1. O. Kirk, T.V. Borchert, and C.C. Fuglsang. Industrial enzyme applications. *Current Opinion in Biotechnology* 13:345–351, 2002.
2. H. von Euler. *General chemistry of the enzymes*. Wiley, 1912.
3. G.A. Tucker, and L.F.J. Woods. *Enzymes in food processing*. Springer Netherlands, 1995.
4. J.R. Whitaker. *Principles of enzymology for the food sciences*. 61st ed. CRC, 1994.
5. Historical introduction, IUBMB Website.

6. F.H. Degnan. (1991). Rethinking the applicability and usefulness of the GRAS concept. *Food and Drug Law Journal* 46:553–582.
7. United States Statutes at Large (59th Congress, Sess. I. Chp. 3. pp., 6-30-1906).
8. G.A. Burdock, and I.G. Carabin. Generally recognized as safe (GRAS): History and description. *Toxicology Letters* 150:3–18, 2004.
9. Federal Food, Drug, and Cosmetic Act (FD&C Act). 1938. 21 U.S.C. 321.
10. P.B. Hutt, R.A. Merrill, and L.A. Grossman. *Food and drug law: Cases and materials*. 3rd ed. New York NY: Foundation Press, 2008.
11. Food Additives Amendment (FAA). 1958. 21 U.S.C. 348.
12. A.M. Rulis, and J.A. Levitt. 2009. FDA's food ingredient approval process: Safety assurance based on scientific assessment. *Regulatory Toxicology and Pharmacology* 53:20–31.
13. Food Additives. 1977a. 21 CFR 170.
14. Substances generally recognized as safe. 1977b. 21 CFR 182.
15. Federal Register Notice – the GRAS Proposal. 4-17-1997a. 62 FR 18938.
16. Exemption of certain food additives from the requirement of tolerances. 10-31-1969. 34 FR 17063.
17. Food additives, eligibility of substances for classification as generally recognized as safe in food. 12-8-1970. 35 FR 18623.
18. GRAS substances (SCOGS) database. http://www.fda.gov/Food/FoodIngredientsPackaging/GenerallyRecognizedasSafeGRAS/GRASSubstancesSCOGSDatabase/default.htm
19. Z.S. Olempska-Beer, R.I. Merker, M.D. Ditto, and M.J. DiNovi. 2006. Food-processing enzymes from recombinant microorganisms – A review. *Regulatory Toxicology and Pharmacology* 45:144–158.
20. M.W. Pariza, and E.A. Johnson. 2001. Evaluating the safety of microbial enzyme preparations used in food processing: Update for a new century. *Regulatory Toxicology and Pharmacology* 33:173–186.
21. R. Porta, A. Pandey, and C. Rosell. 2011. Enzymes as additives or processing aids in food biotechnology. *Enzyme Research*, 2010.
22. M.W. Pariza, and E.M. Foster. 1983. Determining the safety of enzymes used in food-processing. *Journal of Food Protection* 46:453–468.
23. A. Kumar, S. Grover, J. Sharma, and V.K. Batish. 2010. Chymosin and other milk coagulants: Sources and biotechnological interventions. *Critical Reviews in Biotechnology* 30:243–258.
24. E.L. Flamm. 1991. How FDA approved chymosin: A case history. *Nat Biotech.* 9:349–351.
25. GRAS notice inventory. http://www.accessdata.fda.gov/scripts/fcn/fcnNavigation.cfm?rpt=grasListing
26. US Department of Health and Human Services. 2010. Guidance for industry. Enzyme preparations: Recommendations for submission of chemical and technological data for food additive petitions and GRAS notices. http://www.fda.gov/Food/GuidanceComplianceRegulatoryInformation/GuidanceDocuments/FoodIngredientsandPackaging/ucm217685.ht
27. CAS registry website. http://www.cas.org
28. The United States Pharmacopeial Convention. 2008. *Food Chemicals Codex*, 6th Edition, 2008. Rockville, MD.
29. Federal Meat Inspection Act. 1906. 21 U.S.C. § 601.

30. T.N. Nazina, T.P. Tourova, A.B. Poltaraus, E.V. Novikova, A.A. Grigoryan, A.E. Ivanova, et al. (2001). Taxonomic study of aerobic thermophilic bacilli: descriptions of *Geobacillus subterraneus* gen. nov., sp. nov. and *Geobacillus uzenensis* sp. nov. from petroleum reservoirs and transfer of *Bacillus stearothermophilus, Bacillus thermocatenulatus, Bacillus thermoleovorans, Bacillus kaustophilus, Bacillus thermodenitrificans* to *Geobacillus* as the new combinations *G. stearothermophilus*, G. th. *International Journal of Systematic and Evolutionary Microbiology* 51:433.
31. A.S. Deboer, F. Priest, and B. Diderichsen. 1994. On the industrial use of *Bacillus Licheniformis* – A review. *Applied Microbiology and Biotechnology* 40:595–598.
32. Biotechnology program under toxic substances control act (DSCA). 1996. Final microbial assessments. http://www.epa.gov/biotech_rule/rulesupc.htm
33. Current good manufacturing practice in manufacturing, packing, or holding human food. 1986. 21 CFR 110.
34. Food Allergen Labeling and Consumer Protection Act of 2004. 2004. 21 U.S.C. 201.

8

Trace Element Speciation in Food

Paula Berton[1,2], Estefania M. Martinis[1,2] and Rodolfo G. Wuilloud[1,2]

[1]National Council for Scientific and Technical Research (CONICET), Argentina

[2]Analytical Chemistry Research and Development Group (QUIANID), Institute of Basic Sciences, National University of Cuyo, Mendoza, Argentina

Abstract

Food is usually one of the main sources of exposure to toxic and essential metal compounds. However, nutritional and toxicological properties of a chemical element critically depend on the form in which it occurs in food. As a consequence, trace element speciation, particularly for toxic trace elements, is nowadays considered to be the main interest to ensure food safety, and it is becoming an important need worldwide for industrial quality control and regulatory implementation. Furthermore, since trace element bioavailability is highly variable among chemical forms, speciation analysis is essential to estimate nutritional quality. In order to achieve this toxicological and nutritional analysis in foods, robust analytical methods with well-established procedures for food sampling and sample treatment are required to assure the identity of the different chemical species.

In this chapter, an introductory discussion on the issue of trace elemental speciation in food is given. General aspects demonstrating the great relevance that elemental speciation is having in different fields, such as toxicology and nutrition, are critically commented on and discussed. Special emphasis is placed on the species of toxic heavy metals and metalloids (such as arsenic, mercury, tin, chromium, and cadmium) and on the species of essential elements (such as iron, selenium, cobalt, and zinc) occurring in food. Additionally, the impact of industrial food processing and domestic preparation on element speciation and bioavailability in foodstuff is briefly commented on. Lastly, a summary of mostly relevant and applied analytical methods and techniques to develop speciation studies in different foods is exposed.

Visakh P. M., Sabu Thomas, Laura B. Iturriaga, and Pablo Daniel Ribotta (eds.) Advances in Food Science and Technology, (227–264) 2013 © Scrivener Publishing LLC

Keywords: Elemental speciation, food processing, element bioavailability, essential elements, toxic elemental species, functional food, analytical methods

8.1 Introduction

Life sciences obtain more and more benefits from the development of novel analytical methods. At present, and on the subject of trace element determination, this refers to the identification, separation and quantification of different chemical forms (species) under which a chemical element can occur in biological systems, environment and food. Thus, the word "speciation" has become very popular and it is commonly utilized in those studies related to trace elements [1–6]. This concept is extremely relevant within nutritional and contamination studies as it generates crucial information regarding the bioavailability and toxicity of an element. Moreover, speciation studies have demonstrated that these two properties for a specific element depend not only on its chemical nature, but also on its chemical forms and combinations with other more complex molecular structures [5, 7–9]. Some classical examples mentioned in the literature are as follows:

- The higher toxicity of Chromium Cr^{6+} as compared to Cr^{3+} is due to its high bioavailability [10].
- The easiness of organic Mercury (Hg) species to be transported through cell membranes with the consequent bioaccumulation in living organisms, such as fish, thus leads to magnification of Hg in the human food chain [11].
- Although Se has been widely recognized as an essential nutrient for humans, its toxicity is definitively linked to the type of inorganic or organic species occurring in food [6].

Widely accepted definitions of elemental speciation, along with its related terminology, have already been reported by the International Union for Pure and Applied Chemistry (IUPAC) as follows [12]:

Chemical species. Chemical element: specific form of an element defined as to isotopic composition, electronic or oxidation state, and/or complex or molecular structure.

Speciation analysis. Analytical chemistry: analytical activities of identifying and/or measuring the quantitities of one or more individual chemical species in a sample.

Speciation of an element. Speciation: Distribution of an element amongst defined chemical species in a system.

Despite these definitions, many times it is not possible to specifically evaluate the concentration of individual elemental species in a given sample due to insufficient chemical stability, conversion to a different chemical form, changing of oxidation state, etc. Therefore, when total elemental speciation analysis is not achieved, the term "fractionation" is employed and defined as follows:

Fractionation. Process of classification of an analyte or a group of analytes from a certain sample according to physical (e.g., size, solubility) or chemical (e.g., bonding, reactivity) properties.

Trace elements speciation, particularly for toxic trace elements, is nowadays considered to be of main interest to ensure food safety, and it is becoming an important need for industrial quality control and regulatory implementation by many countries around the world. Therefore, the evaluation of total level of trace elements does not guarantee the safety of foods, since species often differ considerably in their adverse effects, which can range from beneficial to highly toxic. The effects on living organisms by essential trace elements, such as iron (Fe), selenium (Se) and zinc (Zn), and traditional toxic elements, for example As and Hg, are defined by their total levels and species distribution in food. In fact, food authorities have drawn attention to the need of establishing proper dietary requirements and upper safe intake limits for essential elements and tolerable dietary intake levels for potentially toxic trace elements. On the other hand, since trace element bioavailability is highly variable among chemical forms as well as total levels in food, speciation analysis is essential to ensure food safety and to evaluate nutritional quality. Therefore, the role of speciation analysis is becoming an increasingly important tool in defining and assuring food safety and nutritional requirements. In order to accomplish these aims, speciation in foods requires robust analytical methods with well-established procedures for food sampling and sample treatment which assure the identity of the different chemical species. However, the availability of standard procedures for trace element speciation is still an important issue within speciation studies, which is illustrated considering the limited number of existing certified reference materials as compared to the broad spectrum of food matrixes to be currently analyzed by most routine laboratories.

In this chapter, an introductory discussion to the issue of trace elemental speciation in food is given. General aspects demonstrating the great relevance that elemental speciation is having for different fields, such as toxicology and nutrition, are critically commented on and discussed. Furthermore, a summary of mostly relevant and applied analytical methods and techniques to develop speciation studies in different foods is exposed.

8.2 Implications of Toxic Elements Speciation for Food Safety

Food safety depends not only on the determination of total levels but also on the speciation of trace elements occurring in foodstuffs. Thus, the biochemical and toxicological properties of a chemical element critically depend on the form in which it occurs in food [13, 14]. Elements can exist in various chemical valence states, forms, and compounds. Some species of an element may have a radical impact on human health (even at extremely low concentrations), therefore, the total element concentration becomes of little value in determining the impact of the trace element. The identification and quantification of elemental species provides information about bioaccumulation, detoxification, and other toxicological implications [13–15]. Bioavailability and metabolism are often highly variable between different chemical forms of the same element, thus, speciation provides an understanding of how the absorption and bioavailability of elements can be reduced for toxic elements.

Human exposure to metal compounds in the general environment is usually greater through food and drink than through air [16]. Elemental species can be present in food due to anthropogenic or natural sources. In the first case it is a result of external contamination because of environmental pollution, food processing or leaching from packaging materials. In the second case it results from an endogenous synthesis by a plant or an animal (methylmercury or organoarsenic species) [17]. The role of elemental speciation and speciation analysis in human health hazard and risk assessment is critical for several toxic heavy metals and metalloids like arsenic (As), Hg, tin (Sn), Cr and cadmium (Cd). For these entire elements, some considerations regarding their sources, presence in food and toxicity are reviewed in the following sections.

8.2.1 Arsenic

Arsenic occurs in food as inorganic, as well as organic, compounds. Toxicity varies greatly between individual species. In general, organic As compounds are significantly less toxic than inorganic As compounds. Mobility in water and in body fluids largely determines species toxicity. It is reported that the toxicity conforms to the following order (highest to lowest toxicity): arsines > inorganic arsenites > organic trivalent compounds (arsenooxides) > inorganic arsenates > organic pentavalent compounds > arsonium compounds > elemental As [18, 19]. For organic species, generally, the toxicity decreases as the degree of methylation increases [20].

People have always been exposed to As from food, drinking water and other sources. As occurs naturally in rocks and soil. However, the mining industry and industrial effluents contribute greatly to its spread in the environment. As its trioxide, As is used in large quantities in the manufacture of glass to eliminate a green color caused by impurities of Fe compounds. Furthermore, elemental As is sometimes added to lead and special alloys to harden them [14, 15].

Total As levels are very high in the marine food chain due to bioaccumulation phenomenon. Marine organisms with the highest concentrations of As are fish and crustaceans [13]. Nevertheless, a high number of organic As species found in seafood, such as arsenobetaine and arsenocholine, are considered to be nontoxic. Likewise, the transformations that As undergoes in marine food chains are still being studied. For example, arsenobetaine is thought to be the final metabolite of As in food chains, although it is not present in all fish species [13]. Seafood is followed by meat and grain based on As concentration. Generally, lower total concentrations have been found in fruits, vegetables, and dairy products [15]. Moreover, high contents of inorganic As have been found in meat, poultry, and cereals [15]. As species commonly found in food are presented in Table 8.1.

Classical syndromes of chronic As exposure include hyperkeratosis, corns, and warts on the feet (blackfoot) and hands. Exposure to inorganic As in drinking water is associated with health risks related to the duration and level of exposure, particularly above

Table 8.1 Common As species occurring in food.

Species	Abbreviation	Formula	Food
Inorganic compounds			
Arsenous acid (arsenite)	As^{3+}	$As(OH)_3$	Fish, shrimp, crab, shellfish, lobster seaweed, rice, grain, meat, meat, poultry, cereals, carrots, edible, mushroom
Arsenic acid (arsenate)	As^{5+}	$AsO(OH)_3$	
Organic compounds			
Monomethylarsenic acid	MMA^{5+}	$CH_3AsO(OH)_2$	tuna fish, freshwater, catfish, freshwater, turbot, freshwater, carp, fresh-water trout, lobster, shrimp, rab, oyster, clam, shellfish, green algae, edible mushroom, seaweed
Dimethylarsenic acid	DMA^{5+}	$(CH_3)_2AsO(OH)$	
Arsenobetaine	AsB	$(CH_3)_3As^+CH_2COOH$	
Arsenocholine	AsC	$(CH_3)_3As^+CH_2CH_2OH$	
Trimethyl arsine oxide	TMAO	$(CH_3)_3AsO$	
p-Arsanilic acid	p-ASA	$C_6H_8AsNO_3$	
Trimethylarsoniopropionate	TMAP	$(CH_3)_3As^+CH_2CH_2COO^-$	
Dimethyldithioarsinic acid	$DMDTA^{5+}$	$(CH_3)_2As(S)(SH)$	

Species	Abbreviation	Formula	Food
Dimethylmonothioarsinic acid	$DMMTA^{5+}$	$(CH_3)_2As(S)(OH)$	tuna fish, freshwater catfish, freshwater turbot, freshwater carp, fresh-water trout lobster, shrimp, crab, oyster, clam, shellfish, green algae, edible mushroom, seaweed
Thio-arsenosugar glycerol	Thio-Gly	$C_7H_{14}AsO_3(S)$ $OCH_2CH(OH)CH_2OH$	
Thio-arsenosugar sulfate	Thio-SO_4	$C_{10}H_{16}AsO_5(S)OSO_3H$	
Thio-arsenosugar phosphate	Thio-PO_4	$C_7H_{14}AsO_3(S)$ $OCH_2CH(OH)CH_2OPO_2$ $-OCH_2CH(OH)CH_2OH$	
Trimethylarsine sulfide	TMAS	$(CH_3)_3As(S)$	
Thio-arsenosugar sulfonate	Thio-SO_3	$C_{10}H_{16}AsO_5(S)SO_3H$	
Thio-dimethylarsenoacetate	Thio-DMAA	$(CH_3)_2As(S)CH_2COOH$	
Thio-dimethylarsinate	Thio-DMA	$(CH_3)_2As(S)(OH)$	
Thio-dimethylarsenoethanol	Thio-DMAE	$(CH_3)_2As(S)CH_2COOH$	

300 μg L^{-1}. Acute poisoning is associated with vomiting, bloody diarrhea, abnormal heart rhythm, esophageal and abdominal pain, and sometimes death because of cardiopulmonary collapse. As may be an indirect carcinogen [14, 16], the US Environmental Protection Agency (EPA) recently reduced the standards for As in drinking water from 50 μg L^{-1} to 10 μg L^{-1} [21]. In contrast to adverse effects of As, small amounts of the metal may be essential to the body. Approximately 10 to 50 μg g^{-1} might be necessary to maintain homeostasis of the body. Also, As (arsenic trioxide) has been used successfully to treat patients with acute promyelocytic leukemia (APL) [14].

8.2.2 Mercury

Hg is one of the most toxic elements impacting human health. Because of its high bioaccumulation, Hg is among the most highly bioconcentrated trace metal in the human food chain. For example, predatory fish can have up to 106-fold higher Hg concentrations than ambient water and up to 95% of this Hg can be in the form of methylmercury [15, 22]. The chemical form of Hg controls its bioavailability, transport, persistence, and impact on the human body [15, 16]. All Hg species are toxic, while organic Hg compounds are generally more toxic than inorganic species [22].

The nervous system is highly sensitive to all forms of Hg. Exposure to high levels of metallic, inorganic, or organic Hg can permanently damage the brain, kidneys, and a developing fetus. Methylmercury and metallic Hg vapors are more harmful than other forms, because these forms reach the brain quickly [14, 16]. Effects on brain functioning may result in irritability, shyness, tremors, changes in vision or hearing, and memory problems. Methylmercury is toxic to cerebral and cerebellum cortices, causing focal necrosis of neurons and destruction of glial cells. In addition, methylmercury is a known teratogen. Short-term exposure to high levels of metallic Hg vapors may cause lung damage, nausea, vomiting, diarrhea, increases in blood pressure or heart rate, skin rashes, and eye irritation [14, 23, 24]. Research studies in animals have shown that mercuric chloride increases several types of tumors in rats and mice, while methylmercury has caused kidney tumors in male mice [14].

Hg emissions from both anthropogenic and natural sources are mainly in the form of elemental Hg (Hg^0) which constitutes >99% of the total Hg in the atmosphere [25]. However, their residence time in the air is very short (minutes) and they are rapidly removed by deposition processes due to their high surface activity and water solubility [22]. Biogeochemical transformations can lead to Hg species in the oxidation states I and II. Most inorganic Hg^+ compounds are sparingly soluble in water. In contrast, inorganic Hg^{2+} forms complexes or compounds with inorganic and/or organic species (e.g., $[HgCl_x]^{2-x}$; $[Hg^{2+}\text{-DOC}]$, DOC: dissolved organic carbon; HgS), depending on the local chemical environment. Inorganic Hg^{2+} also undergoes biomethylation, resulting in the formation of monomethylmercury (MMeHg; CH_3Hg^+) and dimethylmercury (DMeHg; $(CH_3)_2Hg$). These reactions are reversible with demethylation facilitated by microorganisms and/or photolytic decomposition. All of these species are highly mobile [26].

The EPA has set a limit of 2 $\mu g\ L^{-1}$ in drinking water. On the other hand, the US Food and Drug Administration (FDA) has set a maximum permissible level of 1 part of methylmercury in a million parts of seafood (1 $mg\ kg^{-1}$) [14].

8.2.3 Tin

Sn is one of the essential elements at trace levels involved in various metabolic processes in humans. It may be introduced into food either as inorganic or as organotin compounds. Most of the inorganic Sn compounds are nontoxic because of their low solubility and absorption [27]. However, organic Sn compounds are mostly toxic [15].

Canned foods, such as tomato sauce and fruit juices, are known to contain high concentrations of Sn. Other sources of Sn are cereal grains, dairy, meat, vegetables, seaweed, and licorice. When inorganic Sn is introduced to foodstuff, there is a possibility of it turning into an organic Sn compound [28]. Additionally, dietary exposure to organotin compound may result from the consumption of organotin-contaminated meat and fish products. The butyltin and phenyltin compounds accumulate within the marine food chain, eventually accumulating in aquatic food products such as fish, oysters, and crab.

There has been growing concern about the significance and toxicity of this element. It is reported that Sn^{2+}, as stannous chloride, is readily taken up by human white blood cells and can cause damage to DNA [29]. By contrast, Sn^{4+} is not taken up by cells, so it does not cause DNA damage or inhibit stimulation of DNA synthesis in cells [29]. The gastrointestinal absorption of soluble Sn salts is only a few percent of the ingested dose. In chronic exposures, bone is the major storage organ for Sn, and its biological half-life in bone is approximately 100 days. The excretory routes of Sn compounds may vary depending on the type of Sn compounds and the mode of exposure. High intakes of inorganic Sn compounds can cause abdominal pain and anemia [27]. Short-chain alkyltin compounds such as trimethyl and triethyl tins are well absorbed from the gastrointestinal tract, whereas long-chain alkyltin compounds are not much absorbed. The toxicity of organotin compounds differs, depending on their physicochemical properties. Alkyl and aromatic Sn compounds are neurotoxins. Triethyltin can cause encephalopathy and cerebral edema [27]. Organotin compounds can penetrate cell membranes because of their lipophilicity and cause damage to the cell membrane, interrupt oxidative phosphorylation, and damage mitochondria. They can inhibit synthesis of heme oxygenase, and can be immunotoxic and genotoxic [27]. There is no definite evidence that inorganic or organic Sn compounds can cause carcinogenic or teratogenic effects, although in a few studies effects have been reported. Tributyltin and triphenyltin are implicated in endocrine disruptions, and hence, cause reproductive failure in marine organisms [27].

Sn is widely used in industry. Sn compounds are used in food packaging, in some veterinary formulations, in marine antifouling paints on the hulls of ships, in wood preservation, as a stabilizer for polyvinyl chloride, as fungicides for crops, and as electrochemical catalysts. Sn is a component of many soils and may be released in dust from windstorms, roads, and farming activities. Other sources of Sn are processes such as burning of waste or burning of fossil fuels (coal or oil) [16, 17].

8.2.4 Chromium

Cr is extensively used in the chemical industry as a catalyst, pigment, and other applications such as metal plating. As a result, different species of Cr can be released into the environment (soil, surface, and ground waters) and are then available to humans [15, 30].

Cr can exist in several chemical forms, presenting oxidation numbers between 0 and 6+. However, trivalent and hexavalent Cr are the stable states occurring in the environment. Cr^{3+} compounds are essential at trace levels in humans, playing a role in the metabolism of glucose and certain lipids, mainly cholesterol. However, it has been demonstrated that Cr^{3+} is capable of eliciting eczema at low concentrations and of causing DNA damage in cell-culture systems [31]. Because of the high oxidation potential and the capacity to pass through biological membranes, Cr^{6+} compounds are approximately 100-fold more toxic than Cr^{3+} salts for both acute and chronic exposure [14]. Cr^{6+} has been recognized as a highly toxic species which is classified as a human carcinogen by the EPA and a class I human carcinogen by the International Agency for Research on Cancer (IARC) [30]. The toxicological disparity between Cr^{3+} and Cr^{6+} is associated with the chemical properties of each species, which also determine the stability, mobility, and bioavailability of these species in the environment [32].

Concentrations of Cr vary considerably in foodstuffs. Thus, high concentrations of Cr can be found in meat and vegetables. On the other hand, unrefined sugar, white fish, vegetable oil, and fruit contain smaller amounts. Generally speaking, concentrations are reported from non-detectable to approximately 0.5 mg kg^{-1} wet weight for various food items [17].

Furthermore, water is considered one of the most important sources of metal exposure in the normal diet. The Cr concentration in rivers and lakes is usually between 1 and 10 μg L^{-1}, a fraction of which may be in the hexavalent state. Drinking water, in general, contains higher amounts of Cr than river water. The most frequently found Cr species in river water are chromate (CrO_4^{2-}), cationic hydroxo complexes ($Cr(OH)^{2+}$ and $Cr(OH)_2^{+}$, etc.) and organically bound or colloidally sorbed Cr^{3+} [16].

8.2.5 Cadmium

Cd is mainly present in foodstuffs as inorganic Cd salts because organic Cd compounds are unstable [14]. Cd can be found in all types of food, and particularly high amounts occur in organs of cattle, seafood, and some mushroom species. This metal is found in all parts of food plants, but in animals and humans it is found in liver, kidney, and milk. Absorption of Cd from food varies and depends on age, nutritional status, and genetic factors. Adults accumulate less Cd than children. Cd absorption increases when the calcium (Ca) or Fe status is poor. Due to its low excretion rate (biological half-life=0–30 years), Cd accumulates in the body [33]. Exposure to high levels of Cd affects the liver and the erythropoietic system. Cd irritates the stomach, leading to vomiting and diarrhea. Chronic exposure to Cd produces kidney damage and bones become fragile and break easily [14, 34]. Animal studies have shown a relationship between Cd in the drinking water and hypertension, Fe-deficient blood, liver disease, and nerve or brain damage. Studies on humans and animals that had high intakes of Cd did not show an increase in cancer. The IARC has determined that Cd is probably carcinogenic to humans. The EPA has determined that Cd is a probable human carcinogen by inhalation [35].

Cd has been widely distributed in the environment due to extensive industrial use. Cd may be electrolytically deposited as a coating on metals, chiefly Fe on steel, on which it forms a chemically resistant coating. Alloys of Cd with lead and zinc (Zn) are used as a solder for Fe. Cd salts are used in photography and to manufacture fireworks, rubber, fluorescent paints, glass, and porcelain. Cd sulfide is also employed in photovoltaic cells [14].

8.3 Elemental Species and Its Impact on the Nutritional Value of Food

Food is the primary source of essential elements for humans. To exert an effect, essential elements must be bioavailable from food, i.e., available both for absorption and for subsequent utilization by the body. On the other hand, essential elements can also be toxic if taken in excess. The margin between deficiency and toxicity can be narrower for some elements (Fe and Selenium (Se)) than for others (cobalt or Zn). A better understanding of the predominant chemical forms of trace elements in foods and their bioavailability would assist those who have to make decisions concerning food safety, dietary requirements, nutritional quality evaluation, and legislation.

8.3.1 Selenium

Se is an essential trace element for man and animals. It is an integral part of the antioxidant enzymes (gluthatione peroxidase and iodothyronine deiodinase) which protect cells against the effects of free radicals formed during normal oxygen metabolism. Se is also present in the so-called Se-proteins, for which the biological functions are still to be elucidated. The range between adequate Se and toxicity is narrow: 0.1 mg kg^{-1} and 2 mg kg^{-1} of diet, respectively [36]. Even though Se status is determined by dietary intake, its bioavailability and toxicity are defined by Se speciation in the diet.

Accumulated evidence on animals and epidemiological studies indicates an inverse relationship between Se levels/consumption and risk of several cancers, particularly lung, breast, colorectal and prostate cancers [37–41], and other diseases such as diabetes [42]. The anticarcinogenic property and ability to support synthesis of Se-enzymes depend on speciation. Most experiments have employed inorganic forms of Se or organic Se from yeast or garlic (e.g., Se-methylselenocysteine (MeSeCys)). Several Se-synthetic forms (e.g., ebselen, benzyl selenocyanate) have also been shown to be effective. However, it is difficult to assess which products may have a beneficial effect against cancer, since there is a wide variation in the content of Se in foodstuffs. The most frequently consumed food generally has a low Se content. Nuts, particularly Brazil nuts, offal and seafood provide the highest yields. There is also considerable variation in Se content in cereals and grains from region to region, depending upon the extent to which Se is available in soils.

Generally speaking, little information exists on the proportional levels of the various organic and inorganic forms of Se in food. The Se content and species of both plant and animal provisions depend on environmental conditions, in particular, the quantity and species of Se to which the animal/plant is exposed, and with the biosynthetic pathways involved in Se assimilation by plants and how these species are metabolized in animals. Selenate (SeO_4^{2-}) is the most predominant inorganic form found in both animal and plant tissues. Selenomethionine (Se-Met) and smaller amounts of selenocysteine (Se-Cys) are the predominant forms of Se found in cereal grains, soybeans, and grassland legumes. MeSeCys is the predominant form of Se present in Se-accumulating plants and in Se-enriched vegetables, such as garlic, broccoli, onions, and wild leeks. On the other hand, the evidence on the species of Se in dietary sources of animal origin is still scarce. The predominantly organic form of Se in animals is Se-Cys. In fish, SeO_4^{2-} and selenite (SeO_3^{2-}) have also been detected and there appear to be large differences between fish species in relation to selenoproteins. Se-yeast is produced by fermenting yeast in a Se-enriched medium when the Se becomes organically bound to yeast components. A considerable variability also exits in products described as Se-yeast, frequently used for supplementation, which is reflected in the species composition. Thus, Se speciation varies with yeast strain and is still not clearly understood.

Absorption of Se is not homeostatically regulated and is not believed to be affected by nutritional status. Although most dietary Se is absorbed efficiently, the retention of organic forms is higher than that of inorganic ones [43]. This difference is undoubtedly due to the ability of Se-Met from digested organic Se sources to be absorbed through the same enzyme transport system and incorporated in place of methionine (Met) into tissue proteins, erythrocytes and plasma albumin, where it can act as a Se store though it becomes available to the body only upon turnover of tissue proteins. On the other hand, SeO_3^{2-} seems to be absorbed through passive diffusion in the small intestine while SeO_4^{2-} is thought possible to share the same pathway as sulfur. More research into the absorption process as it relates to chemical form and into other factors affecting absorption (positive or negative interactions) is needed.

On the other hand, Se toxicity episodes in humans are scarcer than symptoms of deficiency. The signs of Se intoxication are: respiratory problems, skin infections, enzymatic systems inhibition, chromosomic aberrations, etc.

8.3.2 Iron

Fe is the most abundant transition metal in the human body (4–5 g in a human adult of 70 kg weight), and its deficiency is the most frequent nutritional problem in the world. It is an essential element required for growth and survival because it is involved in a broad spectrum of essential biological functions such as oxygen transport, electron transfer and DNA synthesis.

In man, dietary Fe intake consists of two components: heme Fe (as present in red meat) and non-heme or inorganic Fe (as in vegetables, cereals, etc.). Inorganic Fe is present in the diet as either the ferrous (Fe^{2+}) or the ferric (Fe^{3+}) species. Food non-heme Fe is in high molecular weight species, hence digestive release of Fe is important for Fe absorption. At neutral pH and in the presence of oxygen (physiological conditions), Fe^{2+} is rapidly oxidized to Fe^{3+} that can then precipitate as Fe hydroxide (therefore poorly bioavailable). Numerous diet compounds strongly affect the absorption of dietary Fe. Phytate, polyphenols, Ca, and some proteins present in milk, egg and soybean inhibit Fe absorption [44]. On the other hand, vitamin C and muscle tissue enhance Fe absorption, primarily by reducing Fe^{3+} to Fe^{2+}, thus inhibiting the formation of poorly soluble Fe compounds [44]. Non-heme Fe is absorbed early in digestion mainly in the duodenum, where low pH favors solubility of Fe. Further down the intestine it is likely that formation of insoluble Fe^{3+} complexes reduces bioavailability. Unlike inorganic Fe, heme Fe is highly bioavailable, well absorbed, and there is little influence on its absorption by other dietary factors. The intact Fe-porphyrin is transported across the intestinal brush border membrane. Calculations of heme and non-heme Fe and dietary manipulations of these two categories are believed to offer the means to improve the Fe nutritional status.

Since mammals are not equipped with mechanisms for the excretion of excess Fe, chronic Fe overload is associated with the slow progression of failure of various organs including the heart, liver, and pancreas, and in the absence of effective therapies may result in early death.

8.3.3 Cobalt

Cobalt (Co) is the only essential oligoelement that needs to be supplied in a particular form, that is, cobalamins, to be physiologically active. Cobalamins are molecules with a corrinoid nucleus formed by four pyrrolidine rings and a Co atom coordinated with four nitrogen atoms. Cobalamins are one of the most complex naturally occurring coordination compounds and participate as a co-enzyme in an important series of biological reactions and transformations. They are essential nutrients for cells and their deficiency produces delayed growth. Four common and naturally occurring cobalamins are cyanocobalamin (vitamin B_{12}), hydroxocobalamin (vitamin B_{12b}); 5′-deoxyadenosylcobalamin (coenzyme B_{12}); and methylcobalamin (methylcoenzyme B_{12}), important coenzymes involved in methylation processes [45]. Most of the Co ingested by humans is inorganic, and vitamin B_{12} represents only a small fraction. Human dietary intake of Co is highly variable, generally between 5 and 50 $\mu g\ day^{-1}$. So far, no other physiological role of Co was demonstrated in humans.

Vitamin B_{12} is exclusively synthesized by certain bacteria. Therefore, in humans, most of the vitamin B_{12} is obtained from dietary sources. Vegetables contain inorganic Co but little or no vitamin B_{12} [45]. The main sources of vitamin B_{12} in food are beef liver and kidney [46]. In well-balanced diets, the obtained amounts of vitamin B_{12} are normally quite sufficient and meet the recommended daily allowance (2.4 μg day^{-1} for adults) [47]. Nutritional imbalance (especially among vegans), malabsorption syndromes, and other gastrointestinal problems are the main causes of vitamin B_{12} deficiency. Its deficit primarily gives rise to pernicious anemia. In some elderly patients, neural and mental symptoms may develop prior to the appearance of hematological problems [48].

8.3.4 Zinc

As part of a large number of enzymes, Zn acts as a stabilizer of the molecular structure of cellular constituents and membranes. It plays an essential role in some processes of genetic expression and participates in the synthesis and degradation of carbohydrates, lipids, proteins, and nucleic acids. Zn deficiency can thus provoke health disorders in humans, such as growth retardation, delay in sexual and skeletal maturation, retarded growth and development, low immunity, poor healing, dermatitis, low physical work capacity, abnormal neuro-psychological functions, and other abnormalities. Its deficit is also associated with other pathologies such as rheumatoid arthritis, chronic giardiasis, and tumors.

In the water-soluble fraction from fruits and vegetables, Zn is mainly bound as species with low molecular weight (LMW) non-carbohydrate compounds, smaller than 5 kDa [49]. On the other hand, high molecular weight (HMW) Zn-containing substances larger than 100 kDa were detected in wheat, oats, and nuts [50, 51]. The major Zn species found in pumpkin seeds and Brazil nuts in the water-soluble fraction were identified as isoforms of the water-soluble sulfur-rich 2S-albumin, known as storage proteins [52], and Zn-glutathione in oxidized form (612 Da), indicating that glutathione may play a role as a Zn-binding ligand [50, 53]. More Zn is available from animal and fish sources as these high-protein foods contain amino acids which bind to Zn and make it more soluble. In meat, over 70% of soluble Zn was associated with two components having molecular weights of 65 and 35 kDa [54]. Studies of Zn in cow's milk determined that most of the Zn was associated with HMW fractions, whereas Zn in human milk was associated with LMW fractions [55]. Almost all investigations found Zn-citrate (present in LMW fraction) to be the predominant Zn species in human milk. Several species present in HMW fraction, found of minor importance, were Zn-lactoferrin, Zn-casein, Zn-albumin, and Zn-α-lactalbumin. The high bioavailability of Zn in human milk is believed to be linked to Zn-citrate [56].

A number of factors influence the absorption of Zn from the diet, which occurs in the small intestine. It ranges from less than 10 to more than 90%, with an average of 20–30%. Several compounds present in foods such as phytates, oxalates, fiber and Ca, bind Zn and reduce the amount available for absorption. Food additives and chemicals such as ethylenediaminetetraacetic acid (EDTA), usually employed in food processing, can also reduce Zn absorption. Competition for absorption occurs between Zn and other elements, such as copper (Cu), Fe and Cd. Whole grains are a better source of Zn than refined grains as they have the ability to produce enzymes that can destroy phytic acid. It has been found that increasing intake of vitamins such as Vitamin C, E and B_6 and minerals such as Mg can increase Zn absorption in the body.

Concerning toxicity, poisonous effects of Zn are rare as excessive absorption is usually prevented by abdominal pain, nausea and vomiting caused by very high doses (around 200 mg). Other symptoms include dehydration, lethargy, anemia and dizziness. Long-term use of doses above 150 mg have been reported to cause secondary deficiency of Cu, the suppression of immune function and decreased levels of HDL cholesterol which can lead to heart disease. Excessive use of supplements during pregnancy may be harmful to the fetus.

8.4 Elemental Species in Food Processing

Industrial food processing and domestic preparation have a great influence in element speciation and bioavailability in foodstuff. These processes are responsible for the chemical composition of the final ready-to-eat product and may greatly affect element content [4]. A high number of factors can produce a significant alteration of food chemical composition: chemical reactions between species, interaction with the container and equipment material, microbiological activity, temperature, pH, light action, long-term storage, etc. [4, 57]. It is very important to consider the influence of these factors as they can cause species interconversion or losses. For example, thermal treatment would cause denaturation and precipitation of metalloproteins and decomposition of original metallobiomolecules [58]. However, the extent of element species alteration varied with the nature of the element and stability of the element species [13, 57]. Analytical development in speciation analysis now makes it possible to quantitatively evaluate alteration of individual elemental species during processing of several foods [58]. However, very little research has been done in this area.

The effect of cooking temperatures on chemical changes in organic As species in seafood was studied by Devesa *et al.* [59]. The results obtained by the research group show that, in all the types of seafood studied (sole, dory, hake, sardine, and raw), TMA^+ appeared after cooking, possibly because heating facilitates decarboxylation of AB to TMA^+. Koplíc *et al.* have described changes of solubility and fractions of soluble species of eight elements investigated by size exclusion chromatography (SEC) coupled to ICP–MS in the course of soaking and boiling peas [58]. The analyses by SEC/ICP–MS showed identical element species in soaked and original peas. Thus, they have concluded that soaking does not change the stability of the original elemental species. On the other hand, considerable alterations of elemental contents have occurred as a result of pea boiling. Most of the Co, nickel (Ni) and molybdenum (Mo) contents (approx. 80%) and a half of the Cu content were dissolved. Lower amounts of the element were liberated in water in the cases of phosphorus (P), Zn (approx. 40%), Fe (27%) and manganese (Mn) (<10%) during pea boiling. The amounts of soluble (i.e., extractable to Tris–HCl) compounds of Mn, Cu, Fe, Zn, Mo and P in the boiled peas were decreased compared to values in the original peas. In the case of Mn, the boiling makes this element in peas almost completely insoluble. They have hypothesized that this could be caused by denaturation of original Mn-containing biomolecules or liberation of the metal ions and formation of insoluble inorganic compounds such as MnO_2. In another work, Koplíc *et al.* have studied the effect of technological processing and the maturity stage of seeds on the content and speciation of P and trace elements in peas [60]. They have arrived at some conclusions: the blanching of green peas practically did not change either the total amount or chemical speciation of elements but boiling did; high molecular mass species of all elements were diminished. However, the low molecular mass species of Co, Ni, Zn and Mo mostly persisted and could be considered as stable against thermal treatment. Speciation of Cu was changed during mature pea storage. If the peas were stored as meal or powder, Cu was readily relocated from original species to more stable low molecular mass species.

Furthermore, Crews *et al.* have studied the effect of cooking in Se speciation and bioavailability [61]. They have investigated Se in cooked cod and in enzyme extracts of cooked cod following simulated gastric and gastrointestinal digestion. Se speciation of the extracts by HPLC-ICP-MS enabled identification of only 12% of total Se as SeO_3^{2-}, while the remaining Se eluted at a different retention time from that of any other Se standard measured (Se-Met, Se-Cys, sodium SeO_3^{2-} and sodium SeO_4^{2-}). However, as the retention time was close to that of Se-Met, they suggested that Se-containing species were organic rather than inorganic. Previously, the same approach was applied by Crews to investigate Cd speciation in cooked pig kidney [62]. A metallothionein-like protein containing 20% of the total Cd and able to survive cooking and *in vitro* gastrointestinal digestion was identified.

Very recently, Hart *et al.* have studied the retention of Se species during processing and production of flour and bread using Se-enriched wheat grain as raw material [63]. An average of 80% of the total Se present in Se-enriched whole meal/white flour was Se-Met, and after bread production the Se-Met content was still the largest proportion (78%) of the total extractable forms of Se. They did not detect a large reduction in Se-Met content after the processing and production of bread. Other Se species identified in the Se-enriched flour and bread included Se-Cys (5%), MeSeCys (3%), SeO_3^{2-} (5%) and SeO_4^{2-} (4%). They have concluded that bread has the potential to provide a suitable increase of intake of bioavailable Se by Se-deficient populations. Changes in the chemical form of Se during the manufacture of a Se-enriched sourdough bread for use in human nutrition were also studied by Bryszewska *et al.* [64].

In recent years, research involving speciation has been growing rapidly. However, the application of trace element speciation analysis to evaluate chemical species alteration for a specific food and an industrial process are still scarce. These kinds of studies could be very useful and should be further developed and intensified in order to improve food processing, thereby ensuring the safety and nutritional quality of food. Including the chemical form of the element renders the information gained through careful analysis much more valuable.

8.5 Potential Functional Food Derived from Health Benefits of Elemental Species

Functional or medicinal food refers to any healthy food claimed to have a health-promoting or disease-preventing property beyond the basic function of supplying nutrients. These foods provide health benefits due to certain physiologically active components, which may or may not have been manipulated or modified to enhance their bioactivity. Although many of the nutritional compounds in functional foods are either naturally present or added during processing, some may be the result of agricultural breeding techniques, including conventional crossbreeding and food biotechnology.

8.5.1 Selenium

The interest in Se as a food supplement and its marketing to the public has increased in recent years. Development and commercialization of organic forms of Se has initiated a new era in the availability of Se-enriched products. Some strategies used for this purpose were the result of using Se for soil fertilization or breeding techniques, and supplementation of food staples such as flour. In general, eggs and meat are considered to be good sources of Se in the human diet. It has been shown that egg Se content can easily be manipulated to produce increased levels, especially when organic Se is included in a hen's diet at levels that provide 0.3–0.5 mg kg^{-1} Se in the feed. Se-enriched chicken, pork and beef can also be produced when using organic Se in the diet of poultry and farm animals [65–69].

Se is present in soil (naturally or due to anthropogenic activities) and can enter the food chain through plants. Some plants have the ability not only to grow in the presence of elevated levels of Se, but also to accumulate its species. The antioxidant and anticarcinogenic properties attributed to some selenocompounds justify the increased interest in growing Se-enriched vegetables, which represents an important source of this element in the human diet. The highest chemopreventive activity was observed in vegetables from *Allium* genus such as garlic, onion and ramp. Therefore, these plants are mostly used to study the uptake, incorporation and distribution of Se [70]. The major compounds found in the plant samples enriched with Se^{4+} were Se-Met, selenocystine ($SeCys_2$),

MeSeCys and derivatives such as γ-glutamyl-Se-methylselenocysteine (γ-Glu-MeSeCys) [70]. Recently, lentils have been proposed as a fortified food with Se, Fe and Zn [71]. Other plants that may accumulate Se include broccoli, several species of mushroom, various algae, multiple *Brassica* species, and Brazil nuts [72].

In addition, genetic engineering technology offers considerable potential for increasing the uptake of Se from soils and incorporating the mineral into nontoxic compounds in the edible parts of plants. In recent years, research studies based on genetic engineering reported that plants which normally do not accumulate Se can be transformed to incorporate more Se from soil and convert it to nontoxic MeSeCys as compared to wild type plants [73, 74]. Thus, Se at appropriate concentrations would be safe for the plant and for human consumption. After genetic modification, the accumulation of Se organic forms, particularly MeSeCys and γ-Glu-MeSeCys, may also be increased, which has been shown for the Indian mustard (*Brassica juncea*) [70].

It should be kept in mind that Se is toxic at levels only a little greater than those required in a healthy diet, therefore caution is warranted with supplementation and increased intakes.

8.5.2 Iron and Zinc

As mentioned in Section 8.3, Fe deficiency anemia is one of the most widespread nutritional disease in the world [75]. Fe and Zn are trace minerals that can be deficient in human diets, especially where meat is not consumed. For this reason, the enrichment of primary foods, especially those consumed in poor countries, is one of the top priorities in international agricultural and nutrition research. In rice-eating populations, Fe and Zn deficiencies are caused by insufficient dietary intake, absorption inhibitors (such as phytate), and lack of absorption enhancing factors for Fe (such as ascorbic acid).

In the baby food industry, Fe is frequently added to dairy-based beverages, and regularly helps to reduce the problems associated with Fe deficiency [76]. In order to keep organoleptic properties, research has focused on optimizing the Fe compounds used in fortification, promoting their inclusion in the food while improving the bioavailability of this micronutrient [77]. Notable successes have been achieved by microencapsulation of Fe salts [78–80] or a combination of such salts with other protective compounds such as phytase [81]. In order to reduce phytate concentration, and thus increase non-heme Fe absorption, phytase was successfully added to wheat bread rolls and soymilk [82]. Another approach recently reported was the development of a transgenic rice in cell culture that expressed the gene for human lactoferrin, a milk protein that binds Fe [83]. Recombinant lactoferrin may be a functional alternative to human lactoferrin in infant formula and provide another way to improve Fe availability for infants. The most common Fe-fortified foodstuff is wheat flour, where Fe is added to grains during the milling of flour [84]. Experimentally, foods which can be good vehicles for Fe such as sugar, salt and soy sauce have also been successfully enriched [77].

In cereals, many trace minerals are stored in the husk and subsequently lost during milling and polishing [85]. Therefore, strategies to increase the Fe content of cereals and grains face the challenge of targeting Fe storage in a form and location in the plant where it will be bioavailable when consumed. In order to potentially improve Fe nutrition in rice-eating populations a genetically modified rice was proposed with an increased Fe content, rich in phytase, cysteine-peptide and β-carotene [86]. The bioavailability of Fe in transgenic rice varieties containing the Fe storage protein, ferritin, was shown to be as good as ferrous sulphate, commonly used in Fe supplements [87, 88]. Fe content in the transgenic rice seeds was up to threefold greater than in non-transgenic control plants. Aromatic rice tends to have the highest Fe levels and several varieties have been successfully crossed with elite rice lines having excellent agronomic characteristics and grain qualities. The high-Fe rice which was developed is currently being tested for Fe bioavailability and effects on Fe nutrition status in the Philippines.

Fe transport and uptake in plants is carefully regulated. Fe transporter proteins in transgenic plants have been shown to increase Fe uptake into roots when Fe is deficient [89]. However, the same transporters also transport toxic metals such as Pb or Cd. There is a possibility of engineering plants with the ability to take up desirable minerals while excluding toxic and undesirable ones. Since Fe and Zn levels tend to be present together in many plants, genetic modification of selected varieties to further increase Fe content might also improve Zn levels.

Increasing the Zn content of cereals and grains, especially where soils are low in Zn, may be an effective way to improve human nutrition and at the same time increase plant yields. Recent biotechnological studies, suggest that increasing the production of Zn transporter proteins may be one approach to increase the Zn content of cereals [90]. Fermented milk is a very interesting vehicle for Zn fortification. However the effects of added Zn on the sensory properties of foods should be tested in the combination of vehicle-fortificant at fortification levels. Moreover, previous work has demonstrated that probiotics enhanced Zn bioavailability, and that Zn gluconate stabilized with glycine (suitable to be used in technological processes of industrial food fortification) combined with a probiotic has similar bioavailability compared to Zn sulfate (which is very reactive to the nutritional matrix and changes the color and taste of several foods) [91].

8.6 Analytical Methods for Food Elemental Speciation Analysis

One of the main reasons for the tremendous development of elemental speciation studies has been the advances in instrumentation. The continuous search for lower and lower detection limits in atomic spectrometry and mass spectrometry, allows passing over of the barrier between trace total element and element species. Nowadays, for trace element speciation it is generally necessary to use a combination of efficient separation techniques and highly sensitive detectors, coalescing them into hyphenated techniques. The evolution and advantages (mainly high degree of automation, good reproducibility and short analysis time) of the hyphenated techniques have made these approaches the preferred tool for speciation studies. A summary of different analytical techniques and hyphenation strategies are shown in Figure 8.1. Likewise, a complete overview on elemental speciation hyphenated techniques was made by Cornelis *et al.* in 2003 [92]. Thus, only a brief introduction to the most popular analytical techniques used for elemental speciation analysis will be presented throughout the following sections of this chapter.

8.6.1. Species Separation

The most common separation techniques are gas and liquid chromatography (GC and LC respectively). However, other separation

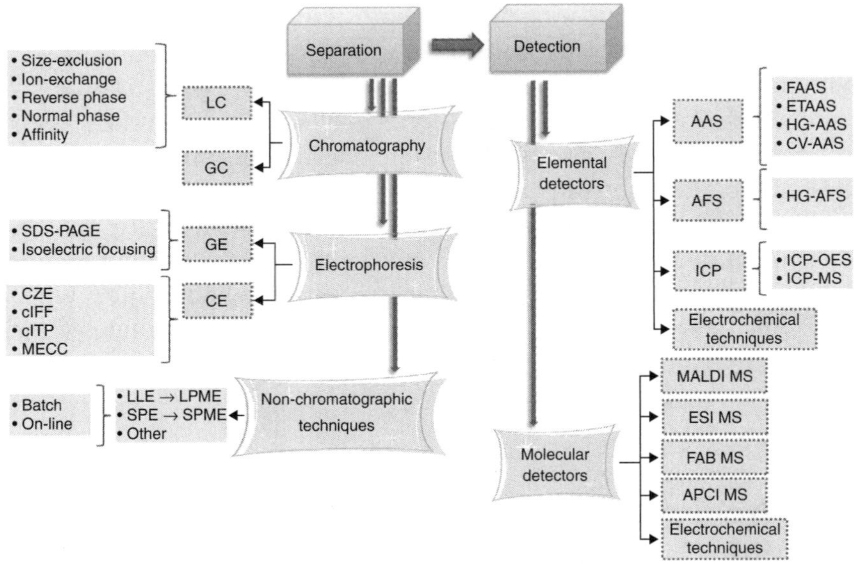

Figure 8.1 Hyphenated techniques for trace element speciation analysis in food.

techniques such as capillary and gel electrophoresis (CE and GE respectively) are also employed. Non-chromatographic methodologies for species determination, its evolution and development, were extensively reviewed [93–95]. The choice will depend on the chemical properties of the species, the available skills and infrastructure in the laboratory, and, last but not least, the available resources.

8.6.1.1. Liquid Chromatography

In this separation technique, the sample is introduced into a chromatographic column filled with a stationary phase while a liquid mobile phase is continuously pumped through the column. The analytes interact to a different extent with the stationary phase and the mobile phase, thus determining the time of residence of each analyte in the column. Usually, the stationary phase is a chemically modified silica or polymer. LC has emerged as one of the most popular separation techniques for elemental speciation analysis due to its versatility: depending on the chemical characteristics of the species of interest, both the stationary and mobile phase can be altered to achieve the desired separation. The majority of LC separations performed currently are part of a subset of LC known as high performance liquid chromatography (HPLC). The stationary phase of HPLC columns has small-diameter particles (3–5 μm) and the mobile phase is pumped under increased pressure. Depending on the type of stationary phase employed in the separation, HPLC separations can be classified as size exclusion chromatography, ion exchange chromatography, affinity chromatography and normal and reversed phase chromatography [96]. Different strategies for species determination are the addition of ion pair reagents (reversed phase ion pair chromatography) or surfactants (micellar chromatography) to the mobile phase. Among element-specific detection methods, inductively coupled plasma mass spectrometry (ICP-MS) is probably the most widely used LC detection method for elemental speciation analyses because of its superior sensitivity and because it is easily interfaced to LC systems [97]. Nowadays, it is also possible to couple an LC system to a soft ionization system, such as electrospray mass spectrometry (ES-MS), in order to obtain structural information.

8.6.1.2 Gas Chromatography

Unlike LC, only volatile and thermally stable species qualify for separation by GC. Very few compounds satisfy these requirements, but fortunately the analyst can resort to chemical reactions known as "derivatization," thus transforming non-volatile compounds into volatile and thermally stable ones. Packed column GC was the first chromatographic technique to be applied for elemental speciation, offering an improved separation of the analytes through interaction with the highly stable columns, combined with separation on the basis of their volatility. Packed columns, however, lack the necessary resolution and cannot be routinely applied. Most extensively employed is the cryogenic trapping and sequential thermal desorption from packed columns. This method is not very selective, but unstable compounds can be preserved for a long time before desorption and analysis. An improvement of resolution is achieved with GC with capillary columns. However, the limiting factors of its employment are their very small loading capacity and the difficulty of coupling to detectors. Electron capture detector (ECD) has been applied for species determination, but it cannot ensure specific detection. On the other hand, due to their high elemental sensitivity and selectivity, atomic spectroscopy detectors are perfectly suited for elemental speciation analysis by GC. Moreover, the matrix influence can be reduced or completely eliminated. Due to the extremely high sensitivity and selectivity, speed and multielemental capabilities, the most common detector is ICP-MS, followed by ICP-Optical emission spectrometry (ICP-OES).

8.6.1.3 Capillary Electrophoresis

CE is less mature but offers exciting possibilities for speciation analysis owing to its high separation efficiency, the nanoliter sample requirement, and the absence of packing susceptible to interact with metal species and to affect speciation originally present in samples [98, 99]. Moreover, CE analysis is faster than an LC separation. The principle of separation by CE is based on differences in the electrically driven mobility of charged analytes, similar to conventional electrophoresis. A high-voltage electrical field (typically 20–30 kV) is applied along an open tube column with a small internal diameter [99]. Different separation modes can be selected in CE: capillary zone electrophoresis (CZE), with separation on the basis of the charge/mass ratio; capillary isoelectric focusing (cIEF), based on the isoelectric point; capillary isotachophoresis (cITP), based on analyte conductivity; and micellar electrokinetic capillary chromatography (MECC), based on hydrophobicity.

CE can be used as a primary or secondary separation technique, for example after HPLC, when it is referred to as a two-dimensional technique. Even though the very small sample volume could be considered as an advantage, the concentration detection limits are, as a consequence, generally two orders of magnitude worse than those for LC separations. Moreover, the high voltage, the buffer/electrolyte composition and nature of additive can alter the integrity of elemental species. Taking into account the very small loading capacity of CE, the two-dimensional approach will yield far more interesting results, bringing the high resolution of CE to its full potential. The detection systems hyphenated with CE are ultraviolet (UV) detection for molecular but nonspecific information, ICP-MS for elemental and isotopes information or electrospray ionization tandem mass spectrometry (ESI-MS/MS) for molecular and structural information. Recently, CE-MS for biospeciation analysis was critically reviewed by Timerbaev [100]. CE analysis offers high resolution and high speed, and it is easily adaptable for automation and quantitative analysis.

8.6.1.4 *Gel Electrophoresis*

The field covered by gel electrophoresis (GE) for elemental speciation consists of charged biomacromolecules to which a metal or semi-metal is bound, covalently or not. Compared to CE, it is an efficient and rapid separation method for complex mixtures; it allows detection with radiotracers; it can be two-dimensional; the amount of material is larger, allows an off-line identification; and the material is always available for further studies. There are practical limitations due to the small amount of material that can be brought onto the gel, and, consequently, the limit of detection of the species [101]. Even though GE remains a semiquantitative method, its resolution is unsurpassable for protein separation. The first prerequisite during the separation procedure is the preservation of the elemental species. This is not evident, considering the nature of the many reagents needed to operate GE. When the metal is covalently bound, denaturing conditions can be used during electrophoresis. This is not the case for more weakly bound elements, for which non-denaturing conditions or native electrophoresis should be applied in order to prevent the loss of the basic structure of the complex and stripping of the metal [102]. Other critical parameters are the choice of buffer and pH. The method can be hyphenated with powerful detection methods, such as laser ablation dynamic reaction cell ICP-MS for elemental detection or matrix-assisted laser desorption/ionization (MALDI) MS for molecular detection [102]. A more tedious way, but reliable for quantitative measurements, consists of cutting out zones of separated proteins in the gel and measuring the element off-line with ICP-MS by using electrothermal vaporization (ETV) as the sample introduction system [103], or direct determination through electrothermal atomic absorption spectrometry (ETAAS).

8.6.2 Species Detection: Elemental and Molecular

Only the most sensitive detectors are suitable for speciation analysis in order to avoid extensive preconcentration steps. Since the trend is to go for online, hyphenated techniques, the most convenient elemental detector for online coupling is ICP-MS. However, due to its high cost, it is certainly worthwhile to consider other methods such as atomic absorption spectrometry (AAS), atomic fluorescence spectrometry (AFS) and optical emission spectrometry (OES).

Additionally, molecular detectors and electrochemical methods are powerful tools for speciation analysis.

8.6.2.1 *Atomic Absorption Spectrometry (AAS)*

Although flame AAS (FAAS) can operate continuously and thus can be used online with separation techniques, it cannot provide the necessary sensitivity for elemental speciation in most cases [104]. On the other hand, even though ETAAS shows higher sensitivity, it cannot be operated continuously over long periods of time, making online methods based on ETAAS less popular for elemental speciation purposes than ICP-MS. When species can be converted to hydrides, such as is routinely done for Hg, Se, As, Sn, Pb and Sb, hydride generation AAS (HG-AAS) is a very interesting, sensitive and inexpensive detection technique. Furthermore, the AAS technique with a quartz tube atomizer is a very sensitive, specific, rugged, and comparatively inexpensive detector for GC. Online solid-phase extraction coupled with ETAAS has also been explored. Finally, cold vapor AAS (CV-AAS) is the most widely used technique for Hg detection.

8.6.2.2 *Atomic Fluorescence Spectrometry (AFS)*

When species can be converted into hydrides, then atomic fluorescence spectrometry becomes a very economical elemental detection technique. It is, however, necessary to keep in mind that the conversion of elemental species into hydrides does not occur to the same extent and at the same rate for all species and elements. However, it is an excellent alternative to more expensive detectors such as ICP-MS in the case of highly toxic elements (i.e., Hg and As).

8.6.2.3 *Inductively Coupled Plasma Optical Emission Spectrometry (ICP-OES)*

Among techniques for emission spectrometry, the most common is ICP-OES, which is also referred to as ICP-atomic emission spectrometry (AES). Elemental speciation based on the plasma source has the advantage of accepting the continuous flow of the HPLC eluent and is therefore easier to hyphenate. This technique offers the most remarkable advantages: multielemental speciation analysis and detection of both metals and nonmetals. The disadvantages are the overall inefficiency of the nebulizer and the sensitivity of plasma to be extinguished upon introduction of mobile phases with high organic solvent concentration. The poor tolerance of plasma sources to common mobile phases, such as ion pair reagents, limits the applicability of ICP-based techniques. The fact that many ion exchange chromatography elutions are not isocratic (i.e., the elution is effected under variable, usually increasing, ionic strength) requires special protocols to circumvent the problem of varying analyte response during the elution [105].

8.6.2.4 Inductively Coupled Plasma Mass Spectrometry (ICP-MS)

Based on the measurement of m/z ratios, ICP-MS offers extremely low detection limits, a wide linear dynamic range, multielemental capabilities, and a high sample throughput for almost all elements. This is due to the very high degree of atomization in the plasma at about 7000 K. This extreme temperature makes it far superior as an atomization source than an electrically-heated graphite tube with temperatures at only 2273 K. However, one of the main disadvantages of the ICP-MS technique is nonspectral and spectral interferences. The former can be fairly easily solved by sample dilution, application of standard additions or isotope dilution for calibration. On the other hand, there exist two modern and major tools to reduce spectral interferences. The first is the dynamic reaction cell, which allows chemical reactions in a collision cell so that interfering isobars are neutralized or analyte is transformed into another, heavier polyatomic compound. Another very reliable, most universal, but very expensive tool to eliminate isobaric interferences is high-mass resolution ICP-MS [106]. Hyphenation of ICP-MS is achieved through the coupling of ICP-MS to a separation technique, normally a chromatographic one. HPLC works well online with ICP-MS, due to the compatibility of the chromatographic effluent and the liquid flow rate required for stable pneumatic nebulization. Similar difficulties due to the influence of the eluent on the plasma can be anticipated and need careful consideration, as mentioned in the previous section on ICP-OES [97, 106]. GC coupled with ICP-MS offers a higher resolving power and 100% introduction efficiency, allows more stable plasma and gives rise to less spectral interference. However, it can be employed only for sufficiently volatile and thermally stable compounds. CE-ICP-MS combines high separation efficiency with the sensitivity of ICP-MS and can be considered as the most important and recent trend in the field of hyphenated techniques [100].

8.6.2.5 *Molecular Detectors*

In order to complement the species characterization, it is becoming extremely important to employ in parallel a molecule-specific detector to obtain structural molecular information about the species under study [107]. Molecular MS offers unique advantages for the identification of metabolites at the sub-nanomolar levels. The preferred method of ionization has been ESI, although the use of fast atom bombardment (FAB), atmospheric pressure chemical ionization (APCI) and MALDI were also reported [108]. They offer soft ionization of metal-containing species followed by MS for the precise determination of the molecular mass of the original species and that of the individual fragments. One of their main drawbacks is that frequently an extensive sample clean-up is needed in order to obtain high sensitivities.

8.6.2.6 *Electrochemical Methods*

Electrochemical methods are based on the measurement of electrical signals associated with the molecular properties or interfacial processes of chemical species. These methods are simple and inexpensive, directly transforming the desired chemical information (concentration, activity) into an electrical signal (potential, current, resistance or capacity). However, the two major drawbacks in the application of these techniques to complex real-world samples have been the lack of selectivity of electrochemistry and the susceptibility of the electrode surface to fouling by surface-active materials in the sample. Town *et al.* have recently reviewed the electroanalytical techniques applied for the quantification of various oxidation states of an element, its organometallic species, or metal complexes in equilibrium with each other [109]. The authors concluded that the ideal is to perform *in situ* measurements with minimal sample perturbation. Despite its many difficulties, the sensitivity of electroanalytical methods makes them very powerful tools for many applications.

8.7 Conclusions

Food is usually one of the main sources of exposure to toxic trace elements and on the other hand the main route for incorporation of essential elements into the human body. However, the sole information of total content of trace elements in food does not provide a complete picture of the potential toxicological effects caused by its ingestion or the real benefits of essential elements consumption. The importance of trace element speciation to evaluate and assure safety and nutritional quality of food is being increasingly recognized. Despite the fact that several analytical methods for speciation studies have been developed, particularly for food, much work is still needed in order to fully evaluate food safety and quality. Thus, the lack of validated speciation methods and certified reference materials are key issues to be solved for correct implementation of trace element speciation as a means to assure food safety.

Finally, accurate information regarding trace element speciation in food allows the industry to improve its manufacturing processes and preservation approaches, design novel and healthier nutritional supplements, and give consumers a useful tool to make the right decision at the time of choosing a healthy food.

References

1. J. Szpunar, R. Lobinski. Multidimensional approaches in biochemical speciation analysis. *Analytical and Bioanalytical Chemistry* 2002, 373, (6), 404–411.
2. C.N. Ferrarello, M.R.F. de la Campa, A. Sanz-Medel. Multielement trace-element speciation in metal-biomolecules by chromatography coupled with ICP-MS. *Analytical and Bioanalytical Chemistry* 2002, 373, (6), 412–421.
3. A. Taylor, S. Branch, D. Halls, M. Patriarca, M. White. Atomic spectrometry update. Clinical and biological materials, foods and beverages. *Journal of Analytical Atomic Spectrometry* 2004, 19, (4), 505–556.
4. F. Cubadda. Inductively coupled plasma-mass spectrometry for the determination of elements and elemental species in food: A review. *Journal of AOAC International* 2004, 87, (1), 173–204.
5. D.M. Templeton. The importance of trace element speciation in biomedical science. *Analytical and Bioanalytical Chemistry* 2003, 375, (8), 1062–1066.
6. A. Sanz-Medel, M. Montes-Bayon, M.L.F. Saanchez. Trace element speciation by ICP-MS in large biomolecules and its potential for proteomics. *Analytical and Bioanalytical Chemistry* 2003, 377, (2), 236–247.
7. B. Michalke. Element speciation definitions, analytical methodology, and some examples. *Ecotoxicology and Environmental Safety* 2003, 56, (1), 122–139.
8. F. Xu, D.R. Qiu, P.Y. Yang, K.J. Hu. Review of chemical and biological speciation analyses for Se. *Spectroscopy and Spectral Analysis* 2002, 22, (2), 331–340.
9. S. Karthikeyan, S. Hirata. Arsenic speciation in environmental samples. *Analytical Letters* 2003, 36, (11), 2355–2366.

10. D.E. Salt, R.C. Prince, I.J. Pickering. Chemical speciation of accumulated metals in plants: Evidence from X-ray absorption spectroscopy. *Microchemical Journal* 2002, 71, (2-3), 255–259.
11. M. Ravichandran. Interactions between mercury and dissolved organic matter – A review. *Chemosphere* 2004, 55, (3), 319–331.
12. D.M. Templeton, F. Ariese, R. Cornelis, L.G. Danielsson, H. Muntau, H.P. Van Leeuwen, R. Lobinski. Guidelines for terms related to chemical speciation and fractionation of elements. Definitions, structural aspects, and methodological approaches (IUPAC recommendations 2000). *Pure and Applied Chemistry* 2000, 72, (8), 1453–1470.
13. L. Ebdon. *Trace element speciation for environment, food and health*. Royal Society of Chemistry: Great Britain, 2001.
14. S.T. Omaye. *Food and nutritional toxicology*. CRC Press: 2004.
15. R. Cornelis, J.A. Caruso, H. Crews, K.G. Heumann. *Handbook of elemental speciation II - Species in the environment, food, medicine and occupational health*. John Wiley & Sons Ltd.: Chichester, 2005; Vol. 2, p 767.
16. G. Nordberg, B.A. Fowler, M. Nordberg, L. Friberg. *Handbook on the toxicology of metals*. 3rd ed. Academic Press: Burlington, 2007; p 992.
17. P. Szefer, J.O. Nriagu. *Mineral components in foods*. CRC Press/Taylor & Francis: 2007.
18. I. Komorowicz, D. Baralkiewicz. Arsenic and its speciation in water samples by high performance liquid chromatography inductively coupled plasma mass spectrometry – Last decade review. *Talanta* 2011, 84, (2), 247–261.
19. B.K. Mandal, K.T. Suzuki. Arsenic round the world: A review. *Talanta* 2002, 58, (1), 201–235.
20. M. Leermakers, W. Baeyens, M. De Gieter, B. Smedts, C. Meert, H.C. De Bisschop, R. Morabito, P. Quevauviller. Toxic arsenic compounds in environmental samples: Speciation and validation. *TrAC Trends in Analytical Chemistry* 2006, 25, (1), 1–10.
21. US Environmental Protection Agency, Interim primary drinking water standards. In Fed.Reg. 40 (1975) 11,990.
22. K. Leopold, M. Foulkes, P. Worsfold. Methods for the determination and speciation of mercury in natural waters – A review. *Analytica Chimica Acta* 2010, 663, (2), 127–138.
23. I.A. Al-Saleh. Health implications of mercury exposure in children. *International Journal of Environment and Health* 2009, 3, (1), 22–57.
24. A. Bhan, N.N. Sarkar. Mercury in the environment: Effect on health and reproduction. *Reviews on Environmental Health* 2005, 20, (1), 39–56.
25. N. Pirrone, R. Mason. *Mercury fate and transport in the global atmosphere: Emissions, measurements and models*. Springer: 2009.
26. L. Friberg, J. Vostal. *Mercury in the environment: An epidemiological and toxicological appraisal*. CRC Press: 1972.
27. M. Nordberg, G.F. Nordberg. Toxicology and biological monitoring of metals. In *General and applied toxicology*, John Wiley & Sons, Ltd: 2009.
28. Y.-H. Li, H. Long, F.-Q. Zhou. Determination of trace tin by catalytic adsorptive cathodic stripping voltammetry. *Analytica Chimica Acta* 2005, 554, (1-2), 86–91.
29. J.R.N. McLean, H.C. Birnboim, R. Pontefact, J.G. Kaplan. The effect of tin chloride on the structure and function of dna in human white blood cells. *Chemico-Biological Interactions* 1983, 46, (2), 189–200.

30. N. Unceta, F. Séby, J. Malherbe, O. Donard. Chromium speciation in solid matrices and regulation: A review. *Analytical And Bioanalytical Chemistry* 2010, 397, (3), 1097–1111.
31. D.A. Eastmond, J.T. MacGregor, R.S. Slesinski. Trivalent chromium: Assessing the genotoxic risk of an essential trace element and widely used human and animal nutritional supplement. *Critical Reviews in Toxicology* 2008, 38, (3), 173–190.
32. J. Kotas, Z. Stasicka. Chromium occurrence in the environment and methods of its speciation. *Environmental Pollution* 2000, 107, (3), 263–283.
33. H.S.H. Seiler. *Handbook on metals in clinical and analytical chemistry.* Marcel Dekker: New York,, 1994; p 283.
34. H.G. Seiler, H. Sigel, *Handbook on toxicity of inorganic compounds.* New York, 1998.
35. R.B. Hayes. The carcinogenicity of metals in humans. *Cancer Causes Control* 1997, 8, 371.
36. S.T. Omaye. *Food and nutritional toxicology.* CRC Press: Boca Raton, United States, 2004; Vol. 1, p 319.
37. G.F. Combs Jr. Status of selenium in prostate cancer prevention. *British Journal of Cancer* 2004, 91, (2), 195–199.
38. G.F. Combs Jr. Current evidence and research needs to support a health claim for selenium and cancer prevention. *Journal of Nutrition* 2005, 135, (2), 343–347.
39. P.D. Whanger. Selenium and its relationship to cancer: An update. *British Journal of Nutrition* 2004, 91, (1), 11–28.
40. K. El-Bayoumy. The protective role of selenium on genetic damage and on cancer. *Mutation Research-Fundamental and Molecular Mechanisms of Mutagenesis* 2001, 475, (1-2), 123–139.
41. K. El-Bayoumy, R. Sinha. Mechanisms of mammary cancer chemoprevention by organoselenium compounds. *Mutation Research - Fundamental and Molecular Mechanisms of Mutagenesis* 2004, 551, (1-2), 181–197.
42. S. Stranges, J.R. Marshall, R. Natarajan, R.P. Donahue, M. Trevisan, G.F. Combs, F.P. Cappuccio, A. Ceriello, M.E. Reid. Effects of long-term selenium supplementation on the incidence of type 2 diabetes: A randomized trial. *Annals of Internal Medicine* 2007, 147, (4), 217–223.
43. S.J. Fairweather-Tait, R. Collings, R. Hurst. Selenium bioavailability: Current knowledge and future research requirements. *American Journal of Clinical Nutrition* 2010, 91, (5), 1484S–1491S.
44. R. Hurrell, I. Egli. Iron bioavailability and dietary reference values. *American Journal of Clinical Nutrition* 2010, 91, (5), 1461S–1467S.
45. G.F. Combs Jr. *The vitamins: Fundamental aspects in nutrition and health.* 3rd ed. Elsevier Academic Press: USA, 2008; p 608.
46. F. Watanabe. Vitamin B_{12} sources and bioavailability. *Experimental Biology and Medicine* 2007, 232, (10), 1266–1274.
47. R. Green, J.W. Miller. Vitamin B_{12}. In *Handbook of vitamins.* 4th ed. J. Zempleni, R.B. Rucker, J.W. Suttie, D.B. McCormick, eds. CRC Press: Boca Raton, 2007; p 608.
48. S.S. Kumar, R.S. Chouhan, M.S. Thakur. Trends in analysis of vitamin B_{12}. *Analytical Biochemistry* 2010, 398, (2), 139–149.

49. K. Günther, B. Kastenholz. Speciation of zinc. In *Handbook of elemental speciation II – Species in the environment, food, medicine and occupational health.* John Wiley & Sons, Ltd: 2005; pp 488–508.
50. J. Naozuka, S.R. Marana, P.V. Oliveira. Water-soluble Cu, Fe, Mn and Zn species in nuts and seeds. *Journal of Food Composition and Analysis* 2010, 23, (1), 78–85.
51. R.G. Wuilloud, S.S. Kannamkumarath, J.A. Caruso. Speciation of nickel, copper, zinc, and manganese in different edible nuts: A comparative study of molecular size distribution by SEC-UV-ICP-MS. *Analytical and Bioanalytical Chemistry* 2004, 379, (3), 495–503.
52. M. Dernovics, P. Giusti, R. Lobinski. ICP-MS-assisted nanoHPLC-electrospray Q/time-of-flight MS/MS selenopeptide mapping in Brazil nuts. *Journal of Analytical Atomic Spectrometry* 2007, 22, (1), 41–50.
53. A. Ovca, J.T. Van Elteren, I. Falnoga, V.S. Selih. Speciation of zinc in pumpkin seeds (Cucurbita pepo) and degradation of its species in the human digestive tract. *Food Chemistry* 2011, 128, (4), 839–846.
54. T. Hazell. Iron and zinc compounds in the muscle meats of beef, lamb, pork and chicken. *Journal of the Science of Food and Agriculture* 1982, 33, (10), 1049–1056.
55. B. Michalke, D.C. Munch, P. Schramel. Contribution to Zn-speciation in human breast milk: Fractionation of organic compounds by HPLC and subsequent Zn-determination by DCP-AES. *Journal of Trace Elements and Electrolytes in Health and Disease* 1991, 5, (4), 251–258.
56. B. Michalke. Trace element speciation in human milk. *Pure and Applied Chemistry* 2006, 78, (1), 79–90.
57. J.L. Gómez Ariza, E. Morales, D. Sánchez-Rodas, I. Giráldez. Stability of chemical species in environmental matrices. *TrAC - Trends in Analytical Chemistry* 2000, 19, (2-3), 200–209.
58. R. Koplík, O. Mestek, J. Komínková, M. Borková, M. Suchánek. Effect of cooking on phosphorus and trace elements species in peas. *Food Chemistry* 2004, 85, (1), 31–39.
59. V. Devesa, A. Martínez, M.A. Súñer, D. Vélez, C. Almela, R. Montoro. Effect of cooking temperatures on chemical changes in species of organic arsenic in seafood. *Journal of Agricultural and Food Chemistry* 2001, 49, (5), 2272–2276.
60. R. Koplík, J. Komínková, M. Borková, O. Mestek, F. Kvasnička, M. Suchánek. Effect of technological processing and maturity stage of seeds on the content and speciation of phosphorus and trace elements in peas. *Food Chemistry* 2004, 87, (3), 423–432.
61. H.M. Crews, P.A. Clarke, D.J. Lewis, L.M. Owen, P.R. Strutt, A. Izquierdo. Investigation of selenium speciation in *in vitro* gastrointestinal extracts of cooked cod by high-performance liquid chromatography-inductively coupled plasma mass spectrometry and electrospray mass spectrometry. *Journal of Analytical Atomic Spectrometry* 1996, 11, (12), 1177–1182.
62. H.M. Crews, J.R. Dean, L. Ebdon, R.C. Massey. Application of high-performance liquid chromatography – Inductively coupled plasma mass spectrometry to the investigation of cadmium speciation in pig kidney following cooking and in vitro gastro-intestinal digestion. *Analyst* 1989, 114, (8), 895–899.

63. D.J. Hart, S.J. Fairweather-Tait, M.R. Broadley, S.J. Dickinson, I. Foot, P. Knott, S.P. McGrath, H. Mowat, K. Norman, P.R. Scott, J.L. Stroud, M. Tucker, P.J. White, F.J. Zhao, R. Hurst. Selenium concentration and speciation in biofortified flour and bread: Retention of selenium during grain biofortification, processing and production of Se-enriched food. *Food Chemistry* 2011, 126, (4), 1771–1778.
64. M.A. Bryszewska, W. Ambroziak, A. Diowksz, M.J. Baxter, N.J. Langford, D.J. Lewis. Changes in the chemical form of selenium observed during the manufacture of a selenium-enriched sourdough bread for use in a human nutrition study. *Food Additives and Contaminants* 2005, 22, (2), 135–140.
65. W. Zhang, S. Xiao, H. Samaraweera, E.J. Lee, D.U. Ahn. Improving functional value of meat products. *Meat Science* 2010, 86, (1), 15–31.
66. V.I. Fisinin, T.T. Papazyan, P.F. Surai. Producing selenium-enriched eggs and meat to improve the selenium status of the general population. *Critical Reviews in Biotechnology* 2009, 29, (1), 18–28.
67. V.I. Fisinin, T.T. Papazyan, P.F. Surai. Producing specialist poultry products to meet human nutrition requirements: Selenium enriched eggs. *World's Poultry Science Journal* 2008, 64, (1), 85–97.
68. E.A. Decker, Y. Park. Healthier meat products as functional foods. *Meat Science* 2010, 86, (1), 49–55.
69. J.B. Taylor, M.J. Marchello, J.W. Finley, T.L. Neville, G.F. Combs, J.S. Caton. Nutritive value and display-life attributes of selenium-enriched beef-muscle foods. *Journal of Food Composition and Analysis* 2008, 21, (2), 183–186.
70. K. Pyrzynska. Selenium speciation in enriched vegetables. *Food Chemistry* 2009, 114, (4), 1183–1191.
71. D. Thavarajah, P. Thavarajah, A. Wejesuriya, M. Rutzke, R. Glahn, G. Combs, A. Vandenberg. The potential of lentil (*Lens culinaris* L.) as a whole food for increased selenium, iron, and zinc intake: preliminary results from a 3 year study. *Euphytica* 2011, 180, (1), 123–128.
72. J.W. Finley. Proposed criteria for assessing the efficacy of cancer reduction by plant foods enriched in carotenoids, glucosinolates, polyphenols and selenocompounds. *Annals of Botany* 2005, 95, (7), 1075–1096.
73. D.L. LeDuc, A.S. Tarun, M. Montes-Bayon, J. Meija, M.F. Malit, C.P. Wu, M. AbdelSamie, C.Y. Chiang, A. Tagmount, M. DeSouza, B. Neuhierl, A. Böck, J. Caruso, N. Terry. Overexpression of selenocysteine methyltransferase in Arabidopsis and Indian mustard increases selenium tolerance and accumulation. *Plant Physiology* 2004, 135, (1), 377–383.
74. D.R. Ellis, T.G. Sors, D.G. Brunk, C. Albrecht, C. Orser, B. Lahner, K.V. Wood, H.H. Harris, I.J. Pickering, D.E. Salt. Production of Se-methylselenocysteine in transgenic plants expressing selenocysteine methyltransferase. *BMC Plant Biology* 2004, 4, (1).
75. M. Hernández Ruiz de Eguílaz, C. Panizo Santos, S. Navas-Carretero, J.A. Martínez Hernández. Ferropenic anaemia: Dietary strategies for its prevention. *Anemia ferropénica: Estrategias dietéticas para su prevención* 2010, 14, (2), 67–71.
76. B.H. Özer, H.A. Kirmaci. Functional milks and dairy beverages. *International Journal of Dairy Technology* 2010, 63, (1), 1–15.

77. R.F. Hurrell. Fortification: Overcoming technical and practical barriers. *The Journal of Nutrition* 2002, 132, (4), 806S–812S.
78. F.M. Hilty, A. Teleki, F. Krumeich, R. Büchel, R.F. Hurrell, S.E. Pratsinis, M.B. Zimmermann. Development and optimization of iron- and zinc-containing nanostructured powders for nutritional applications. *Nanotechnology* 2009, 20, (47), 475101.
79. D. Moretti, M.B. Zimmermann, S. Muthayya, P. Thankachan, T.-C. Lee, A.V. Kurpad, R.F. Hurrell. Extruded rice fortified with micronized ground ferric pyrophosphate reduces iron deficiency in Indian schoolchildren: A double-blind randomized controlled trial. *The American Journal of Clinical Nutrition* 2006, 84, (4), 822–829.
80. M. Roe, R. Collings, J. Hoogewerff, S. Fairweather-Tait. Relative bioavailability of micronized, dispersible ferric pyrophosphate added to an apple juice drink. *European Journal of Nutrition* 2009, 48, (2), 115–119.
81. B. Troesch, I. Egli, C. Zeder, R.F. Hurrell, S. de Pee, M.B. Zimmermann. Optimization of a phytase-containing micronutrient powder with low amounts of highly bioavailable iron for in-home fortification of complementary foods. *The American Journal of Clinical Nutrition* 2009, 89, (2), 539–544.
82. V. Kumar, A.K. Sinha, H.P.S. Makkar, K. Becker. Dietary roles of phytate and phytase in human nutrition: A review. *Food Chemistry* 2010, 120, (4), 945–959.
83. Y.A. Suzuki, S.L. Kelleher, D. Yalda, L. Wu, J. Huang, N. Huang, B. Lönnerdal. Expression, characterization, and biologic activity of recombinant human lactoferrin in rice. *Journal of Pediatric Gastroenterology and Nutrition* 2003, 36, (2), 190–199.
84. H.J. Watzke. Impact of processing on bioavailability examples of minerals in foods. *Trends in Food Science and Technology* 1998, 9, (8-9), 320–327.
85. P.B. Holm, K.N. Kristiansen, H.B. Pedersen. Transgenic approaches in commonly consumed cereals to improve iron and zinc content and bioavailability. *Journal of Nutrition* 2002, 132, (3), 514S–516S.
86. P. Lucca, R. Hurrell, I. Potrykus. Genetic engineering approaches to improve the bioavailability and the level of iron in rice grains. *Theoretical and Applied Genetics* 2001, 102, (2-3), 392–397.
87. L.E. Murray-Kolb, F. Takaiwa, F. Goto, T. Yoshihara, E.C. Theil, J.L. Beard. Transgenic rice is a source of iron for iron-depleted rats. *Journal of Nutrition* 2002, 132, (5), 957–960.
88. F. Goto, T. Yoshihara, N. Shigemoto, S. Toki, F. Takaiwa. Iron fortification of rice seed by the soybean ferritin gene. *Nature Biotechnology* 1999, 17, (3), 282–286.
89. D. Eide, M. Broderius, J. Fett, M.L. Guerinot. A novel iron-regulated metal transporter from plants identified by functional expression in yeast. *Proceedings of the National Academy of Sciences of the United States of America* 1996, 93, (11), 5624–5628.
90. S.A. Ramesh, S. Choimes, D.P. Schachtman. Over-expression of an Arabidopsis zinc transporter in Hordeum vulgare increases short-term zinc uptake after zinc deprivation and seed zinc content. *Plant Molecular Biology* 2004, 54, (3), 373–385.
91. F. Tesán, F. Hernández, H. Torti, F. Massot, M. Huarte, E.R. de Celis, M.L.A. Barreiro, R. Weill, G. Cremaschi, J. Boccio, M.J. Salgueiro. Glycine-stabilized zinc gluconate has similar bioavailability than zinc sulfate in a zinc fortified probiotic food. *Open Nutraceuticals Journal* 2011, 4, 136–143.

92. R. Cornelis. *Handbook of elemental speciation: Techniques and methodology*. John Wiley and Sons: Chichester, England, 2003; Vol. 1, p 670.
93. A. Gonzalvez, S. Armenta, M.L. Cervera, M. de la Guardia. Non-chromatographic speciation. *TrAC - Trends in Analytical Chemistry* 2010, 29, (3), 260–268.
94. A. Gonzalvez, M.L. Cervera, S. Armenta, M. de la Guardia. A review of non-chromatographic methods for speciation analysis. *Analytica Chimica Acta* 2009, 636, (2), 129–157.
95. M.A. Vieira, P. Grinberg, C.R.R. Bobeda, M.N.M. Reyes, R.C. Campos. Non-chromatographic atomic spectrometric methods in speciation analysis: A review. *Spectrochimica Acta - Part B Atomic Spectroscopy* 2009, 64, (6), 459–476.
96. J. Szpunar. Bio-inorganic speciation analysis by hyphenated techniques. *Analyst* 2000, 125, (5), 963–988.
97. A.A. Ammann. Inductively coupled plasma mass spectrometry (ICP MS): A versatile tool. *Journal of Mass Spectrometry* 2007, 42, (4), 419–427.
98. J. Szpunar, R. Lobinski, A. Prange. Hyphenated techniques for elemental speciation in biological systems. *Applied Spectroscopy* 2003, 57, (3), 102A–112A.
99. S.S. Kannamkumarath, K. Wrobel, C. B'Hymer, J.A. Caruso. Capillary electrophoresis-inductively coupled plasma-mass spectrometry: An attractive complementary technique for elemental speciation analysis. *Journal of Chromatography A* 2002, 975, (2), 245–266.
100. A.R. Timerbaev. Capillary electrophoresis coupled to mass spectrometry for biospeciation analysis: Critical evaluation. *TrAC - Trends in Analytical Chemistry* 2009, 28, (4), 416–425.
101. C.C. Chéry. Gel electrophoresis for speciation purposes. In *Handbook of elemental speciation: Techniques and methodology*, R. Cornelis, ed. John Wiley and Sons: Chichester, England, 2003; Vol. 1, pp 224–239.
102. S. Mounicou, J. Szpunar, R. Lobinski. Metallomics: The concept and methodology. *Chemical Society Reviews* 2009, 38, (4), 1119–1138.
103. C.C. Chéry, H. Chassaigne, L. Verbeeck, R. Cornelis, F. Vanhaecke, L. Moens. Detection and quantification of selenium in proteins by means of gel electrophoresis and electrothermal vaporization ICP-MS. *Journal of Analytical Atomic Spectrometry* 2002, 17, (6), 576–580.
104. B. Welz, M. Sperling. *Atomic absorption spectrometry*. 3rd ed. Wiley-VCH Weinheim, Germany, 1999.
105. X. Zhang, C. Zhang. Atomic absorption and atomic emission spectrometry. In *Handbook of elemental speciation: Techniques and methodology*, R. Cornelis, ed. John Wiley and Sons: Chichester, England, 2003; Vol. 1, pp 241–260.
106. J. Szpunar. Trace element speciation analysis of biomaterials by high- performance liquid chromatography with inductively coupled plasma mass spectrometric detection. *Trac-Trends in Analytical Chemistry* 2000, 19, (2-3), 127–137.
107. R. Lobinski, J. Szpunar. Biochemical speciation analysis by hyphenated techniques. *Analytica Chimica Acta* 1999, 400, 321–332.
108. R. Lobinski, D. Schaumlöffel, J. Szpunar. Mass spectrometry in bioinorganic analytical chemistry. *Mass Spectrometry Reviews* 2006, 25, (2), 255–289.
109. R.M. Town. Speciation analysis by electrochemical methods. In *Handbook of elemental speciation: Techniques and methodology*, R. Cornelis, ed. John Wiley and Sons: Chichester, England, 2003; Vol. 1, pp 427–460.

9

Bionanocomposites for Natural Food Packing

Bibin Mathew Cherian[1], Gabriel Molina de Olyveira[2], Ligia Maria Manzine Costa[2], Alcides Lopes Leão[1], Marcia Rodrigues de Morais Chaves[3], Sivoney Ferreira de Souza[2] and Suresh Narine[4]

[1]Department of Natural Resources, College of Agricultural Sciences, Sao Paulo State University, Sao Paulo, Brazil
[2]Department of Nanoscience and Advanced Materials, Federal University of ABC, Sao Paulo, Brazil
[3]Center of Applied Sciences, University of Sagrado Coração, Bauru, Sao Paulo, Brazil
[4]Trent Center for Biomaterials Research, Departments of Physics & Astronomy and Chemistry, Trent University, Ontario, Canada

Abstract

Food packaging is essential for preserving food during the period between production and ultimate consumption. Considering the current problems associated with food production, such as global warming, rising demand for food, occasioned by increased population, reduced arable land, competition between food and fuel production, it is necessary to adopt measures aimed at reducing food losses. Nanotechnology applied to packaging emerges as an effective alternative to minimize losses and increase food security. Nanomaterials confer greater chemical, physical and biological resistance to packaging, and increase food shelf life. Moreover, packaging represents an environmental problem after use since it is produced from petroleum-based polymers, and is nonrenewable and non-biodegradable. It also contributes to the vast amount of waste disposal as well. In this context, the development of packaging based on renewable and biodegradable materials such as starch and cellulose, is critical to the sustainability of the food system. Due to the technological problems of the matrices, nanomaterials play a fundamental role in obtaining biodegradable packaging with efficiency similar or superior to traditional packaging. In this chapter we will present an overview of recent scientific studies related

Visakh P. M., Sabu Thomas, Laura B. Iturriaga, and Pablo Daniel Ribotta (eds.) Advances in Food Science and Technology, (265–300) © 2013 Scrivener Publishing LLC

to obtaining bionanocomposites for application in food packaging, especially in films, considering its properties and relations between different nanomaterials and matrices. The toxicological aspects of bionanocomposites are also briefly discussed.

Keywords: Bionanocomposites, food packing, polysaccharide films, nanoreinforcements, food nanoparticle additives, nanocrystals, nanofibers, toxicology, surface modification

9.1 Introduction

With the new awareness in searching for the use of environmentally friendly products and new applications, the production of biodegradable packaging has proven very promising and important for the future of a more sustainable world. Much of the world's packaging is derived from synthetic polymers. The polymers are formed by repetition of a large number of units linked together. By changing the type of unit, or how to arrange these units in the polymer, materials with very different properties are obtained. Due to its high physical and chemical stability, the durability means that after being discarded, it remains for a long time in the environment, with the degradation time on the order of 100 years. In addition, its decomposition can lead to harmful substances such as furans and phthalates, among others, that affect human health and the environment. This fact increases environmental pollution, which is one of the factors that is contributing to global warming. In order to reduce the environmental impacts resulting from the accumulation of plastics derived from synthetic polymers, research is being developed in the production of packaging polymers derived from renewable sources that degrade over time through natural mechanisms. These compounds, called polymers, can be easily found in nature within the group of polysaccharides (e.g., starch, cellulose), proteins (e.g., soy protein isolates, gelatin), polyesters (e.g., polyhydroxyalkanoates, PHAs), among others. Materials obtained only with the raw material properties are unsatisfactory. To this end, some additives are needed for the polymer matrix to improve its mechanical properties (tensile strength, elongation, and modulus), water absorption (solubility, vapor barriers, swelling), and morphology (homogeneity, porosity). With further studies, the possibility is also opened to add package active agents with antibacterials, antivirals, and antioxidants, among others, called active packaging.

In this review, special attention will be given to bionanocomposites with natural fillers obtained from plants, and modifications aimed at their applications in novel biodegradable packaging.

9.2 Natural Biopolymer-based Films

Biopolymers' naturally occurring polymers can be divided into two classes: natural biodegradable polymers (produced by biological systems such as animals, plants and microorganisms), and biodegradable synthetic polymers (derived from biological precursors producing amino acids, sugars, and natural oils) [1]. To be called a biodegradable material it should be completely degradable by living microorganisms and/or enzymes, generating natural compounds such as CO_2, water, methane, and hydrogen [2, 3, 4]. Many studies are being carried out within the group of natural polymers, with emphasis on proteins and polysaccharides, because studies indicate that good film-forming properties exhibit satisfactory values of the barrier to gases, as well as low cost and feasibility of material [5, 6]. However, the permeability water vapor is often high due to the hydrophilic character of the polymer. To this end, studies are being conducted in the production of films based on proteins and polysaccharides in order to improve the quality of packaging for food preservation.

One of the most widely used techniques in the development of biofilms is called casting, which uses the preparation of a colloidal solution of the macromolecule without additives, and the implementation of this solution on a suitable medium, followed by drying under controlled conditions. The formation of films begins with the formation of the gel, involving inter- and intramolecular crosslinks between polymer chains, forming a rigid three-dimensional matrix in the presence of solvent. After drying polymer films are obtained. The formulation of films needs the use of at least one component capable of forming a structural matrix with a sufficient cohesiveness. Only high molecular weight polymers, owing to their sufficient cohesive strength and capacity for coalescence, can produce such film structure. The degree of cohesion of the polymer matrix affects film properties such as density and compactness, porosity and permeability, flexibility and brittleness [7]. The uniform distribution of polar groups along the chain increases cohesion by interchain hydrogen bonds and ionic interactions. In general, the cohesion is achieved with polar polymers, long chains and crystalline structures. In this section, natural biopolymer films with polysaccharides and proteins, and natural fillers and active agents are discussed.

9.2.1 Polysaccharide Films

Polysaccharides are natural polymers of carbohydrates, formed by the union of numerous monosaccharides with the structural formula $C_n(H_2O_n)$ such as glucose $C_6H_{12}O_6$. Starch is one of the most abundant polysaccharides in nature and can be found in corn, wheat, cassava, rice, yams and potatoes [8, 9]. Starch has unique features like films and coatings that present possibilities for physical or genetic chemical modification [9]. These properties are due to its composition with two types of glucose: amylose and amylopectin, which has different proportions depending on their botanical origin.

The starch is located in the cells of plants and is stored in the form of granules. These granules of native starch have hydrophilic properties, but its processing is impaired, because its melting temperature is above the temperature of degradation. Due to its low cost and high availability, starch has been extensively studied in order to be modified or mixed with other chemicals to improve its processing and produce a versatile family of bioplastics (Figure 9.1). To improve its properties, starch has been modified by chemical methods in order to replace OH groups of amylose and amylopectin by ether or ester groups producing modified starches [10].

According to Lu *et al.* [11] the application of starch in the preparation of biofilms is based on the chemical, physical and functional amylose to form gels and films. The amylose molecules in solution, due to their linearity, tend to be oriented parallel, nearly enough for them to form hydrogen bonds between adjacent hydroxyl polymers. As a result, the affinity of the polymer for water is reduced which produces opaque films and less brittleness. This occurs when starch is subjected to heat in aqueous solution, where the hydrogen bonds of the amorphous region are disrupted, causing destruction of molecular order and irreversible changes in its properties, such as crystallization [11].

According to Lawton [12], depending on the source, starch has different properties attributed to the amylose in the starch content; which ranges from 18–30%, and higher amylose content has improved properties [12]. However, due to their hydrophilic

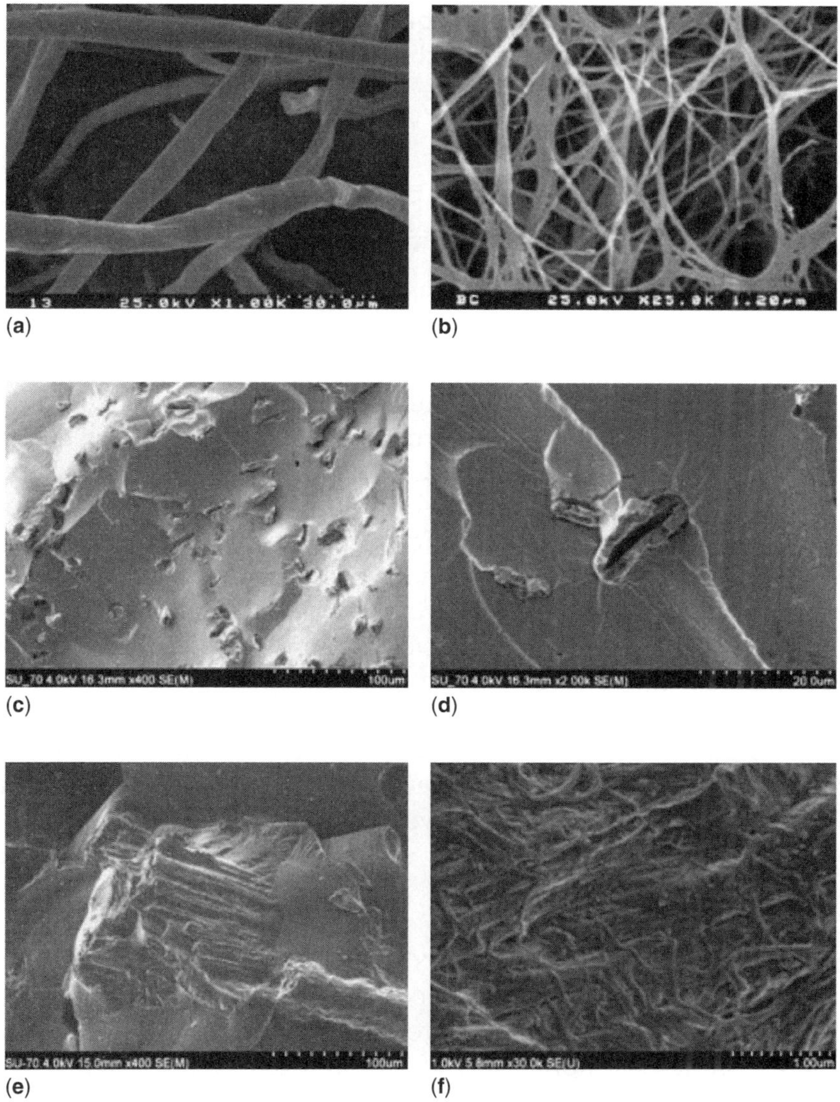

Figure 9.1 SEM micrograph of vegetable and bacterial celluloses and the fragile fractured surface of TPS filled with VC and BC: (A) vegetable cellulose; (B) bacterial cellulose; (C) and (D) TPS/VC composites (5 wt. %); (E) and (F) TPS/BC composites (5 wt. %). Reproduced with permission [10] Copyright © 2009, Elsevier Ltd.

character, these films have low barrier properties to water vapor but also have low permeability to gases such as CO_2 and O_2. Mechanical property is also a limiting factor, compared with synthetic films; it has limited flexibility because starch has strong polar bonds that create brittleness. Cellulose derivatives, chitosan, alginate, pectin and carragenan are other examples of polysaccharides which are important features in the production of films [13].

Yu *et al.* reported that some films of polysaccharides when applied in the form of gels may decrease moisture loss of certain foods, which evaporates before the dehydration of coated foods. It can also promote the effective protection of food on the changes caused by oxygen action [14]. Despite several advantages, properties obtained in films of polymers limit their production on a large scale. To this end, surveys are being conducted to improve their properties with different additions to the polymer matrix, making them competitive with conventional synthetic polymers.

Chitin is the second most abundant natural polymer in nature which is found in the shell of crustaceans, cuticles of insects, and cell walls of fungi [15, 16, 17]. Chitin has bacteriostatic and fungiostatic activities, which are favorable for promoting rapid dermal regeneration and accelerating wound healing (Figure 9.2) [18]. However, applications of chitin have been limited due to its insolubility in water and in most common organic solvents.

Chitosan is a polysaccharide obtained by alkaline deacetylation of chitin [18, 19]. This polymer has interesting properties, including biodegradability, bioadhesiveness, bacteriostatic, fungistatic and haemostatic activities [18]. Besides, its chemical structure allows the introduction of desired properties into chitosan by its chemical modification or its conjugation with other polymers [18, 19].

9.2.2 Protein Films

Proteins are polymers of complex structure, which are synthesized by living organisms through the condensation of several molecules of α-amino acids. There are a diversity of proteins found in nature, due to variable combinations of amino acids giving them different activities and properties. The protein derived from soybeans has become a big focus in the production of biodegradable films for their suitability as adhesives, plastics, among others, creating the possibility of producing films from renewable sources without causing damage to the environment. The soy protein isolates is made up of different structures formed from a set of different amino acids [20]. This can change the spatial structure of noncovalent intramolecular bonds, causing the opening of the polymer and producing greater interactions between chains of amino acids giving greater stability to the polymer matrix and allowing interactions

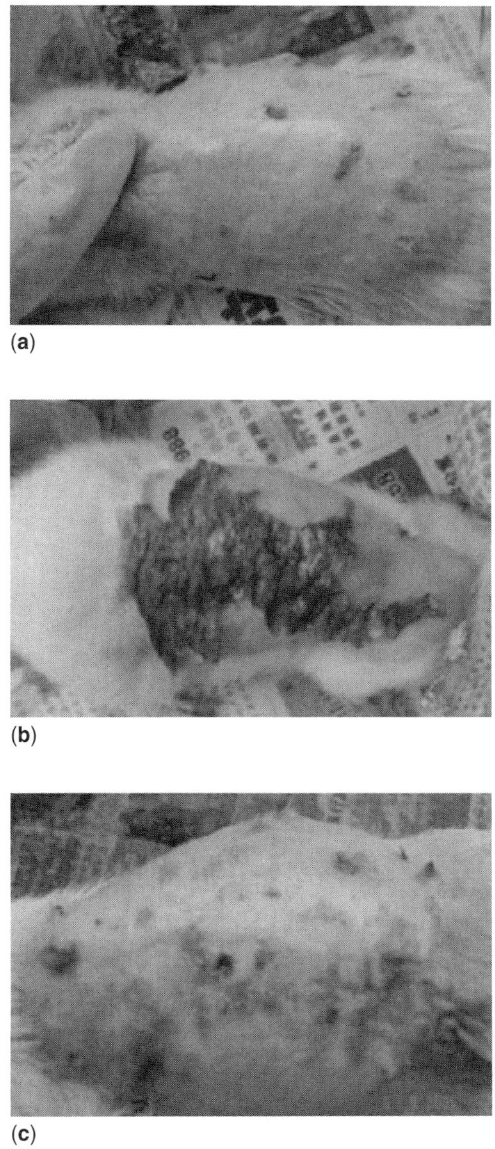

Figure 9.2 Chitosan for Wound healing Applications (a) Ag nanoparticles-chitosan dressing group; (b) Ag-sulfadiazine group; (c) chitosan film group. Reproduced with permission [18]. Copyright © 2009, Elsevier Ltd.

with other molecules to improve the properties of the films. Other proteins such as zein, derived from corn, wheat gluten protein, and animal proteins such as collagen, gelatin, casein, and whey are being studied for the formation of films [21, 22]. Zein protein has a hydrophobic character due to the high concentration of nonpolar amino acids, which produces hard and transparent films with stability to moisture and heat.

9.2.2.1 Polysaccharide and Protein Interactions

Mixed systems of globular proteins and polysaccharides have been widely used to control the structure, texture and stability of food products [23, 24]. Also, the interaction between natural polymers of different chemical structure through hydrogen bonding or that are electrostatic in nature may reinforce the mechanical properties of the materials obtained from such mixtures.

The major forces responsible for polymer interactions are electrostatic in nature but other common interactions such as hydrogen bonding or hydrophobic interactions may be significant in the stabilization of the interactions [25, 26].

Depending on the polymer's characteristics (molecular weight polysaccharide/protein ratio and charge density), and on the solution conditions (pH, ionic strength, total concentration), the association of biomacromolecules may result in the formation of a complex or a phase separation [27].

9.2.2.2 Composite Films – Functional Materials

Scientists and industry stakeholders have already identified potential uses of nanotechnology in virtually every segment of the food industry (Figure 9.3), from agriculture (e.g., pesticide, fertilizer or vaccine delivery; animal and plant pathogen detection; and targeted genetic engineering) to food processing (e.g., encapsulation of flavor or odor enhancers; food textural or quality improvement; new gelation or viscosifying agents) to food packaging (e.g., pathogen, gas or abuse sensors; anticounterfeiting devices, UV-protection, and stronger, more impermeable polymer films) to nutrient supplements (e.g., nutraceuticals with higher stability and bioavailability). Undeniably, the most active area of food nanoscience research and development is packaging: the global nano-enabled food and beverage packaging market was 4.13 billion US dollars in 2008 and has been projected to grow to 7.3 billion by 2014, representing an annual growth rate of 11.65%. This is likely connected to the fact that the public has been shown in some studies to be more willing to embrace nanotechnology in "out of food"

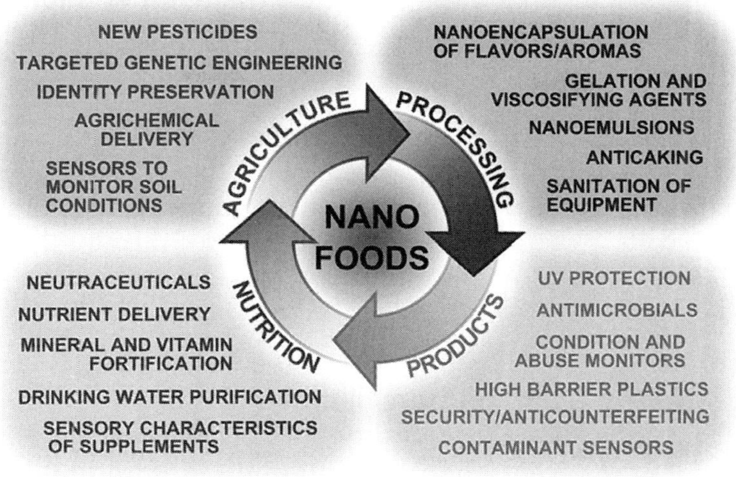

Figure 9.3 Nanotechnology has applications in all areas of food science, from agriculture to food processing to security to packaging to nutrition and neutraceuticals. Some potential applications are shown here. The applications which will be reviewed in this article are those in the orange quadrant, which are the most likely to be marketed in the near term. Reproduced with permission [29] Copyright © 2011, Elsevier Ltd.

applications than those where nanoparticles are directly added to foods [28, 29].

Bioactive food ingredients, or so-called nutraceuticals, are a new class of food supplements with biological added value, containing prophylactic and therapeutic agents for the improvement of human health. The active agents are antioxidants (enzymatic or non-enzymatic), different kinds of vitamins, essential fatty acids, phospholipids, minerals, phytochemicals, etc. A wide variety of delivery systems has been developed to encapsulate functional ingredients with recent applications in polysaccharide and protein, like edible films using nanolamite films. However, many bioactive compounds have a lot of unsaturated bonds in their molecules, and they need to be protected against oxidation and degradation under several conditions [30].

The driving force for adsorption of a substance to a surface depends on the nature of the surface and the nature of the adsorbing substance. The force itself could be electrostatic, hydrogen-bonding, hydrophobic interactive, thermodynamically incompatible, and so on, but it would usually be electrostatic attraction of oppositely charged substances [31].

9.3 Modification of Film Properties

The introduction of polymeric and filler additives is intended to improve certain characteristics of the films produced by the potential change in physical and/or mechanical properties, and generates the possibility of production of active packaging.

9.3.1 Natural Nanoreinforcements

Composites represent a class of materials where two or more substances are combined to display unique properties that are not likely to be obtained from its individual components. When at least one of the constituent phases of the composite has dimensions on the nanometer scale, it is now called nanocomposite. Nanocomposites can be formed by combining different materials, like inorganic-inorganic, organic, or organic-organic (being in the latter case, also called hybrid materials). It is from this scale size that effects can be observed in material properties. Responsible for the emergence of these different properties in nanostructures are: 1) the surface effects, and 2) the effects of quantum confinement [32]. The uniform dispersion of these nanoparticles can lead to a high interfacial area between the constituents; in addition to a large interfacial area, the distance between the nanoelements begins to approach the molecular dimensions in extremely low amounts of nanoparticles. This large interfacial area and nanoscopic dimensions between the constituent polymer nanocomposites differ from traditional composites and loaded plastics. On the other hand, the spatial confinement of charge carriers in nanomaterials provides very significant variations in optical and electronic properties due to changes in the density of electronic states. The arrangement of the constituents is critical in determining the behavior of the material. Conceptually, the spatial arrangement of nanoparticles of different shapes (spherical, cylindrical or flat) in positional arrangements (1-, 2- or 3-dimensions) with various degrees of orientation will be manifest in a variety of systems [33].

Nanocomposites show properties very different from ordinary composites. A great variety of material has been tested for production of nanocomposites. The search for biodegradability and reduction of environmental impact lead to the concept of bionanocomposites, on which all components are from a renewable source. Since the discovery in the early 1990s that dispersion of clay mineral nanoparticles in a polymer matrix significantly improved the mechanical properties of the material [34], a high demand began for so-called nanocomposites or, that is, composites in which at least one of the phases presents with nanometric dimensions. The presence of a phase composed of nanoparticles or nanofibers gives these materials very different characteristics from those of the composite components that come in dimensions on the order of micrometers or larger. Various types of materials, both organic and inorganic, have been tested in the production of nanocomposites. Among them, we can include clay minerals [33, 35, 36] and cellulose fibers obtained from plants [37, 38]. The latter are given special attention because they are biodegradable and renewable, with less impact on the environment than their synthetic counterparts [39].

9.3.2 Cellulose-based Nanoreinforcements

Cellulose is a polymer of long chains that is found in most plants and can also be produced by bacteria. The cellulose ethers and esters are cellulose derivatives that are most known and sold today. The plant cellulose fibers of nanoscale materials have been recently discovered, and are widely explored for technologies in bionanocomposites with numerous applications.

Cellulose fiber plants and their composites with cellulose nanofibers have offered a highly attractive line of research in recent years. The cellulose nanofibers have generated great interest as a source of nanofillers because of their sustainability, accessibility, and also because of their large surface area relative to the volume, which gives the composite excellent mechanical, electrical and thermal properties.

Cellulose fibril morphology is part of the composition of the fibers. Over the past few years, several researchers have been involved in investigating the exploitation of natural fibers as load-bearing components in composite materials [40]. The use of composite materials has increased due to its low price relative to its recyclability and the fact that they can compete well in terms of strength per weight of material.

Natural fibers are considered natural compounds consisting mainly of cellulose fibrils embedded in a matrix of lignin. The cellulose fibrils are aligned along the length of the fiber, which creates maximum tensile and flexural strength, and provides rigidity. The efficiency of building with natural fibers is related to the nature of cellulose and its crystallinity [41]. The structure, microfibrillar angle, the crystal cell dimensions, defects and chemical composition of the fibers are the most important variables that determine the general properties of the fibers [42]. Generally, the tensile strength and modulus of fiber increases with increased fiber content, which in turn depends on the vegetable fiber which has been extracted. This implies that each type of plant can generate microfibers with different characteristics and applications. Polymer composites with wood fiber are being used in a large number of applications such as platforms, docks, window frames and molded panel components [43]. It has been reported that $750 million of polymer composite wood fibers were produced in 1999. Statistics show that the production of these compounds in 2001 increased to 1 billion dollars. In the last three decades, considerable research has been engaged in finding an alternative fiber to replace asbestos in building products and automotive brakes. Asbestos is a naturally-occurring mineral fiber commonly used as a reinforcing material in construction and automobile brakes. It produces dust that comes off vehicle brakes and mineral processing industries causing disease in thousands of human beings and other animal species, and its residue is toxic to the environment. Australian studies focused on natural fibers, and so the fibers of wood pulp were used as a replacement for asbestos in industry [44]. Also other researchers have explored the use of other fibers (bamboo, hemp, eucalyptus, sisal and coconut) as a substitute for asbestos [45, 46]. As these fibers are inexpensive and readily available, the energy required for the processing of these composites is low, biodegradable and nontoxic, and they have been shown to be great as a substitute for asbestos.

Cellulose can be chemically modified to produce derivatives that are widely used in different industrial sectors, in addition to conventional applications. For example, in 2003, 3.2 million tons of pulp were used as feedstock in the production of regenerated fibers and films, in addition to cellulose derivatives, which are still used as coatings, laminates, optical films and absorbents [47]. Moreover, these cellulose derivatives can be found as additives in building materials and also in foods, pharmaceuticals and cosmetics.

Nowadays, cellulose nanofibers obtained from plants have their field of application with other biocompatible and biodegradable materials producing nanocomposites suitable for medical, textile and natural composite applications. Pineapple and banana fibers have a higher cellulose content, which is related to the relatively higher weight of the fruit they support. Other fiber sources such as corn stover, bagasse, wheat, rice and barley straw, all contain nearly the same amount of cellulose. Fibers in these examples support relatively smaller weights in comparison with bananas and pineapples [48, 49]. These compounds have high cellulose stiffness and strength combined with biodegradability and can be used in applications such as food packing, blood bags and barrier materials [50].

9.3.2.1 *Factors Affecting Performance of Cellulose Nanoreinforcements*

Agronomic factors such as crop variety, seed density, soil quality, fertilization, location of the plantation, climate and weather conditions, and timing of the harvest (age of the plant) affect final fiber quality and their overall properties [51]. The mechanical properties of plant fibers do not only depend on the factors mentioned.

The cellulose of natural fibers contains different natural substances such as lignin and waxes. The fibers are made up of cellulose microfibrils with lignin. The physical properties of natural fibers are basically influenced by the chemical structure such as cellulose content, degree of polymerization, orientation, and crystallinity, which are affected by conditions during growth of plants as well as extraction methods used. More importantly, the fiber separation process significantly determines fiber quality and its mechanical properties.

A major disadvantage of cellulose fibers is their highly polar nature, which makes them incompatible with nonpolar polymers. Also, the poor resistance to moisture absorption makes the use of natural fibers less attractive for exterior applications. The resulting properties of nanocomposites with cellulose fibers have been reported to be strongly related to the dimensions and consequent aspect ratio of the fibers, as well as to geometric and mechanical percolation effects [52, 53]. Aspect ratios are related to the origin of the cellulose used and whisker preparation conditions [54].

9.3.2.2 *Improving Compatibility between Cellulose Nanofibers and Hydrophobic Matrices*

Strongly polarized cellulose fibers are not compatible with hydrophobic polymers. The compatibility and dispersability of fiber and matrix can be improved by physical methods, like plasma technique and chemical methods, like mercerization and coupling agents. Some chemical and natural compatiblizations have brought great results with polymer properties in final applications [55, 56].

Dusfrene *et al.* changed the surface of cellulose whiskers with N-Octadecyl isocyanate ($C_{18}H_{37}NCO$), and significant differences were reported according to the nature of the nanoparticle and amount of nanofillers used as reinforcement. It was also proven that the chemical treatment clearly improves the ultimate properties of the nanocomposites [57].

9.3.2.3 *Applications and Effects on Polymer Matrices*

Plant-based cellulose nanofibers have generated a great deal of interest as a source of nanometer-sized fillers because of their sustainability, easy availability, and related characteristics such as a very large surface-to-volume ratio, high-tensile strength, high stiffness, high flexibility, good dynamic, mechanical, electrical and thermal properties as compared with other commercial fibers [58]. The reinforcement is regarded as a nanoparticle only when at least one of the dimensions is lower than 100 nm. The use of nanoreinforcements in the polymer matrix has been predicted to give improved properties compared to polymers and micro composites based on the same fibers [59]. Therefore, it is of great interest to examine the possibilities of cellulose-based nanofibers as reinforcing elements.

In this scope, in the automotive industry cotton fibers embedded in the polyester matrix were used in the body of a car in East Germany. Daimler-Benz has been exploring the idea of replacing the glass fibers in natural fibers in automotive components since 1991. A subsidiary of Mercedes-Benz pioneered this concept with a project in this area titled the "Beleem project" based in Sao Paulo. In this case, coconut fibers were used in commercial vehicles over a period of nine years. Mercedes also used natural fiber in the door panels of its vehicle class in 1996. In September 2000, Daimler Chrysler also began to use natural fibers for its production of vehicles. Almost all major car manufacturers in Germany (Daimler Chrysler, Mercedes, Volkswagen, Audi Group, BMW, Ford and Opel) now use biocomposites in various applications. Several plant-based cellulose fibers, like curuaua fibers, banana fibers and pineapple fibers, have been tested with significant results,.

Deepa *et al.* showed that banana nanofibers obtained from steam explosion had its cellulose content increased from 64% to 95% due to the application of alkali and acid treatments; and surface morphological studies using SEM and AFM revealed that there was a reduction in fiber diameter during the steam explosion followed by acid treatments [60].

In this scope, nanofibers from pineapple leaves are special because they have shown many entanglements, very hygroscopic with various characteristics desired for biomedical applications, such as high crosslinking, uncomplicated chemical structure and nontoxicity [61]. Besides this, pineapple leaves also showed high chitinase activity with antifungal activity relative to other tropical plants, because they adapt to stronger light and dry climate, and it is believed that chitinases derived from leaves of pineapple exhibit unique characteristics [62]. Recently, one study has presented an evaluation of the developmental toxicity of pineapple-leaf extract in rats. This study concluded that orally administered EPL is safe in rats during embryonic development. The present developmental toxicity study has proven the safety of orally administered pineapple leaf in the embryos, which is beneficial to the development and dissemination of pineapple leaf [63]. In Brazil, pineapple is one of the contributors to the agricultural economic activity of the country, and has the potential to produce about 19,600 tons of fiber from about 1011 leaves produced on 58,794 ha.

Cellulose nanofibers were added to improve tensile properties, water vapor permeability, and glass transition temperature of mango puree films [64]. Tensile strength increased (4.09 to 8.76 MPa) with the increase in CNF concentration from 0% to 36%. It was proposed that due to the formation of fibril network within the matrix, there was an effective increment in tensile strength, and Young's modulus, especially at higher concentrations of CNF. The addition of CNF was also effective in improving water vapor barrier of the films (2.66 to 1.67 g.mm/kPa.h.m2). The water vapor permeability was significantly decreased when CNF was incorporated at loadings of at least 10% (10 g/100 g).

Recently, processed nanobiocomposites were produced with cellulose nanoparticles and glycerol plasticized-starch; the tensile strength increased from 3.15 to 10.98 MPa when CN content increased from 0 to 5 wt.%, and water vapor permeability decreased from 5.75×10^{-10} to 3.43×10^{-10} $gm^{-1}s^{-1}Pa^{-1}$. The improvements in these properties may be attributed to the good interaction between CN filler and GPS matrix because of the similar polysaccharide structures of cellulose and starch [65].

Another type of cellulose that is produced by bacteria, have attracted researchers because of major applications in the medical field. However, new research using bacterial cellulose-like addictives in polymer composites are growing. Narkato *et al.* produced bacterial cellulose composites with excellent mechanical strength of cellulose membranes impregnated in phenolic resin at a pressure of 100 MPa. The authors credited these results to the tapes that have uniform size, are extremely thin and are packaged in cellulose microfibrils arranged linearly [66].

Simonsen *et al.* developed a bionanocomposite based on thermoplastic starch and bacterial cellulose nanofibers. The bacterial cellulose was obtained from Acetobacter xylinum cultures [67]. Cassava starch and glycerol were used for the production of thermoplastic starch films. X-ray diffractometry of the films showed the development of starch crystallinity induced by the fibers, which may contribute to improve mechanical properties. Electron scanning microscopy of the disrupted films showed good adhesion between fiber and matrix and good dispersion of the nanofibers.

Hisano developed a new biocomposite based on hydrated BC membranes, and PU resins were prepared. An improvement of the interface between the BC and the PU resin was obtained from the solvent exchange process [68]. Results obtained by FTIR revealed the presence of main bands of urethane bond and disubstituted urea in the biocomposites. Additionally, the observed reduction of the hydroxyl band (3500 cm^{-1}) suggests an interaction between the BC and the NCO-free groups in the resin. The biocomposites presented a noncrystalline character, while the thermal characterization indicates a significant increase in the glass transition temperature.

Mixing a polymer solution and a BC suspension followed by solvent casting is another common method used to prepare BC nanocomposites. Due to the synthesis and nature of thermoplastic polymers, this approach has been more common for preparing BC/thermoplastic nanocomposites and has involved both natural and synthetic polymers.

Dammstrom *et al.*'s preparation of the BC/xylans nanocomposites consisted of first homogeneizing the bacterial cellulose in a blender after which the xylan solutions were added in different ratios, and the blends were allowed to interact for 30 min and solution casted [69]. Xylans were found to aggregate on BC to produce a laminated structure. Besides this, the incorporation of xylans in the composites reduced the tensile strength of homogenized bacterial cellulose from ca 110 MPa to 65 MPa in nanocomposites containing 50% xylans. However, Young's modulus increased from ca 4 GP to 6.5 Gpa when the xylan content increased to 30% after which the modulus was found to decrease again.

Chitosan has also been used in several works to create BC/chitosan nanocomposites. While it has been shown that incorporation of chitosan in the culture medium of bacterial cellulose leads to the incorporation of N-acetyl glucosamide into the cellulose chain, other studies [70, 71] have shown that true nanocomposites can be formed by immersing a purified BC pellicle in a chitosan solution followed by solvent casting. The resulting nanocomposites were considered ideal for wound dressing applications. Chitosan lowered the mechanical properties of the membrane from a tensile strength of 74 MPa to 54 MPa while elongation at break increased from 6.8% to 7.4%.

Tomé *et al.* [72] produced modified bacterial cellulose membranes with tailored properties in regards to their surface and barrier properties. It was prepared by controlled heterogeneous esterification with hexanoyl chloride.

Grande *et al.* [73] developed self-assembled nanocomposites of cellulose synthesized by Acetobacter bacteria and native starch. Potato and corn starch was added into the culture medium and partially gelatinized in order to allow the cellulose nanofibrils to grow in the presence of a starch phase. The BC-starch gels were hot pressed into sheets that had a BC volume fraction higher than 90%. Structural properties determined by XRD and ATR-FTIR showed that the crystallinity of BC was preserved in spite of the presence of starch; hence, the mechanical properties of the nanocomposites showed no significant decrease.

Bacterial cellulose has shown very promising characteristics for reinforcement material for composites with optical functions. Recently, a paper entitled "Optically Transparent Composites Reinforced with Bacterial Cellulose Nanofibers," reported that the characteristics of the composite formed, such as transparency and low coefficient of expansion, are due primarily to networks of chains of semicrystalline nanofibers produced by the bacterium

Acetobacter xylinum [74]. Ifuku *et al.* obtained acetylated BC sheets to enhance the properties of optically transparent composites of acrylic resin reinforced with the nanofibers [75].

9.3.3 Starch Nanocrystals/Starch Nanoparticles

Starch is one of the most promising natural polymers because of its inherent biodegradability, overwhelming abundance and renewability. It is composed of a mixture of glycans that plants synthesize and deposit in the chloroplasts as their principal food reserve. Starch is stored as insoluble granules composed of α-amylose (20–30%) and amylopectin (70–80%) [76]. α-Amylose is a linear polymer of several thousands of glucose residues linked by α(1→4) bonds. The α-glycosidic bonds of α-amylose cause it to adopt a helical conformation (left-handed helix) [76]. Amylopectin consists mainly of α(1→4)-linked glucose residues, but it is a branched molecule with α(1→6) branch points every 24 to 30 glucose residues on average. Amylopectin molecules contain up to 106 glucose residues, making them some of the largest molecules in nature [76].

First of all, it is important to clarify the terms commonly used. Starch crystallites, starch nanocrystal, microcrystalline starch, all refer to the crystalline part of starch obtained by hydrolysis but to a different extent (from the most to the least). It has to be distinguished from starch nanoparticles, which can be amorphous. Most reinforced materials present poor matrix-filler interactions, which tend to improve with decreasing filler dimensions. The use of fillers of a nanometric scale produces nanocomposites with new properties. Nanoparticles have proportionally larger surface area than microparticles, which favors the filler-matrix interactions and the performance of the resulting material [77].

Only a limited number of articles concerning starch nanocrystal production have been published during the past decade. Most of them relate to the use of acid hydrolysis, and even though a variety of starch sources have been used, they all refer to the same two processes: 1) Dufresne *et al.*'s process using HCl, and 2) Angellier *et al.*'s optimization of the process using H_2SO_4 [78].

In the most recent studies, new processes have been tried out to produce starch nanoparticles by i) precipitation of amorphous starch by Ma *et al.* [79] and Tan *et al.* [80], ii) combining complex formation and enzymatic hydrolysis by Kim and Lim [81] yielding

V6I type nanocrystals (i.e., complexed with lipids), and iii) microfluidization by Liu *et al.* [82].

Starch has been extensively investigated as a choice material for food packaging applications due to its wide availability and low cost [83, 84]. The addition of inorganic materials and synthetic polymers [85] has been proposed to improve water resistance of starch. More recently, blends of starch with nanoclays have been investigated. MMT addition reduced water uptake of starch films, possibly due to the tortuous structure formed by the exfoliated clay. Recently, a starch/ZnO–carboxymethylcellulose sodium nanocomposite was prepared using ZnO nanoparticles stabilized by carboxymethylcellulose sodium (CMC) as the filler in glycerol plasticized-pea starch [86].

Plasticizers showed differents results; because of decreased exfoliation in starch-MMT nanocomposites but increased film properties in thermoplastic starch-starch nanocrystals, the storage modulus of the composite material increases, with respect to the unfilled film, by 470% at 50°C, while the permeability increases by 70%.

Yue *et al.* obtained organic-soluble starch nanocrystal (SN); the acetylated starch nanocrystals could reduce their surface energy and showed good solubility in organic solvents such as acetone, chloroform and ethyl acetate. Also, the acetylated starch nanocrystals exhibited unique hydrophobicity [87].

9.3.4 Chitin/Chitosan Nanoparticles

Chitosan is a cationic polymer obtained from chitin comprising copolymers of $\beta(1\rightarrow4)$-glucosamine and N-acetyl-D-glucosamine. Chitin is a natural polysaccharide found particularly in the shell of crustaceans, cuticles of insects and cell walls of fungi, and is the second most abundant polymerized carbon found in nature [88, 89].

The isolation of chitosan fibers and its subsequent processing produce nanoparticles, hydrogels, nanofibers and scaffolds with different surface chemistry and surface morphology, and each one is chosen depending on its application. Nowadays, principal chitosan applications are in biomedical and food packing applications [90, 91]. Lu, Weng, and Zhang [92] prepared chitin whiskers by acid hydrolysis of chitin. Sriupayo *et al.* [93] added chitin whiskers to chitosan films, and observed that the whiskers improved chitosan tensile strength in bionanocomposite.

Another processing alternative is nanoparticles. Chitosan nanoparticles can be obtained by ionic gelation, where the positively charged amino groups of chitosan form electrostatic interactions with polyanions employed as crosslinkers, such as tripolyphosphate [94]. Chitosan/tripolyphosphate nanoparticles were prepared and incorporated in hydroxypropyl methylcellulose films. Chitosan concentration for nanoparticle preparation was 2.14 and 3.15 mg/mL, and tripolyphosphate concentration was 0.3 and 0.6 mg/mL. The mechanical properties, water vapor permeability, thermal stability and scanning electron microscopy of the films were analyzed. The authors showed that chitosan nanoparticles tend to occupy the empty spaces in the pores of the matrix, increasing the collapse of the pores thereby improving film tensile properties and water vapor permeability.

Starch and chitosan are abundant naturally-occurring polysaccharide. Both of them are cheap, renewable, nontoxic, and biodegradable [95]. The starch/chitosan blend exhibits good film forming property, which is attributed to the inter- and intramolecular hydrogen bonding that formed between amino groups and hydroxyl groups on the backbone of two components. The mechanical properties, water barrier properties, and miscibility of biodegradable blend films are affected by the ratio of starch and chitosan [96].

Chang *et al.* [97] produced glycerol plasticized-potato starch (GPS) that was combined with CNP to prepare all-natural nanocomposites by casting and evaporation. The morphological, structural, thermal and mechanical properties of the nanocomposites were evaluated by electron microscopy, X-ray diffraction, dynamic mechanical thermal analysis, and tensile tests. At low loading levels, CNP was uniformly dispersed in the GPS matrix and had good interaction between the filler and matrix, which led to improvements in the tensile strength, storage modulus, glass transition temperature, and water vapor barrier properties of the GPS/CNP composites.

Chitosan is also a bioadhesive material. The adhesive properties of chitosan in a swollen state have been shown to persist well during repeated contacts of chitosan and the substrate [98] which implies that, in addition to the adhesion by hydration, many other mechanisms, such as hydrogen bonding and ionic interactions might also have been involved. Moreover, chitosan exhibits a pH-sensitive behavior as a weak poly-base due to the large quantities of amino groups on its chain.

Chitosan dissolves easily at low pH while it is insoluble at higher pH ranges. The mechanism of pH-sensitive swelling involves the protonation of amine groups of chitosan under low pH conditions. This property has held chitosan to be widely investigated as a delivery matrix. Crosslinking is often used to tailor chitosan-based materials properties. The most common crosslinkers used to crosslink chitosan are dialdehydes such as glyoxal [99] and glutaraldehyde [100].

9.3.5 Plant-Protein Nanoparticle

Biopolymers such as proteins, lipids or polysaccharides are commonly used to encapsulate drugs in order to protect them from rapid degradation by environmental stress. Nanoparticles can be formed from a variety of materials, including synthetic polymers and biopolymers, such as proteins, lipids and carbohydrates. Natural macromolecules from vegetable sources appear to be a very promising alternative to synthetic polymers, mainly in food packing applications. They can also be prepared under soft conditions, without the use of toxic organic solvents or materials. Recently there has been research on the use of storage proteins from pea (legumin and vicilin) and wheat (gliadins) used as a structural material to prepare nanoparticles and their possible applications [101].

Plant proteins are characterized by their three-dimensional organization. Two classes can be distinghed: fibrous proteins composed of polypeptide chains joined together along a linear axis, and globular proteins composed of one or several polypeptide chains rolled up to give a three-dimensional structure. Globulins are the main storage proteins in pea seeds and are complex molecules with an amino acid composition similar to albumins. However, their solubility needs an electrolyte medium. On the other hand, glutelins are the main storage protein of wheat, and glutelins cannot be dissolved in any solvents, due to their high molecular mass and the presence of disulfide bonds [102].

Several methods have been reported in the literature for the preparation of nanoparticles from protein raw materials. Coacervation or controlled desolvatation methods have been developed using solvent or electrolyte as the coacervation agent or by adjusting the pH or ionic strength. In the coacervation methods promoted by solvents, the first step consists of dispersing macromolecules in an adequate solvent, then adding the mixture to a second solvent which is a nonsolvent of the macromolecules [103].

Animal derived proteins used in commercial applications are mainly casein, whey protein, collagen, egg white, and fish myofibrillar protein [104]. Plant-based proteins under consideration include soybean protein, zein (corn protein), and wheat gluten [105, 106]. Compared with nonionic polysaccharide films, protein films have better oxygen barrier properties and lower water vapor permeability [107]. However, serious concerns remain regarding their performance in food packaging, including their high modulus, high-water adsorption, and high gas permeability. Significant efforts have been made to improve the properties of various proteins applying nanocomposite technology, mainly using nanoclays.

Whey protein has received significant attention as edible film and coating material. Sothornvit and Krochta [108] reported the formation of whey protein transparent films, which also acted as an oxygen barrier. TiO_2 was added to form a nanocomposite with improved antimicrobial properties. Mill [109] has developed a promising photoactivated indicator ink for in-package oxygen detection based upon nanosized TiO_2 or SnO_2 particles and a redox-active dye (methylene blue); this detector gradually changes color in response to even minute quantities of oxygen, as shown in Figure 9.4. Soy protein has been of great interest to researchers for its thermoplastic properties and its potential as a biodegradable plastic. However, because of its poor response against moisture and high rigidity, its biodegradability has not been exploited effectively [110]. Similarly to starch, soy protein is also blended with plasticizers to overcome brittleness. However, the use of plasticizers further decreases barrier properties.

Zein, a relatively hydrophobic protein found in corn kernels, is known to form films easily [111]. Zein is used in the food industry as a coating agent and has shown potential as biodegradable polymer [82]. However, zein products, although less water sensitive than other biopolymers, still shows high-water vapor permeability and low tensile strength when compared with commodity polymers. As was the case for other biopolymers, its inherent brittleness may be ameliorated by the use of plasticizers which, on the other hand, further decrease water vapor and gas barrier properties.

9.3.6 Plasticizers

Plasticizers are defined as compounds added to other materials under certain conditions to modify some physical and mechanical properties. Low volatility plasticizers can be added to give flexibility to a polymer film [113].

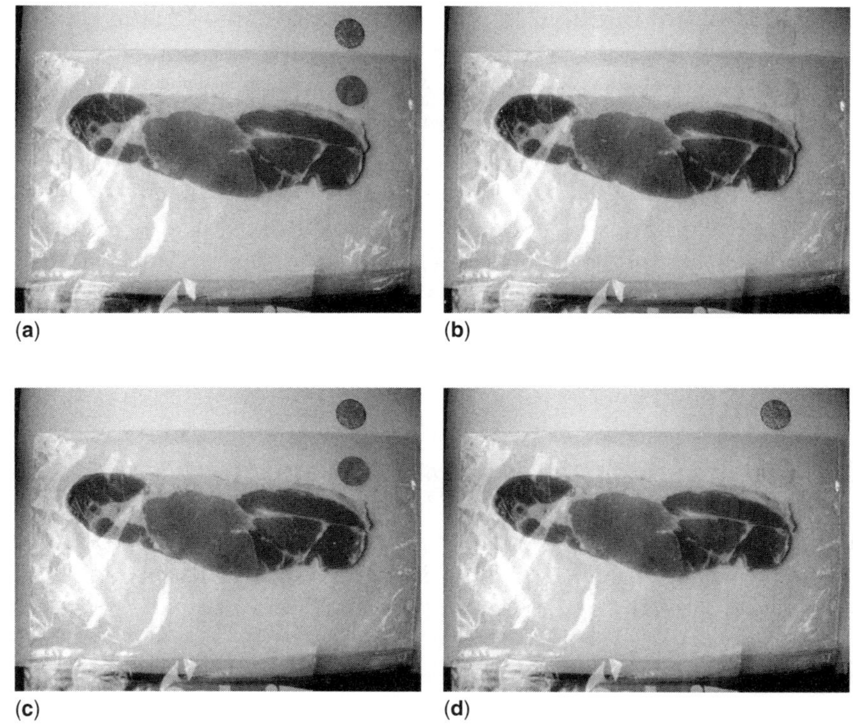

Figure 9.4 Photographs of two typical blue-coloured UV-activated oxygen indicators with the formulation: MB/TiO_2/TEOA/HEC, one placed inside and the other outside a plastic package flushed with CO_2 and sealed. In (a) the package had just been sealed and the two indicators are blue. The two indicators were then bleached by a short (2.5 min) burst of UVA light (b). The indicator outside the package regained its original colour within minutes, whereas, 48 h later, the indicator inside remained bleached (c). Finally, upon opening the package, the indicator within regained its original colour in response to the ingress of oxygen (d). Reproduced with permission from [109]. Copyright © 2005, Royal Society of Chemistry.

The reduction of intermolecular forces between polymer chains as a result of the cohesion facilitates the elongation of the film and decreases its glass transition temperature, but that reduces the barrier properties against gases, vapors and solutes. The addition of these plasticizers increases the mobility of polymer chains and thus gas permeability. The most commonly used plasticizers are monosaccharide, disaccharide and oligosaccharide in addition to the use of polyols. The choice of plasticizer used should be performed according to the compatibility with polymer and solvent [114].

Biofilms derived from proteins and polysaccharides generally have low elasticity and are brittle, and the introduction of plasticizers has been a great alternative to solve this problem. Plasticizers are substances with a high melting point and low volatility, which should be compatible with the polymer to ensure its efficiency. The most widely used plasticizers in film-based proteins and polysaccharides are polyols such as glycerol and sorbitol, which have good interaction with the polymer due to its structure and hydrophilic character [115]. The increase in the amount of plasticizer can also lead to an increase in permeability to gases hydrophilic film, because it reduces the density of the molecules, facilitating the diffusion of gases through the material.

9.3.7 Clays

Clays are natural materials of earthy texture and fine grain, and their particles are constituted of lamellar or fibrous clay minerals. These clay minerals are hydrated silicates with a lamellar structure of the tetrahedron SiO_4 arranged in the hexagonal form, mainly by condensed layers of aluminium [116].

A large group of interest is the smectite clays composed of aluminum, magnesium, iron, sodium and calcium. This type of clay is plastic and has very high-water retention. Furthermore, they are known as swelling clays due to their ease of separation and lamellar volume increase. The plates are irregular and no more than 1 mM [117].

This type of clay has a negative total charge on its surface resulting from the interaction of clay minerals known as isomorphic substitutions. This charge is neutralized by the presence of a cation located in the interlayer space, if this cation is sodium clay it is known as sodium clay smectite [116].

The interest in this material is exactly because of its expansive behavior that allows for the incorporation of other components in the interlayer space. Montmorillonite (MMT) in its natural state is hydrophilic, and through a process of exchange of cations, usually Na + is changed to be easier due to the monovalent or cation organic, usually an alkyl ammonium (surfactant). This method is known as organophilization [117].

This treatment of the clay is essential to decrease surface energy and to obtain a good dispersion and exfoliation of clay in the polymeric matrix, and only after organophilization does clay change its interface and allows for its dispersion in a polymer matrix nanocomposite [118].

Clay, as potential filler, has been chosen for improving the properties of TPS in such applications [119, 120]. It has been shown that both the tensile strength and the elongation at break of TPS were increased with the presence of small amounts (less than 5%) of sodium montmorillonite [121]. In addition, the decomposition temperature was increased while the relative water vapor diffusion coefficient of TPS was decreased [122]. Recently, starch/clay nanocomposite films were obtained by dispersing montmorillonite nanoparticles via polymer melt processing techniques [123]. Mechanical characterization results show an increase of modulus and tensile strength. In addition, the conformity of the resulting material samples with actual (2005) regulations and European directives on biodegradable materials was verified by migration tests [123].

Lin *et al.* [124] reported on a novel method for the preparation of a chitosan/montmorillonite nanocomposite using a solvent casting method. First, they prepared potassium persulfate (KPS), intercalated MMT by dissolving purified MMT in 0.5% KSP, and freeze-dried the mixture and pulverized it to KPS-MMT powder (less than 75 μm). A chitosan solution (1 wt %) was prepared separately by dissolving chitosan (degree of deacetylation = 85%) in 0.17 M acetic acid. After removing the non-exfoliated MMT, solutions were cast to form a film of a chitosan/MMT nanocomposite. TEM images of the chitosan/KPS-MMT nanocomposite films showed that partially and fully exfoliated MMTs were observed with the layers flattened out in parallel to the surface.

Xu *et al.* [125] prepared chitosan-based nanocomposite films with Na-MMT and Cloisite 30B using a solvent casting method. Structural properties tested using XRD and TEM indicated that the nanoclay was exfoliated along with the chitosan matrix with small amounts of Na-MMT, and that the intercalation with some exfoliation occurred with up to 5 wt% Na-MMT.

Chen and others [126] investigated the mechanism of interaction between soy protein and MMT clay by correlating structure and properties. The surface electrostatic interaction between the soy protein (+ charged) and the MMT layers (– charge), as well as the hydrogen bonding between the -NH and Si-O groups, were understood to be the interacting mechanism for the protein/MMT system. Such a mechanism resulted in the improved mechanical strength of the nanocomposite. Young's modulus (E) increased from 180.2 to 587.6 MPa with an increase of the MMT content from 0–20 wt%.

Dean and Yu [127] also prepared soy protein-based nanocomposite films and tested their microstructure and mechanical properties. They prepared the nanocomposite films by blending 400 g of water with 400 g of glycerol followed by adding 60 g of Cloisite Na+, after which the mixture was treated with a point source ultrasonic device for one hour. This mixture was combined drip-wise to 1200 g of soy protein isolates (Profam 974, Archer Daniels Midland) using a high speed mixer for five minutes, then extruded using a twin-screw extruder (Theysohn 30) at the set temperature of 140°C.

9.3.8 Active Agents

In order to produce biodegradable plastics, innovations such as active packaging to preserve the quality and safety of food are necessary. This idea is based on the principle of the interaction of product packaging with the observable need of each food.

Along with the incorporation of several active agents, research is also found on the application of biosensors, conducting polymers, properties with antimicrobial effects, antioxidants, flavors, pigments, vitamins, among others [128, 129]. Olyveira *et al.* obtained polymer nanocomposites using Ag/TiO_2 nanoparticles as an antimicrobial agent [130]. The results showed that incorporation of silver/titanium dioxide particles on composites obtained systems with different dispersions. The Ag/TiO_2 particles showed uniform distribution of Ag on TiO_2 particles as observed by SEM-EDX, and antimicrobial tests according to JIS Z 2801 shows excellent antimicrobial properties. In addition, Costa *et al.* obtained a new biocomposite with natural antimicrobial properties using the electrospinning technique [131]. This bionanocomposite has pineapple nanofibers and natural antimicrobial extract. SEM images showed equal distribution of pineapple nanofibers. DSC and TGA showed higher thermal properties and changes in crystallinity of the developed bionanocomposite.

9.4 Environmental Impact of Bionanocomposites Materials

Nanomaterials used in the cultivation, preparation, storage and packaging of food and drink has enabled the obtainment of products with better characteristics, such as materials for the controlled release of medicines and agrochemicals, containers with higher mechanical strength and antimicrobial properties, smart packaging capable of preserving food for longer periods of time, among others [132].

On one hand these materials are a breakthrough in technology that ensure the supply of food and materials, on the other hand, questions have been raised about the safety to human health and the environment as a result of these materials [133]. Consequently, studies have been conducted to obtain information on the characteristics of the nanoparticles and their relationship with adverse health effects in order to establish subsidies for the development of standards and regulatory parameters for nanoparticle use [134].

Considering the diverse applicability of the nanoparticles (NPs), their release into the environment will increase the extent that its use increases. The NPs have multiple routes of entry into the environment, including domestic and industrial solid and liquid waste, accidental spills, and atmospheric emissions. These routes allow the wide dispersion of NPs in the environment [134]. The fate and transport of nanoparticles in the environment are very important for safety assessment. The toxic effects of NPs are determined by their availability and reactivity with organic matter. The availability and reactivity of NPs are modulated by many parameters which affect the physico-chemical properties of these particles, such as the geochemical pathway during their transport, association with other chemical species, deposition, adsorption, change in redox state, environmental conditions (e.g., pH, ionic strength, salinity), and others. Thus, the environmental impact should be evaluated for each type of nanomaterial [133, 134].

9.4.1 Safety and Toxicology

Nanotechnology is increasingly being used in agriculture, food processing, and food packaging. Nanomaterials as nanoparticles, nanoemulsions and nanocapsules are found in agricultural chemicals, processed foods, food packaging and food contact materials, including food storage containers, cutlery and chopping boards [132]. Despite rapid developments in food nanotechnology, little is known about the occurrence, fate, and toxicity of NPs [135].

Nanoparticles represent a toxicological challenge issue. The size and shape of NPs regulate their toxicity. It is known that the smaller the particle, the larger the specific surface area, which leads to the higher reactivity of NPs and increase their interaction with the cell membrane [133, 134]. Miller and Senjen (2010) discussed how much a particle needs to be nanosized in order to show the desired characteristics (e.g., antimicrobial) and, at the same time, be enough of a size to not show cytotoxicity [132]. According to Garnett and Kallinteri (2006), particles < 300 nm in size can be taken up into individual cells, leading to damage effects, and < 70 nm is able to enter into the DNA structure [136]. Thus, more research is needed to find the size to reach the equilibrium between working properties and toxicity. The NPs toxicity is also influenced by chemical composition, shape, surface structure and charge, catalytic behavior, and particle aggregation [137, 138, 139].

Nanotechnology for food packing is based on organic and inorganic nanomaterials added into a polymer matrix. Nanoparticles such as metals and metal oxides, cellulose nanofibers, chitin and chitosan, and exfoliated clay are used as mechanical reinforcing, barriers to gas diffusion, and antimicrobial additives [140].

Clay nanoparticle toxicology data is still lacking, as are developments in strategies to detect and categorize clay and other nanoparticles in complex food matrices [29]. One study determined that exfoliated silicate nanoclays exhibited low cytotoxicity and genotoxicity, even when part of a diet fed to rats (measured acute oral toxicity, median lethal dose, LD50 > 5700 mg/kg body weight under the conditions probed) [141, 142] .

Polysaccharide nanoparticles such as cellulose nanofibers and nanowiskers are known to be usually nontoxic materials, acting as reinforcing agents. In the toxicological study, it was reported that nanofibers derived from cotton (white, green, and brown) and curaua could cause alterations in plant cells and be genotoxic in animal cells (human lymphocytes and mouse fibroblasts). However, the ruby cotton nanofibers did not present a genotoxic effect on plant and animal cells [143]. This fact demonstrates that the toxicity needs to be determined for each type of nanomaterial, and the toxicity behavior cannot be generalized for a specific class of material. In addition, this also indicates that even though the nanofibers toxicity cannot lead to cell death, the nanoparticles can affect genetic material. This is potentially dangerous since damage to the DNA cannot be repaired properly, causing health issues [143].

Nanoparticles of Ag, ZnO, TiO_2 and SiO_2 are commonly used in food plastic wrapping, in a polymer-based nanocomposite. These

NPs present excellent UV blocking and gas diffusion barrier, but the main characteristic of their use is antimicrobial action [135].

Mechanisms of NPs-biologic interaction explain the excellent antimicrobial behavior of metal and metal oxide. They include dissolution and release of toxic ions, disturbance of electron/ion cell membrane transport activity, oxidative damage through catalysis, lipid peroxidation or surfactant properties, and production of reactive oxygen species (ROS) [133].

ROS are considered mainly responsible for the NPs toxic effects, leading to secondary process that can cause cell damage or death. In addition, ROS are produced by ZnO and TiO2 due to their semiconductor property, confirming their highest antimicrobial behavior [133, 144].

9.4.2 Biodegradability and Compostability

Food packaging materials are the express source of pollution, due to the high amount disposed of in the environment in the world. The problem is aggravated once these materials are usually made from nonbiodegradable and nonrenewable sources, such as petroleum-based polymers [132].

Biocomposite materials based on starch, cellulose and chitin/chitosan are biodegradable, being a suitable alternative to the petroleum-based polymer materials for food packaging [145]. However, these materials are more sensitive to physico-chemical degradation and suitable to be attacked by microorganisms. Thus, additives are incorporated in these materials to increase their mechanical, chemical and biological resistance.

Nanoparticles are increasingly used as an additive in food packaging and food contact materials due to their antimicrobial property [135]. After use, these materials need to be discarded in the environment. The effect on the biodegradability and compostability is related to the microbial toxicity of NPs.

The biodegradation process occurs through microorganisms. The use of antimicrobial additives (e.g., Ag, TiO_2, ZnO, and SiO_2) in large scale may be hazardous to the microbes in the environment [144, 146]. Thus, the biodegradation process will be severely compromised, and it may be completely inhibited, affecting the decomposition of these materials in the landfill and composting units.

9.5 Conclusions and Future Perspectives

Bionanocomposites have very strong future prospects because of their degrability and better mechanical properties with filler in nanometric sizes. However, a better choice in polymer matrices or knowledge between proteins and polysaccharides is necessary. Biopolymers and their inherent brittleness may be ameliorated by the use of plasticizers which, on the other hand, further decrease water vapor and gas barrier properties. Nowadays, such problems have been solved with the addition of clay and new applications with protein and polysaccharide nanoparticles. Otherwise, active agents appear to have a very bright future for a wide range of applications.

References

1. D.S. Rosa, B.L.M. Franco, and M.R. Calil. *Polímeros: Ciência e Tecnologia* Vol. 11, p. 82, 2001.
2. A. Bhatnagar, and M. Sain. *Journal of Reinforced Plastics and Composites* Vol. 24, p. 1259, 2005.
3. H. Danner, and R. Braunn, *Chemical Society Reviews* Vol. 28, p. 395, 1999.
4. M.E. Gomes, R.L. Reis, A.M. Cunha, C.A. Blitterswijk, and J.D.D. Bruijn. Vol. 22, p. 883, 2001.
5. G.J.L. Griffin. *Chemistry and technology of biodegradable polymers*. London, Blackie Academic & Professional, 1994.
6. M. Salame. Barrier polymers. In M. Bakker, *The Wiley encyclopedia of packaging technology*, New York, pp. 48–54, 1986
7. R.V. Nonato, P.E. Mantelato, and C.E.V. Rossell. *Applied Microbiology Biotechnology* Vol. 57, p. 1, 2001.
8. J. Plank. *Applied Microbiology and Biotechnology* Vol. 66, p. 1, 2004.
9. M.A. Huneault, and H. Li. *Polymer* Vol. 48, p. 270, 2007.
10. I.M.G. Martins, S.P. Magina, L.Oliveira, C.S.R. Freire, A.J.D. Silvestre, C.P. Neto, and A. Gandini. *Composites Science and Technology* Vol. 69, p. 2163, 2009.
11. D.R. Lu, C.M. Xiao, and S.J. Xu. *Polymer Letters* Vol. 3, p. 366, 2009.
12. J.W. Lawton. *Carbohydrate Polymers* Vol. 29, p. 203, 1996.
13. S.J. Klahorst. *Food Product Design* p.1, 1999.
14. L. Yu, K. Dean, and L. Li. *Progress in Polymer Science* Vol. 31, p. 576, 2006.
15. M.N.V.R. Kumar. *Reactive & Functional Polymers* Vol. 46, p. 1, 2000.
16. M.N.V.R. Kumar, R.A.A. Muzzarelli, C. Muzzarelli, H. Sashiwa, and A.J. Domb. *Chemical Reviews* Vol.104, p. 6017, 2004.
17. K. Kurita, *Progress in polymer science*, Vol. 26, p. 1921, 2001.
18. M. Prabaharan, P.T. Sudheesh Kumar, S.V. Nair, H. Tamura. *Biotechnology Advances* Vol. 29, p. 322, 2011.

19. I.Y. Kim, S.J. Seo, H.S. Moon, M.K. Yoo, I.Y. Park, B.C. Kim, and C.S. Cho. *Biotechnology Advances* Vol. 26, p. 1, 2008.
20. X.D. Guo, Q.X. Zheng, J.Y. Du, S.H. Yang, H. Wang, Z.W. Shao, and E.J. Sun. *Journal Wuhan University Technology* Vol. 17 , p. 30, 2002.
21. A. Chilkoti, T. Christensen, and J.A. MacKay. *Current Opinion in Chemical Biology* Vol. 10, p. 652, 2006.
22. A. Patel, B. Fine, M. Sandig, and K. Mequanint. *Cardiovascular Research* Vol. 71, p.40, 2006.
23. R.M. Musampa, M.M. Alves, and J.M. Maia. *Food Hydrocolloids* Vol. 21, p. 92, 2007.
24. M.E. Berthand, and S. L. Turgeon. *Food Hydrocolloids* Vol. 21, p. 159, 2007.
25. D. Feldman. *Journal of Macromolecular Science - Part A: Pure and Applied Chemistry* Vol. 42, p. 587, 2005.
26. D.J. McClements. *Biotechnology Advances* Vol. 24, p. 621, 2006.
27. S.L. Turgeon, M. Beaulieu, C. Schmitt, and C. Sanchez. *Current Opinion in Colloid and Interface Science* Vol. 8, p. 401, 2003.
28. [B] Market attitude research services, australian community attitudes about nanotechnology – 2005–2009. Department of Industry, Innovation, Science and Research, Australia, 2009.
29. [C] T.V. Duncan. *Journal of Colloid and Interface Science* Vol. 363, p. 1, 2012.
30. G.E. Remondetto, E. Beyssac, and M. Subirade. *Journal of Agricultural and Food Chemistry* Vol. 52, p. 8137, 2004.
31. K.P. Velikov, and E. Pelan. *Soft Matter* Vol. 4, p. 1964, 2008.
32. Y.W. Mai, and Z.Z. Yu. *Polymer nanocomposite.* Cambridge, Woodhead Publishing Limited, 2006.
33. C. Bréchignac, P. Houdy, and M. Lahmani. *Nanomaterials and nanochemistry.* France, Springer, 2006.
34. A. Usuki, Y. Kojima, M. Kawasumi, A. Okada, Y. Fukushima, T. Kurauchi, O. Kamigaito. *Journal of Materials Research* Vol. 8, p. 1179, 1993.
35. H.M. Wilhelm, M.R. Sierakowski, G.P. Souza, and F. Wypych. *Carbohydrate Polymers* Vol. 52, p. 101, 2003.
36. B. Chen, and J.R.G. Evans. *Carbohydrate Polymers* Vol. 61, p. 455, 2005.
37. L. Mazzola. *Nature Biotechnology* Vol. 21, p. 1137, 2003.
38. C.M. Stewart, R.B. Tompkin, and M.B. Cole. *Innovative Food Science & Emerging Technologies* Vol. 3, p. 105, 2002.
39. S.Y. Yoon, and Y. Deng. *Journal of Applied Polymer Science* Vol. 100, p. 1032, 2006.
40. K. Jayaraman. *Composites Science and Technology* Vol. 63, p. 367, 2003.
41. M.J. John, and S. Thomas. *Carbohydrate Polymers* Vol. 71, p. 343, 2008.
42. K.G. Satyanarayana, K.K. Ravikumar, K. Sukumaran, P.S. Mukherjee, S.G.K. Pillai, and A.K. Kulkami. *Journal of Material Science* Vol. 21, p. 57, 1986.
43. Q. Li, and L.M. Matuana. *Journal of Applied Polymer Science* Vol. 88, p. 278, 2002.
44. R.S.P. Coutts. *Cement and Concrete Composites* Vol. 27, p. 518, 2005.
45. K. Ghavami. *Cement and Concrete Composites* Vol. 27, p. 637, 2005.
46. V. Agopyan, H. Savastano, V.M. John, and M.A. Cincotto. *Cement and Concrete Composites* Vol. 27, p. 527, 2005.

47. D. Klemm, B. Heublein, H.P. Fink, and A. Bohn. *Angewandte Chemie International* Vol.44, p. 3358, 2005.
48. B.M. Cherian, A.L. Leao, S.F. Souza, L.M.M. Costa, G.M. Olyveira, M. Kottaisamy, E.R. Nagarajan, S. Thomas. *Carbohydrate Polymers* Vol. 86, p. 1790, 2011.
49. P.K. Sukumaran, B. Sangani, C. Mahadik, H Yagnik, S. Telang, F. Vas, R.A. Oberroi, B. Modell, S.M. Merchant. *Metals Materials Processes* Vol. 13, p. 121, 2001.
50. B.C. Suddell, and W.J. Evans. Natural fiber composites in automotive applications: Natural fibers. In A.K. Mohanty, M. Misra and L.T. Drza, *Biopolymers and their biocomposites*, pp. 231, CRC Press, 2005.
51. S.J. Eichhorn, C.A. Baillie, N. Zafeiropoulos, L.Y. Mwaikambo, M.P. Ansell, A. Dufresne, K.M. Entwistle, P.J. Herrera-Franco, G.C. Escamilla, L. Groom, M. Hughes, C. Hill, T.G. Rials, and P.M. Wild. *Journal of Materials Science* Vol. 26, p. 2107, 2001.
52. D. Dubief, E. Samain, and A. Dufresne. *Macromolecules* Vol. 32, p. 5765, 1999.
53. M.A. Hubbe, O.J. Rojas, L.A. Lucia, and M. Sain, *Bioresources*, Vol. 3, p. 929, 2008.
54. M.A. Azizi Samir, F Alloin, and A. Dufresne. *Biomacromolecules* Vol.6, p. 612, 2005.
55. R.G. Raj, B.V. Kokta, and C. Daneault. *Macromolecular Symposia* Vol. 28, p. 187, 1989.
56. J. George, S.S. Bhagawan, and S. Thomas. *Composite Interfaces* Vol. 5, p. 201, 1998.
57. G. Siqueira, J. Bras, and A. Dufresne. *Biomacromolecules* Vol. 10, p. 425, 2009.
58. P. Wambua, J. Ivens, and I. Verpoest. *Composites Science and Technology* Vol. 63, p. 1259, 2003.
59. K. Wötzel, R. Wirth, and M. Flake. *Angewandte Makromolekulare Chemie* Vol. 272, p. 121, 1999.
60. B. Deepa, E. Abraham, B.M. Cherian, A. Bismarck, J.J. Blaker, L.A. Pothan, A.L. Leão, S.F. de Souza, and M. Kottaisamy. *Bioresource Technology* Vol. 102, p. 1988, 2011.
61. B.M. Cherian, A.L. Leão, S.F. de Souza, S. Thomas, L.A. Pothan, and M. Kottaisamy. *Carbohydrate Polymers* Vol. 81, p.720, 2010.
62. J. Hu, H. Lin, J. Shen, J. lan, C. Ma, Y. Zhao, F. Lei, D. Xing, and L. Du. *Food and Chemical Toxicology* Vol. 49, p. 1455, 2011.
63. K. Satyanarayana, G.G.C. Arizaga, and F. Wypych. *Progress in Polymer Science* Vol. 34, p. 982, 2009.
64. H.M.C. Azeredo, L.H.C.Mattoso, D. Wood, T.G.Williams, R.J. Avena-Bustillos, and T.H. McHugh. *Journal of Food Science* Vol. 74, 2009.
65. P.R. Chang, R. Jian, P. Zheng, J. Yu, and X. Ma. *Carbohydrate Polymers* Vol. 79, p. 301, 2010.
66. A.N. Nakagaito, S. Iwamoto, and H. Yano, *Applied Physics A* Vol. 80, p. 93, 2005.
67. J. Simonsen. Bio-based nanocomposites: Challenges and opportunities, http://woodscience.oregonstate.edu/faculty/simonsen/Nanocomposites, 2007.
68. C. Hisano. Desenvolvimento de materiais compósitos baseados em celulose-bacteriana produzida por *Acetobacter xylinum*, 100 f., Dissertação (Mestrado) – Instituto de Química, Universidade Estadual Paulista, Araraquara, 2006.

69. S. Dammstrom and P. Gatenholm. Preparation and properties of cellulose/ xylan nanocomposites. In D. Stokke, and L.H. Groom, *Characterization of the cellulosic cell wall*, Willey-Blackwell Publishing, pp. 53–66, 2006.
70. P.F. Hamlyn, J. Crighton, M.G. Dobb, and A. Tasker. Cellulose product, GB Patent 2314856, January 14, 1998.
71. V. Dubey, L.K. Pandey, and C. Saxena. *Journal of Membrane Science* Vol. 251, p. 131, 2005.
72. L.C. Tomé, L. Brandão, A.M. Mendes, A.J.D Silvestre, C.P. Neto, A. Gandini, C.S.R. Freire, and I.M. Marrucho. *Cellulose* Vol. 17, p. 1203, 2010.
73. C.J. Grande, F.G. Torres, C.M. Gomez, O.P. Troncoso, J. Canet-Ferrer, and J. Martinez-Pastor. *Materials Science and Engineering C* Vol. 29, p. 1098, 2009.
74. H. Yano, J. Sugiyama, A.N. Nakahaito, M. Nogi, T. Matsuura, M. Hikita, and K. Handa. *Advanced Materials* Vol. 17, p. 153, 2005.
75. S. Ifuku, M. Nogi, K. Abe, K. Handa, F. Nakatsubo, and H. Yano. *Biomacromolecules* Vol. 8, p. 1973, 2007.
76. D. Le Corre, J. Bras, and A. Dufresne. Starch nanoparticles: A review. *Biomacromolecules* Vol. 11, p. 1139, 2010.
77. A. Dufresne, J.Y Cavaille, and W. Helbert. *Macromolecule* Vol. 29, p. 7624, 1996.
78. D. French. Organization of starch granules. In R.L. Whistler, J.N. BeMiller, and E.F. Paschall, *Starch: Chemistry and technology*, New York, Academic Press pp. 183–247, 1984.
79. X. Ma, R. Jian, P.R. Chang, and J. Yu. *Biomacromolecules* Vol. 9, p. 3314, 2008.
80. Y. Tan, K. Xu, L. Li, C. Liu, C. Song, and P. Wang. *ACS Applied Materials and Interfaces* Vol. 1, p. 956, 2009.
81. J.Y. Kim and S.T. Lim. *Carbohydrate Polymers* Vol. 76, p. 110, 2009.
82. X. Liu, W. Sun, H. Wang, L. Zhang, and J.Y. Wang. *Biomaterials* Vol. 26, p. 109, 2005.
83. R.P. Singh, J. Pandey, D. Rutot, P. Degee, and P. Dubois. *Carbohydrate Research* Vol. 338, p. 1759, 2003.
84. S. Sinha Ray, and M. Okamoto. *Progress in Polymer Science* Vol. 28, p. 1539, 2003.
85. J.C. Huang, Y. Xiao, K.Y. Mya, X.M. Liu, C.B. He, J. Da, and Y.P. Siow. *Journal of Materials Chemistry* Vol. 14, p. 2858, 2003.
86. J. Yu, J. Yang, B. Liu, and X. Ma. *Bioresource Technology* Vol. 100, p. 2832, 2009.
87. Y. Xu, W. Ding, J. Liu, Y. Li, J.F. Kennedy, Q. Gu, and S. Shao. *Carbohydrate Polymers* Vol. 80, p. 1078, 2010.
88. E. Khor and L.Y. Lim. *Biomaterials* Vol. 24, p. 2339, 2003.
89. Y. Huang, S. Onyeri, M. Siewe, A. Moshfeghian, and S.V. Madihally. *Biomaterials* Vol. 26, p. 7616, 2005.
90. S. Pielka, D. Paluch, J.S Kus, B. Zywicka, L. Solski, L. Szosland, and E. Zaczynska. *Fibres and Textiles in Eastern Europe* Vol. 11, p. 79, 2003.
91. Y.W. Cho, Y.N. Cho, S.H. Chung, G. Yoo, and S.W. Ko. *Biomaterials* Vol. 20, p. 2139, 1999.
92. Y. Lu, L. Weng, and L. Zhang. *Biomacromolecules* Vol. 5, p. 1046, 2004.
93. J. Sriupayo, P. Supaphol, J. Blackwell, and R. Rujiravanit. *Carbohydrate Polymers* Vol. 62, p. 130, 2005.
94. T. Lopez-Leon, E.L.S. Carvalho, B. Seijo, J.L. Ortega-Vinuesa, and D. Bastos-Gonzalez. *Journal of Colloid Interface Science* Vol. 283, p. 344, 2005.

95. A. Domard. *Carbohydrate Polymers* Vol. 84, p. 696, 2011.
96. R. Jayakumar, D. Menon, K. Manzoor, S.V. Nair, and H. Tamura. *Carbohydrate Polymers* Vol. 82, p. 227, 2010.
97. P.R. Chang, R. Jian, J. Yu, and X. Mab. *Food Chemistry* Vol. 120, p. 736, 2010.
98. M. George, and T.E. Abraham. *Journal of Controlled Release* Vol. 114, p. 1, 2006.
99. V.R. Patel, and M.M. Amiji. *Pharmacological Research* Vol. 13, p. 588, 1996.
100. P.B. Malafaya, A. Pedro, A. Peterbauer, C. Gabriel, H. Redl, and R. Reis. *Journal of Materials Science: Materials in Medicine* Vol. 16, p. 1077, 2006.
101. S. Goin. *Trends in Food Science and Technology* Vol. 15, p. 330, 2004.
102. R. Bodmeier, H. Chen, and E. Paeratakul. *Pharmaceutical Research* Vol. 6, p. 413, 1989.
103. M.S. El-Samaligy and P. Rohdewald. *Journal of Pharmacy and Pharmacology* Vol. 35, p. 537, 1983.
104. R.X. Zhao, P. Torley, and P.J. Halley. *Journal of Materials Science* Vol. 43, p. 3058, 2008.
105. A.H. Brandenburg, C.L. Weller, and R.F. Testin. *Journal of Food Science* Vol. 58, p. 1086, 1993.
106. C. Lee, D.A. Scheufele, and B.V. Lewenstein. *Science Communication* Vol. 27, p. 240, 2005.
107. K.S. Miller and J.M. Krochta. *Trends in Food Science and Technology* Vol. 8, p. 228, 1997.
108. R. Sothornvit and J.M. Krochta. Plasticizers in edible films and coatings. In J.H. Han, *Innovation in food packaging*, New York, Elsevier Publishers, 2005.
109. A. Mills. *Chemical Society Reviews* Vol. 34, p. 1003, 2005.
110. H. Zheng, F. Ai, P.R. Chang, J. Huang, and A. Dufresne. *Polymer Composites* Vol. 30, p. 474, 2009.
111. J.W. Lawton. *Cereal Chemistry* Vol. 79, p. 1, 2002.
112. X. Liu, W. Sun, H. Wang, L. Zhang, and J.Y. Wang. *Biomaterials* Vol. 26, p. 109, 2005.
113. B. Cuq, N. Gontard, and S. Guilbert. Edible film and coating as active layers. In M.L. Rooney, *Active food packaging*, London, Blackie Academic and Professional, p. 111, 1995.
114. F. Debeaufort, J.A. Quezada-Gallo, and A. Voilley. *Critical Reviews in Food Science and Nutrition* Vol. 38, p. 299, 1998.
115. H.M.C. Azeredo, L.H.C. Mattoso, R.J. Aven-Bustillos, G.C. Filho, M.L. Munford, D. Wood, and T.H. McHugh. *Journal of Food Science* Vol. 75, 2010.
116. L.B. Paiva, A.R. Morales, and T.R. Guimaraes. *Polímeros* Vol. 16, p. 136, 2006.
117. Y.S. Chun, Y.J. Kyung, H.C. Jung, and W.N Kim. *Polymer* Vol. 41, p. 8729, 2000.
118. L.B. Paiva, A.R. Morales, F.R.V. Díaz. *Cerâmica* Vol. 54, p. 213, 2008.
119. E.P. Giannelis, R. Krishnamoorti, and E. Manias. *Advances in Polymer Science* Vol. 138, p. 107, 1999.
120. M. Alexandre and P. Dubois. *Materials Science and Engineering* Vol. 28, p. 1, 2000.
121. H.M. Park, X. Li, C.Z. Jin, C.Y. Park, W.J. Cho, and C.S. Ha. *Macromolecular Materials and Engineering* Vol. 287, p. 553, 2002.
122. H.M. Park, W.K. Lee, C.Y. Park, W.J. Cho, C.S. Ha. *Journal of Materials Science* Vol. 38, p. 909, 2003.

123. M. Avella, J.J. De Vlieger, M.E. Errico, S. Fischer, P. Vacca, and M.G. Volpe. *Food Chemistry* Vol. 93, p. 467, 2005.
124. K.F. Lin, C.Y. Hsu, T.S. Huang, W.Y.M. Chiu, Y.H. Lee, and T.H. Young. *Journal of Applied Polymer Science* Vol. 98, p. 2042, 2005.
125. Y. Xu, X. Ren, and M.A. Hanna. *Journal of Applied Polymer Science* Vol. 99, p. 1684, 2006.
126. P. Chen, and L. Zhang. *Biomacromolecules* Vol. 7, p. 1700, 2006.
127. K. Dean and L. Yu. *Biodegradable polymers for industrial application*. Boca Raton, CRC Press, 2005.
128. J.W. Rhim. *Critical Reviews in Food Science and Nutrition* Vol. 47, p. 411, 2007.
129. A. Arora and G.W. Padua. *Journal of Food Science* Vol. 75, 2010.
130. G.M. de Olyveira, L.M.M. Costa, A.L. Leão, S.F. de Souza, B.M. Cherian, A.J.F. de Carvalho, L.A. Pessan, and S. Narine. *Molecular Crystals and Liquid Crystals* Vol. 556, p. 168, 2012.
131. L.M.M. Costa, G.M. de Olyveira, B.M. Cherian, A.L. Leão, S.F. de Souza, and M. Ferreira. *Industrial Crops and Products* Vol. 41, p. 198, 2013.
132. G. Miller, and R. Senjen. Nanotechnology in food and agriculture. In *Nano meets macro: Social perspectives on nanoscience and nanotechnology*. Pan Stanford Publishing, p.417–444, 2010.
133. A. Elsaesser, C.A. Howard. *Advanced Drug Delivery Reviews* Vol. 64, p. 129, 2012.
134. A. Lapresta-Fernández, A. Fernández, J. Blasco. *Environment International* Vol. 39, p.148, 2012.
135. S.B. Sekhon. *Nanotechnology, Science and Applications* Vol. 3, p. 1, 2010.
136. M.C. Garnett, P. Kallinteri. *Occupational Medicine* Vol. 56, p. 307, 2006.
137. C. Sayes, R. Wahi, P. Kurian, Y. Liu, J. West, K. Ausman, D. Warheit, and V. Colvin. *Toxicological Sciences* Vol. 92, p. 174, 2006.
138. J. Fabrega, S. N. Luoma, C.R, Tyler, T.S. Galloway, J.R. Lead. *Environment International* Vol. 37, p. 517, 2011
139. C. Fajardo, L.T. Ortíz, M.L. Rodríguez-Membibre, M. Nande, M.C. Lobo, M. Martin. *Chemosphere* Vol. 86, p. 802, 2012.
140. P. Das, M.A. Xenopoulos, C.J. Williams, Md.E. Hoque, and C.D. Metcalfe. *Environmental Toxicology and Chemistry* Vol. 31, p. 122, 2012.
141. P.R. Li, J.C. Wei, Y.F. Chiu, H.L. Su, F.C. Peng, J.J. Lin. *ACS Applied Material Interface* Vol. 2, p. 1608, 2010.
142. P. Simon, Q. Chaudhry, D. Bakoš. *Journal of Food and Nutrition Research* Vol. 47, p. 105, 2008.
143. R. De Lima, L.O. Feitosa, C.R. Maruyama, M.A. Barga, P.C. Yamawaki, I.J. Vieira, E.M. Teixeira, A.C. Corrêa, L.H.C. Matoso, L.F. Fraceto. *International Journal of Nanomedicine* Vol. 7, p. 3555, 2012.
144. D. Sharma, J. Rajput, B.S. Kaith, M. Kaur, S. Sharma. *Thin Solid Films* Vol. 519, p. 1224, 2010.
145. V. Siracusa, P. Rocculi, S. Romani, M. Dalla Rosa. *Trends in Food Science & Technology* Vol. 19, p. 634, 2008.
146. C. Levard, E.M. Hotze, G. Lowry, G.E. Brown Jr. *Environmental Science and Technology* Vol. 46, p. 6900, 2012.

Index

Acid
- acetyl salicylic, 175–177
- amino acids, 162, 169, 172
- arachidonic acid, 164
- ascorbic, 175–177
- benzoic, 164
- caffeic, 164
- citric, 175–177
- docosahexaenoic, 165
- docosapentaenoic, 164
- eicosapentaenoic, 164
- fatty acid, 161–165, 167, 169–170
- ferrulic, 164
- gentisic, 164
- hydroxybenzoic, 164
- hydroxy-cinnamic, 164
- lactic acid, 167
- lactic acid bacteria, 167
- linoleic, 164
- p-anisic, 164
- phenolic acids, 162–164
- sinapic, 164
- α-linolenic, 164
- ω-3 fatty acids, 161, 164–165, 170
- ω-6 fatty acids, 164

Active packaging, 290
- antimicrobial nanocomposites, 112
- carbon nanotubes, 113
- release, 112
- titanium dioxide, 113

Additives, 169–170
Amino acids, 162, 169, 172
Anthocyanins, 176–177
Anticarcinogenic, 168, 175
Anti-clotting agents, 163
Antioxidants, 162–163, 169–170, 175
Antiviral, 175
Aroma, 169, 172
Aromatic plants, 162
Arsenic, 231
Atherosclerosis, 165
Atopic diseases, 168
Bile, 166
Bioactive food ingredients, 273
Bioadhesive, 284
Biodegradable packaging, 266
Bionanocomposites, 280
B-vitamin, 161
Cadmium, 237
Calcium, 154, 161, 175–177
Cancer, 154, 163, 165, 168, 176
Carbohydrates, 154, 163–164, 166, 169, 173
Carbonyl groups, 176
Carboxylic group, 164
Carcinogenic processes, 174
Cardiovascular, 163, 170, 176
Carotene, 175
Catalase, 175
Catechins, 164

Causes of food insecurity, 27
access to land, 33
conflicts, 35
population growth and urbanisation, 30
poverty, 28
Cellulose,167, 173
applications, 278
bacterial, 280
fibrils, 278
mechanical properties, 277
nanofibers, 278
surface modification, 276
Chitin and chitosan
carbohydrates, 270
nanoparticles, 283
Cholesterol, 163–164, 168, 170, 174
Chromium, 236
Clays, 288
Clays and silicates
applications, 109
cation exchange capacity, 109
montmorillonite, 108
nanocomposites, 107–109
structure, 107–109
types of composite, 107–109
Coating material, 286
Cobalt, 241
Conjugated linoleic acid, 161
Contaminants, 169
Copper, 175
Cytokines, 165
DHA, 165
Dietary, 158–159, 162, 164, 173
DPA, 164–165
Economic Issues of food security
finance aid, 36
trade, 38
Eicosanoids, 165
Elemental speciation in food, 227, 229, 243, 245, 249- 250, 257
Elemental species in food processing, 243
Environmental issues of food security
biodiversity and genetic resources, 47
climate change and natural disasters, 41
pests and pesticide impacts, 49
soil and forest degradation, 44
water resources, 45
Enzyme preparations as food ingredients
affirmed as GRAS, 206, 208–210
approved as food additives, 206–207
generally recognized as safe notices, 210–215
regulatory history, 206–216
safety evaluations by FDA, 216–223
Enzymes, 175–176
antioxidant, 175
digestive, 166
EPA, 164–165
Ethylene production, 176
Fatty Acids, 161–165, 170
Fibers, 161
Films
biopolymers-based, 267
edible, 286
properties, 274
protein, 270
Flavonoids, 162
Folate, 162
Food allergens, 161
Food elemental speciation analysis
Food formulations
alginates, 105
encapsulation, 105
liposomes, 105
nanocapsules, 105

Food ingredients
 1958 Food Additives Amendment, 203–204
 enzyme preparations, 201–225
 food additives, 203, 206
 the Federal Food, Drug, and Cosmetics Act, 203–204
Food insecurity dimension
 economic crisis, 55
 food prices volatility, 65
 global food production and trade, 72
 global level, 50
Food production
 cereal, 188–192
 functional foods, 190
 meat, 186, 188, 193–196
 milk, 188, 193
Food properties
 conjugated linoleic acid, 196
 water activity, 196–197
Food quality
 food safety, 197
Food security
 definitions and basic concepts, 20
Freezing and frozen storage
 color, 144–145
 drip loss, 143
 flavor, 144–145
 freeze cracking, 142
 microbiological aspects, 145–146
 moisture migration, 142–143
 nutritional quality, 145
 recrystallization, 143
 texture, 144–145
Freezing methods and equipment
 batch air blast freezers, 131–132
 combination of freezing methods, 137–139
 contact with cold liquid, 135
 contact with cold surfaces, 135–136
 continuous air blast freezers, 132–134
 cryogenic, 136–137
 fluidized bed freezers, 134–135
 innovations in freezing, 137–139
Freezing process, 129–131
Freshness, 169
Fructooligo-saccharides, 167
Functional food, elemental species
Functional materials, 272
Glutathione peroxidase, 175
Glycerol, 164
Gut, 168
HDL, 163
Hydrocarbonated chain, 164
Intelligent packaging
 conducting polymer nanocomposites, 114
 metal oxide gas sensors, 114
 nano-based sensors, 114
Inulin, 167
Iron, 161, 240, 247
Isoflavones, 162
Isothiocyanates, 162
Lactose intolerance, 168
Lecithin, 162
Lignin, 162
Lipid, 169–170
Lipid oxidation, 170
Lutein, 161
Lysine, 171
Manganese, 175
Margarine, 161
Market, 104
Mercury, 234
Microbial, 162–163, 166
Minerals, 153, 163, 169, 171
MUFAs, 162
Nanocomposites
 biodegradation, 293
 compostability, 293
 use, 274

Nanofillers
  barrier properties, 111
  nanowhiskers, 110
  release, 110
Nanoparticles
  antimicrobial properties, 286
  filler additives, 274
  plant-protein interaction, 285
  polymeric additives, 274
  safety and toxicology, 291
Nanotechnology, 103–107, 112, 115–116
Natural reinforcements, 274
Nitric oxide, 165
Nutraceuticals, 151, 168
Nutrient requirements, 166
Nutrients, 166, 170–171
Odor, 173
Oils, 161, 163, 170, 172
Oligosaccharides, 162, 167
Oxygen, 175
Peptides, 161
Permeability, 107, 110–111, 113
Phenolic compounds, 162–164, 174–176
Phenols, 162, 164, 175–176
Phenylalanine, 176
Phospholipids, 165, 165
Pigments, 176–177
Plants, 164, 170, 173, 175, 177
Plasticizers, 286
Polypeptide, 285
Polyphenolic compounds, 163
Polyphenols, 162, 175
Polysaccharides, 268, 164
Potassium, 154
Prebiotics, 151, 162, 166–167, 169
Pre-freezing treatments
  fish products, 127–128
  fruits and vegetables, 125–127
  meat products, 128–129
Preservatives, 170
Probiotics, 151, 162, 166–169
Processing of food, 168–169
Protein, 169–174
PUFA, 162, 164
Radical, 162, 165, 175
Reactive oxygen species, 175
Regulation
  consumers, 116
  migration limit, 115
Resistant starch, 167
Saccharides, 162, 164, 167
Selenium, 238, 246
Sodium, 154
Soybean, 163, 170–172
Species detection, 253
Species separation, 249
Starch
  carbohydrates, 268
  nanocrystals, 282
  potato, 284
Starches, 173
Stilbenes, 162
Sugar, 161, 163, 169, 173
Synergistic effect, 168, 174
Tannins, 162
Terpenes, 162
Texture, 169, 173–174
Tin, 235
Tocopherols, 162, 175
Toxic elemental species in food
Unsaturated fatty acids, 164, 170
Vitamin
  vitamin B, 161
  vitamin C, 154, 161, 175
  vitamin D, 154
  vitamin E, 175
  vitamins, 153, 169, 171, 174–175
Water insoluble polysaccharides, 164
Watermelon, 163, 177
Wheat, 161, 163, 173
Xanthan gum, 173
Xylitol, 161
Zinc, 175, 242, 247